# PROPENSITY SCORE ANALYSIS

# Propensity Score Analysis

## FUNDAMENTALS AND DEVELOPMENTS

edited by
**Wei Pan**
**Haiyan Bai**

THE GUILFORD PRESS
New York    London

© 2015 The Guilford Press
A Division of Guilford Publications, Inc.
370 Seventh Avenue, Suite 1200, New York, NY 10001
www.guilford.com

All rights reserved

No part of this book may be reproduced, translated, stored in a retrieval system, or transmitted, in any form or by any means, electronic, mechanical, photocopying, microfilming, recording, or otherwise, without written permission from the publisher.

Printed in the United States of America

This book is printed on acid-free paper.

Last digit is print number:   9   8   7   6   5   4   3   2   1

**Library of Congress Cataloging-in-Publication Data**

Propensity score analysis : fundamentals and developments / edited by Wei Pan, Haiyan Bai.
   pages cm
  Includes bibliographical references and index.
  ISBN 978-1-4625-1949-1 (hardback)
  1. Social sciences—Statistical methods.   I. Pan, Wei, 1958–
  HA29.P764 2015
  001.4′22—dc23
                                                            2015000367

*With gratitude to the contributing authors
for their remarkable cooperation
and commitment to the advancement
of propensity score methodology*

# Preface

Researchers often use observational data to estimate treatment effects because randomized controlled trials or experimental designs are not always feasible. The use of observational data poses a threat to the validity of causal inference by introducing selection bias into the treatment assignment. To tackle this problem, in 1983, Paul R. Rosenbaum and Donald B. Rubin theorized propensity score analysis, which balances the distributions of observed covariates between the treatment and control groups, as a means of mimicking characteristics of randomized controlled trials and, therefore, reducing selection bias. Over the past three decades, propensity score methods have become increasingly popular in the social, behavioral, and health sciences for making causal inferences based on observational studies.

However, both methodological and practical challenges persist in the use of propensity score analysis. These include what estimation method should be used to estimate propensity scores, under what conditions propensity score matching is appropriate, how to assess matching quality, how to implement propensity score analysis effectively on complex data, what should be considered after implementing propensity score analysis, and what computer program is appropriate for a specific data condition. This edited book introduces new methodological developments that address these challenges encountered in practice. We do not intend to solve all the challenges in this single volume but rather hope to stimulate further discussions and, therefore, advance its use. The book is written for statisticians, methodological and practical researchers, and graduate students preparing for careers as statisticians and researchers in the social, behavioral, and health sciences.

The volume includes 15 chapters organized in five parts. Beginning with fundamentals of propensity score analysis, Part I includes an overview of propensity score analysis underlying concepts and current issues (Chapter 1), as well as a review of computer programs for propensity score analysis (Chapter 2). The next three parts encompass the main body of the book, introducing new developments that address current issues in propensity score estimation and matching in Part II (Chapters 3–5), outcome analysis after matching in Part III (Chapters 6–8), and use of propensity score analysis on complex data in Part IV (Chapters 9–11). The last section, Part V, includes discussions on missing data in propensity scores (Chapter 12), sensitivity of unobserved confounding in propensity score analysis (Chapters 13 and 14), and the extension of propensity score analysis to prognostic score analysis for causal inference (Chapter 15).

Chapter 1 provides a comprehensive overview of propensity score analysis and the basic concepts of propensity score methods. By summarizing the existing propensity score matching methods, the steps in propensity score analysis, analysis after matching, and the current issues, Wei Pan and Haiyan Bai present a complete set of road maps for researchers to understand the fundamentals of propensity score analysis. They also build connections for readers between these concepts and the other chapters for further exploration of specific topics of interest.

Modern technology makes statistical computing a less demanding task. Positioned for both methodological and practical researchers, this book allows an overall understanding of the availability of statistical programs that can be used for propensity score analysis. In Chapter 2, Megan Schuler reviews the range of statistical software from which researchers will be able to find one that is appropriate and familiar to conduct propensity score analysis.

Providing that the strong ignorability assumption stands, propensity score as a single score is used to balance the selection bias between the treatment and control groups. It is essential to understand the procedures for propensity score estimation and its new developments to solve some critical problems in propensity score estimation. In Chapter 3, Lane F. Burgette, Daniel F. McCaffrey, and Beth Ann Griffin describe the propensity score estimation steps and provide an illustrative example of how to estimate propensity scores using generalized boosted models.

## Preface

Propensity score matching is one of the most important propensity score methods; however, it is usually a daunting task for practical researchers to identify which matching method works best for their data. Researchers often struggle with deciding if matching should be done with replacement, how much common support is sufficient, and whether sample size ratio is influential for bias reduction results. Haiyan Bai, in Chapter 4, helps address these methodological considerations in implementing propensity score matching by providing a systematic investigation with 60 experimental trials to assist researchers in selecting an appropriate matching method, and to aid methodologists in initiating further investigations into these intricate issues.

Evaluating the quality of covariate balance is a critical procedure for verifying the validity of using a propensity score method. In Chapter 5, Cassandra W. Pattanayak focuses on how to evaluate balance results on key background covariates after matching. She demonstrates best practices for evaluating balance and addresses the related issues of missing data, generalizability, and an occasional need for using matching or subclassification in randomized experiments.

In Chapter 6, M. H. Clark discusses how to use propensity score methods (or propensity score adjustment methods) to reduce selection bias in quasi-experimental studies. Through both a literature review and a case study, she describes and compares four propensity score adjustment methods in their capability to balance covariates and reduce selection bias in treatment effects for both continuous and categorical outcome variables. She provides guidance and useful information for researchers to understand the conditions under which each method is most appropriate.

Chapter 7 describes an alternative propensity score method, the matching weight. This method was developed to reduce the complexity of using the existing propensity score matching methods. Liang Li, Tom H. Greene, and Brian C. Sauer illustrate how the matching weight method is simple to implement and generally more efficient than the pair matching estimator, while producing accurate variance estimation, improved covariate balance, and double robust estimation.

Chapter 8 focuses on the design and analysis of matched pairs in observational studies. Scott F. Kosten, Joseph W. McKean, and Bradley E. Huitema provide a general overview of the role of propensity scores in the design and analysis of observational studies. They also introduce a newly developed method of outcome analysis and provide an example to illustrate the advantages of the new method over competing approaches. Input and output for new software that computes this analysis, and competing alternatives are also provided.

In this era of easier access to data, researchers are increasingly faced with more complex datasets that are challenging to analyze. In Chapter 9, Walter L. Leite offers an overview of the use of propensity score matching methods in longitudinal studies. He presents a set of growth models that can be used to analyze the matched longitudinal dataset. He demonstrates the application of the methods for researchers to better understand how to apply propensity score methods to longitudinal data and the use of statistical programs in such situations. In Chapter 10, Qiu Wang provides researchers with useful and critical information for applying propensity score matching methods to clustered or multilevel data. He introduces the dual-matching method for reducing selection bias due to both individual and cluster covariates when clusters are the intervention units.

Researchers may be engaged in analyzing data from complex samples, rather than a simple random sample, such as with national or international surveys. In Chapter 11, Debbie L. Hahs-Vaughn provides a general review of the literature on this topic and enables readers to understand the applications of propensity score analysis to complex samples and the impact of ignoring the sampling design on parameter estimation.

Issues of missing data cannot be ignored in data analysis. In propensity score analysis, missing data can significantly influence propensity score estimation. In Chapter 12, Robin Mitra addresses the problem of missing covariate data and the existing imputation approaches. Multiple imputation procedures are illustrated for researchers to understand possible ways to handle missing covariates in propensity score estimation.

Evaluation of the impact of potential uncontrolled confounding is an important component for causal inference in observational studies: the propensity score methods do not deal with unobserved confounders. In Chapter 13, Rolf H. H. Groenwold and Olaf H. Klungel introduce propensity score calibration for directly controlling for unobserved confounding and discuss the extent to which propensity score methods indirectly control for unobserved confounding. They also illustrate how the sensitivity analysis can be used as a diagnostic tool for unobserved confounding. In Chapter 14, Lingling Li, Changyu Shen, and Xiaochun Li introduce two additional sensitivity analysis approaches that are based on the inverse probability weighting estimator, but extend it to accounting for uncontrolled confounding from an alternative perspective. In addition, they demonstrate a real-life example for applying the two sensitivity analyses.

## Preface

It is always helpful for researchers to know extensions to the existing methods. In Chapter 15, Ben Kelcey and Christopher M. Swoboda introduce prognostic score analysis as a complement to propensity score analysis and applications of prognostic score analysis to clustered or multilevel settings. They also illustrate the use of prognostic score analysis using an empirical example to investigate the treatment effects. This last chapter exposes readers to an extension of propensity score analysis in an effort to keep a wide vision toward new approaches.

The chapters are logically ordered with basic contents presented in the early chapters. Thus, the fundamentals part (Part I) assists readers with limited knowledge of or experience with propensity score analysis to learn basic concepts and understand the current issues in propensity score analysis. Readers who have mastered the fundamentals and those with some prior knowledge of propensity score analysis can benefit from reading the later chapters for cutting-edge discussions about developments and extensions in propensity score analysis. The chapters also can be used independently because each one focuses on a specific topic. This book will serve as an excellent supplemental text for advanced research methods courses.

This book has both methodological and practical value. Methodologists can use this book to further explore new directions and improvement of propensity score methods. Also, it can help practical researchers to use propensity score analysis both appropriately and directly to improve the validity of their research on causal claims. In addition, this book provides necessary statistical program codes and application examples for practical researchers to follow.

Given that this is our first edited book, we greatly appreciated the chapter authors' extensive involvement. Without their remarkable cooperation, flexibility, and dedication, this book would not be possible. They not only contributed their own excellent chapters to this book, but many also spent their precious time peer-reviewing others' chapters. Along with three ad hoc chapter reviewers who kindly lent their expertise to the project, the chapter reviewers were:

Lane F. Burgette, RAND Corporation

Haiwen Chen, Global Assessment Department, Educational Testing Service

M. H. Clark, Department of Educational and Human Sciences, University of Central Florida

Beth Ann Griffin, RAND Corporation

Rolf H. H. Groenwold, Julius Center for Health Sciences and Primary Care, University Medical Center Utrecht, The Netherlands

Debbie L. Hahs-Vaughn, Department of Educational and Human Sciences, University of Central Florida

Walter L. Leite, Research and Evaluation Methodology Program, University of Florida

Liang Li, Department of Biostatistics, The University of Texas MD Anderson Cancer Center

Joseph W. McKean, Department of Statistics, Western Michigan University

Daniel F. McCaffrey, Educational Testing Service

Robin Mitra, Mathematical Sciences, University of Southampton, United Kingdom

Megan Schuler, Department of Mental Health, Johns Hopkins Bloomberg School of Public Health

Elizabeth A. Stuart, Departments of Mental Health and Biostatistics, Johns Hopkins Bloomberg School of Public Health

Christopher M. Swoboda, School of Education, University of Cincinnati

Qiu Wang, Department of Higher Education, Syracuse University

Rebecca Zwick, Statistical and Psychometric Theory and Practice, Educational Testing Service

We express our deepest thanks to these reviewers as well as the initially anonymous reviewers—Suzanne E. Graham, Department of Education, University of New Hampshire, and Xitao Fan, Chair Professor and Dean, Faculty of Education, University of Macau, China—who made the book more rigorous and readable. We particularly appreciate our valued colleagues M. H. Clark, Sharron Docherty, Debbie Hahs-Vaughn, Judith Hays, Janet Levy, Marilyn Oermann, and Susan Silva for their generous professional assistance and support. We also thank C. Deborah Laughton and her team at The Guilford Press for their support and advice through the entire process of the project. Last, but not least, we are grateful to our families, who, as always, gave us continuous and strong support while we were editing the book.

# Contents

**PART I. Fundamentals of Propensity Score Analysis**

1. Propensity Score Analysis: Concepts and Issues    3
   *Wei Pan and Haiyan Bai*

2. Overview of Implementing Propensity Score Analyses    20
   in Statistical Software
   *Megan Schuler*

**PART II. Propensity Score Estimation, Matching, and Covariate Balance**

3. Propensity Score Estimation with Boosted Regression    49
   *Lane F. Burgette, Daniel F. McCaffrey, and Beth Ann Griffin*

4. Methodological Considerations in Implementing    74
   Propensity Score Matching
   *Haiyan Bai*

5. Evaluating Covariate Balance    89
   *Cassandra W. Pattanayak*

## PART III. Weighting Schemes and Other Strategies for Outcome Analysis after Matching

**6.** Propensity Score Adjustment Methods — 115
*M. H. Clark*

**7.** Propensity Score Analysis with Matching Weights — 141
*Liang Li, Tom H. Greene, and Brian C. Sauer*

**8.** Robust Outcome Analysis for Propensity-Matched Designs — 168
*Scott F. Kosten, Joseph W. McKean, and Bradley E. Huitema*

## PART IV. Propensity Score Analysis on Complex Data

**9.** Latent Growth Modeling of Longitudinal Data with Propensity-Score-Matched Groups — 191
*Walter L. Leite*

**10.** Propensity Score Matching on Multilevel Data — 217
*Qiu Wang*

**11.** Propensity Score Analysis with Complex Survey Samples — 236
*Debbie L. Hahs-Vaughn*

## PART V. Sensitivity Analysis and Extensions Related to Propensity Score Analysis

**12.** Missing Data in Propensity Scores — 267
*Robin Mitra*

**13.** Unobserved Confounding in Propensity Score Analysis — 296
*Rolf H. H. Groenwold and Olaf H. Klungel*

**14.** Propensity-Score-Based Sensitivity Analysis — 320
*Lingling Li, Changyu Shen, and Xiaochun Li*

**15.** Prognostic Scores in Clustered Settings — 348
*Ben Kelcey and Christopher M. Swoboda*

Author Index — 377
Subject Index — 385
About the Editors — 399
Contributors — 401

---

The data and software code for the book's examples are available at *www.guilford.com/pan-materials*.

# PART I

# Fundamentals of Propensity Score Analysis

# CHAPTER 1

# Propensity Score Analysis
## Concepts and Issues

**Wei Pan**
**Haiyan Bai**

Since the seminal paper by Rosenbaum and Rubin (1983b) on propensity score analysis, research using propensity score analysis has grown exponentially over three decades. Nevertheless, some methodological and practical issues still remain unresolved. This introductory chapter describes these issues along with an introduction to basic concepts of propensity score analysis. The remaining chapters in this book represent a collective effort to further address these issues and provide demonstrations and recommendations on how to use propensity score analysis appropriately and effectively for various situations.

The rest of this chapter proceeds as follows: It starts with a general introduction to propensity score analysis based on the theoretical framework of causal inference, followed by a detailed description of four major steps in propensity score analysis, and concludes with a brief discussion of current issues in propensity score analysis.

## CAUSAL INFERENCE AND PROPENSITY SCORE ANALYSIS

Suppose one has $N$ units (e.g., subjects). Denote $z$ as a treatment condition and $r$ as a potential response. For each unit $i$ ($i = 1, \ldots, N$), $z_i = 1$ indicates that the unit $i$ is in the treatment group with a corresponding potential response $r_{1i}$, and $z_i = 0$ indicates that the unit $i$ is in the control group with a corresponding potential response $r_{0i}$. In the counterfactual framework for modeling causal effects (Holland, 1986; Rubin, 1974; Sobel, 1996; Winship & Morgan, 1999), the quantity of interest is the treatment effect for each unit $i$, which is defined as $\Delta_i = r_{1i} - r_{0i}$.

Unfortunately, for each unit $i$, $r_{1i}$ and $r_{0i}$ are not observable at the same time because the same unit cannot simultaneously be in both the treatment and control groups. Alternatively, one can estimate the *average treatment effect* (ATE; Holland, 1986; Rubin, 1974; Winship & Morgan, 1999) for the population, which is defined as ATE = $E(r_1 - r_0) = E(r_1) - E(r_0)$, where $E(r_1)$ is the expected value of $r$ for all the units in the treatment group and $E(r_0)$ is the expected value of $r$ for all the units in the control group. In randomized controlled trials (RCTs), ATE is an unbiased estimate of the treatment effect because the treatment group does not, on average, differ systematically from the control group on their observed and unobserved background characteristics, due to randomization (Rubin, 1974). In non-RCTs or observational studies, ATE could be biased because the treatment and control groups may not be comparable, resulting from group selection bias in the observational data.

Selection bias can be overt, hidden, or both (Rosenbaum, 2010). Fortunately, propensity score analysis set forth by Rosenbaum and Rubin (1983b) can reduce overt bias in observational studies by balancing the distributions of observed characteristics (or covariates) between the treatment and control groups. Therefore, propensity score analysis allows one to obtain an unbiased estimate of ATE from observational studies under the assumption of "no unobserved confounders," which is referred to as the *strong ignorability* in treatment assignment, described in the next section of this chapter.

In fact, ATE is not always the quantity of interest (Heckman, Ichimura, & Todd, 1997; Heckman & Robb, 1985; Rubin, 1977). For example, one may be interested in the treatment effect of a specific physician-supervised weight-loss program for obese people who volunteered to participate in the program, not all obese people in the population. In this instance, one wants to estimate the *average treatment effect for the treated* (ATT; Imbens, 2004; Winship & Morgan, 1999), which is defined as ATE = $E(r_1 - r_0|z = 1)$ = $E(r_1|z = 1) - E(r_0|z = 1)$. This still encounters the counterfactual problem that one can never observe $r_0$ when $z = 1$. To tackle this problem, one can analyze matched data on propensity scores. The matched units in the control group have similar probabilities of $z = 1$ to those of the corresponding units in the treatment group and, therefore, propensity score analysis allows one to estimate ATT (Imbens, 2004). Chapters 6, 7, and 8 in this book discuss various methods of estimating ATT using propensity scores.

## PROPENSITY SCORE AND ITS ASSUMPTIONS

Suppose each unit $i$ has, in addition to a treatment condition $z_i$ and a response $r_i$, a covariate value vector $X_i = (X_{i1}, \ldots, X_{iK})'$, where $K$ is the number of covariates. Rosenbaum and Rubin (1983b) defined a propensity score for unit $i$ as the probability of the unit being assigned to the treatment group, conditional on the covariate vector $X_i$, that is, $e(X_i) = \Pr(z_1 = 1|X_i)$. The propensity score is a balancing score with two assumptions about the strong ignorability in treatment assignment (Rosenbaum & Rubin, 1983b):

1. $(r_{1i}, r_{0i}) \perp z_i|X_i$;
2. $0 < e(X_i) < 1$.

The first assumption states a condition that treatment assignment $z_i$ and response $(r_{1i}, r_{0i})$ are conditionally independent, given $X_i$; and the second one assumes a common support between the treatment and control groups.

Rosenbaum and Rubin (1983b, Theorem 3) further demonstrated that ignorability conditional on $X_i$ implies ignorability conditional on $e(X_i)$, that is,

$$(r_{1i}, r_{0i}) \perp z_i|X_i \Rightarrow (r_{1i}, r_{0i}) \perp z_i|e(X_i) \tag{1.1}$$

Thus, under the assumptions of the strong ignorability in treatment assignment, when a unit in the treatment group and a corresponding matched unit in the control group have the same propensity score, the two matched units will have, in probability, the same value of the covariate vector $X_i$. Therefore, analyses on the matched data after matching, or on the original data using related methods (e.g., subclassification, weighting, or adjustment) tend to produce unbiased estimates of the treatment effects due to the reduced selection bias through balancing the distributions of observed covariates between the treatment and control groups.

In order to make a causal inference in observational studies using propensity scores, another assumption has to be met: the *stable unit treatment value assumption* (SUTVA; Rubin, 1980, 1986). This assumption means that "the observation on one unit should be unaffected by the particular assignment of treatments to the other units" (Cox, 1958, p. 19). This assumption is not always attainable in practice. For example, a participant in a diabetes self-management treatment group may like to share his or her experience of the treatment with his or her friends who happen to be in the control group. Such contamination would affect the friends' performance on the outcome. However, we can reduce such between-group contamination by improving designs (Stuart, 2010). Thus, we could ensure that this assumption can be satisfied, in addition to emerging discussions in the literature about strategies to relax the assumptions (e.g., Hong & Raudenbush, 2006; Hudgens & Halloran, 2008; Sobel, 2006).

## STEPS IN PROPENSITY SCORE ANALYSIS

There are four major steps in propensity score analysis in observational studies: propensity score estimation, propensity score matching or related method, matching quality evaluation, and outcome analysis after matching or related method. These steps are discussed in the following four subsections.

### Propensity Score Estimation

A propensity score for a unit $i$, $e(\mathbf{X}_i)$, can be estimated from logistic regression of the treatment condition $z_i$ on the covariate vector $\mathbf{X}_i$ (Agresti, 2013):

$$\ln\left(\frac{e(\mathbf{X}_i)}{1-e(\mathbf{X}_i)}\right) = \beta \mathbf{X}_i \qquad (1.2)$$

where $\beta$ is a vector of the regression coefficients. The logit of propensity scores, rather than the propensity score $\hat{e}(\mathbf{X}_i)$ itself, is commonly used to achieve normality. If there are more than two treatment conditions, multinomial logistic regression or discriminant analysis can be used. There are some other estimation methods for obtaining propensity scores. See Chapter 3 in this book for a detailed discussion on this topic.

### Propensity Score Matching and Related Methods

A number of different propensity score matching methods can be used to match units on their propensity scores. The basic method of propensity score matching is *nearest neighbor matching* (Rosenbaum & Rubin, 1985), which matches each unit $i$ in the treatment group with a unit $j$ in the control group with the closest absolute distance between their propensity scores, expressed as $d(i, j) = \min_j\{|e(X_i) - e(X_j)|\}$. Alternatively, *caliper matching* (Cochran & Rubin, 1973) matches each unit $i$ in the treatment group with a unit $j$ in the control group within a prespecified caliper band $b$; that is, $d(i, j) = \min_j\{|e(X_i) - e(X_j)| < b\}$. Based on work by Cochran and Rubin (1973), Rosenbaum and Rubin (1985) recommended that the prespecified caliper band $b$ should be less than or equal to 0.25 of the standard deviation of the propensity scores. Later, Austin (2011) asserted that $b = 0.20$ of the standard deviation of the propensity scores is the optimal caliper bandwidth. A variant of caliper matching is *radius matching* (Dehejia & Wahba, 2002), which is a one-to-many matching and matches each unit $i$ in the treatment group with multiple units in the control group within a prespecified band $b$; that is, $d(i, j) = \{|e(X_i) - e(X_j)| < b\}$.

Other propensity score matching methods include *Mahalanobis metric matching* (Rosenbaum & Rubin, 1985), *Mahalanobis caliper matching* (Guo, Barth, & Gibbons, 2006; Rubin & Thomas, 2000), and *genetic matching* (Diamond & Sekhon, 2013). In Mahalanobis metric matching, each unit $i$ in the treatment group is matched with a unit $j$ in the control group, with the closest Mahalanobis distance calculated based on proximities of the variables; that is, $d(i, j) = \min_j\{D_{ij}\}$, where $D_{ij} = (V_i^T - V_j^T)^T S^{-1}(V_i^T - V_j^T)$, $V_\bullet$ ($\bullet = i$ or $j$) is a new vector $(X_\bullet, e(X_\bullet))$, and $S$ is the sample variance–covariance matrix of the new vector for the control group. Mahalanobis caliper matching and genetic matching are two variants of Mahalanobis metric matching. Mahalanobis caliper matching uses $d(i, j) = \min_j\{D_{ij} < b\}$, where $D_{ij} = (X_i^T - X_j^T)^T S^{-1}(X_i^T - X_j^T)$; genetic matching also uses the same distance as Mahalanobis metric matching uses, but with a weighted distance $D_{ij} = (V_i^T - V_j^T)^T W S^{-1}(V_i^T - V_j^T)$ or $D_{ij} = (X_i^T - X_j^T)^T W S^{-1}(X_i^T - X_j^T)$, where $W$ is a weight matrix. Diamond and Sekhon (2013) provide various ways to specify $W$.

The propensity score matching methods discussed thus far can be implemented by using either a *greedy matching* or *optimal matching* algorithm (Rosenbaum, 1989). In greedy matching, once a match is made, the matched units cannot be changed. Each pair of matched units is the best matched pair currently available. In optimal matching, previous matched units can be changed before making the current match to achieve the overall minimum or optimal distance. Both matching algorithms usually produce similar matched data when the size of the control group is large; however, optimal matching gives rise to smaller overall distances within matched units (Gu & Rosenbaum, 1993; Ho, Imai, King, & Stuart, 2007, 2011). Thus, if the goal is simply to find well-matched groups, greedy matching may be sufficient; if, instead, the goal is to find well-matched pairs, then optimal matching may be preferable (Stuart, 2010).

There are propensity-score-matching-related methods that do not strictly match individual units. For example, *subclassification* (or *stratification*) (Rosenbaum & Rubin, 1984; Schafer & Kang, 2008) classifies all the units in the entire sample into several strata based on the corresponding number of percentiles of the propensity scores and matches units by stratum. Cochran (1965) observed that five strata would remove up to 90% of selection bias. A particular type of subclassification is *full matching* (Gu & Rosenbaum, 1993; Hansen, 2004; Rosenbaum, 1991) that produces subclasses in an optimal way. A fully matched sample consists of matched subsets, in which each matched set contains one treated unit and one or more controls, or one control unit and one or more treated units. Full matching is optimal in terms of minimizing a weighted average of the estimated distance measure between each treated subject and each control subject within each subclass. Another propensity score matching-related method is *kernel matching* (or *local linear matching*) (Heckman et al., 1997), which combines matching and outcome analysis into one procedure with one-to-all matching, a variant being *difference-in-differences matching* (Heckman et al., 1997).

In addition to propensity score matching and subclassification, one can also incorporate propensity scores directly into outcome analysis with propensity score weighting or adjustment. Chapters 4, 5, and 6 in this book present more extensive discussions of various propensity score matching and related methods. It is also worth noting, however, that selecting a specific method is in general less important than selecting covariates used to estimate the propensity scores (Steiner & Cook, 2013).

## Matching Quality Evaluation

After a matching method is implemented, it is important to evaluate the quality of covariate balance. This evaluation can be statistical or graphical. In statistical evaluation, three commonly used statistical criteria can be evaluated: selection bias ($B$) with a significance test, standardized bias ($SB$), and percent bias reduction ($PBR$).

The selection bias associated with a covariate $X_k$ ($k = 1, \ldots, K$) is defined as the mean difference in the covariate between the treatment conditions; that is, $B = M_1(X_k) - M_0(X_k)$, where $M_1(X_k)$ and $M_0(X_k)$ are the means of the covariate for the units in the treatment and control groups, respectively. If the covariate is dichotomous, $B$ can be expressed as the proportion difference; that is, $B = p_1(X_k) - p_0(X_k)$, where $p_1(X_k)$ and $p_0(X_k)$ are the proportions of the dichotomous covariate in the treatment and control groups, respectively. An independent-samples $t$-test or $z$-test under

$H_0: B = 0$ can follow, respectively, to test the significance of the selection bias. However, statistical significance testing used for evaluating covariate balance is discouraged because statistical significance testing is sensitive to sample size (Austin, 2011; Imai, King, & Stuart, 2008).

An alternative way to evaluate covariate balance is to examine the standardized bias for each covariate, which is defined as (Rosenbaum & Rubin, 1985)

$$SB = \frac{B}{\sqrt{\frac{V_1(X_k) + V_0(X_k)}{2}}} \times 100\% \tag{1.3}$$

where $V_1(X_k)$ is the variance of the covariate for all the units in the treatment group and $V_0(X_k)$ is the variance of the covariate for all the units in the control group. For a dichotomous covariate, $SB$ can be expressed as

$$SB = \frac{B}{\sqrt{\frac{p_1(X_k)(1-p_1(X_k)) + p_0(X_k)(1-p_0(X_k))}{2}}} \times 100\% \tag{1.4}$$

According to Caliendo and Kopeinig (2008), if $SB$ is reduced to below 5% after matching, the matching method is considered effective in balancing the distributions of the covariate.

The *PBR* or percent reduction in bias (Cochran & Rubin, 1973) on the covariate is another criterion to assess the effectiveness of matching. It is defined as

$$PBR = \frac{B_{\text{before matching}} - B_{\text{after matching}}}{B_{\text{before matching}}} \times 100\% \tag{1.5}$$

Although there is no established cutoff value for *PBR*, an 80% of *PBR* can be reasonably regarded as a sufficient amount of bias reduction based on the examples in Cochran and Rubin (1973) showing that most of satisfactory matched samples had a *PBR* value of 80% or higher.

In terms of graphical evaluation of the quality of covariate balance between the treatment and control groups, common graphs revealing sample distributions, such as histograms, box plots, Q–Q plots, and so on, can be utilized to compare the distributions of the covariates and the propensity scores between the treatment and control groups for the matched data. See Chapter 5 for an extensive discussion about graphical evaluation of the quality of covariate balance.

## Outcome Analysis after Matching or Related Method

In general, outcome analysis after matching can be done on the matched data as if it had been done on the entire original data. In fact, there are some variations in outcome analysis after matching or related method, depending on the appropriateness of propensity score methods. The rest of this section describes four ways of conducting outcome analysis after matching or related method.

### Outcome Analysis on the Matched Data after Propensity Score Matching

Intuitively, a mean difference between the treated and control units in the matched data would be a sufficient estimate of ATT as $\widehat{ATT} = \bar{r}_1 - \bar{r}_0$. Nonetheless, to control chance imbalances after matching, because in practice propensity score matching cannot produce perfectly matched data, Rosenbaum and Rubin (1985) recommended using regression with controlling for some unbalanced covariates, denoted as $X_{i1}^*, \ldots, X_{iq}^*$, that may have remaining selection bias after matching. Then, ATT can be estimated as $\widehat{ATT} = \hat{\beta}_1$ where $\hat{\beta}_1$ is an estimated regression coefficient of $z_i$ in the following regression model on the matched data with controlling for those unbalanced covariates:

$$r_i = \beta_0 + \beta_1 z_i + \beta_2 X_{i1}^* + \ldots + \beta_{q+1} X_{iq}^* + \varepsilon_i \qquad (1.6)$$

Therefore, for nearest neighbor matching, caliper matching, Mahalanobis metric matching, and the like that produce one-to-one matched pairs, $\widehat{ATT} = \hat{\beta}_1$ can be obtained using the regression model with controlling for the unbalanced covariates on the matched data (Equation 1.6). However, if a matching method produces variable numbers of treated and control units within matched subsets, such as exact matching, radius matching, and full matching, a *weighted* regression model with controlling for the unbalanced covariates on the matched data (similar to Equation 1.6) should be used to estimate ATT. The weights are created automatically in most matching programs such as *MatchIt* (Ho et al., 2007, 2011) by assigning 1 to each treated unit and a proportion (i.e., [number of treated units]/[number of control units]) to each control unit within each matched subset.

Outcome analysis after matching on the matched data is usually used for estimating ATT as randomized controlled trials do. One can also conduct outcome analysis after matching on the entire original data to estimate ATT or ATE, using propensity-score-matching-related methods, such as subclassification, kernel matching, and other specific propensity score weighting techniques, such as the inverse-probability-of-treatment-weighted (IPTW) estimator (Robins, Hernán, & Brumback, 2000).

## Outcome Analysis on the Entire Original Data after Subclassification

In subclassification, denote $S$ as the number of subsets; $n_s$ as the number of all units in the $s$th subset ($s = 1, \ldots, S$; $\Sigma_s n_s = N$); $n_{s1}$ as the number of the treated units in the $s$th subset; $N_1$ as the total number of the treated units in the entire original data ($\Sigma_s n_{s1} = N_1$); and $\bar{r}_{s1}$ and $\bar{r}_{s0}$ as the means of the responses for the treated and control units in the $s$th subset, respectively. There are two steps in outcome analysis after subclassification. One can first run regression with controlling for the unbalanced covariates (Equation 1.6) (or simply calculate the mean difference if $n_s$ is too small) within each subset. Then, the second step is to compute a weighted average of the regression coefficients $\hat{\beta}_{s1}$ (or mean differences ($\bar{r}_{s1} - \bar{r}_{s0}$)) by the number of the treated units in the subsets, $n_{s1}$, for estimating ATT as $\widehat{\text{ATT}} = \sum_s (n_{s1}\hat{\beta}_{s1}/N_1)$ (or $\widehat{\text{ATT}} = \sum_s (n_{s1}(\bar{r}_{s1} - \bar{r}_{s0})/N_1)$); or a weighted average of the regression coefficients (or mean differences) by the number of the total units in the subsets, $n_s$, for estimating ATE as $\widehat{\text{ATE}} = \sum_s (n_s \hat{\beta}_{s1}/N)$ (or $\widehat{\text{ATE}} = \sum_s (n_s (\bar{r}_{s1} - \bar{r}_{s0})/N)$).

## Outcome Analysis on the Entire Original Data with Propensity Score Weighting

For kernel matching as an example of propensity score weighting, which combines matching and analysis into one step, one can calculate the weighted average of the mean differences between each treated unit and a linear combination of all the control units as an estimate of ATT as

$$\widehat{\text{ATT}} = \frac{1}{N_1} \sum_{i=1}^{N_1} \left( r_{1i} - \sum_{j=1}^{N_0} w_{ij} r_{0j} \right) \quad (1.7)$$

where

$$w_{ij} = \frac{K\left(\frac{e(X_j) - e(X_i)}{h}\right)}{\sum_{l=1}^{N_0} K\left(\frac{e(X_l) - e(X_i)}{h}\right)} \quad (1.8)$$

$K(\bullet)$ is a kernel function, $h$ is a bandwidth, and $N_1$ and $N_0$ are the total numbers of the treated and control units, respectively, in the entire original data $(N_1 + N_0 = N)$. See Guo et al. (2006) for the specification of $K(\bullet)$ and $h$.

Another example of propensity score weighting is IPTW that can be used in two ways for estimating treatment effects. One can directly estimate ATE on the entire original data as

$$\widehat{\text{ATE}} = \frac{1}{N} \sum_{i=1}^{N} \left[ \frac{z_i r_i}{e(X_i)} - \frac{(1-z_i) r_i}{1-e(X_i)} \right] \quad (1.9)$$

which is the estimator from Horvitz and Thompson (1952). IPTW can also be used in a weighted regression with controlling for the unbalanced covariates (Equation 1.6), with regression weights as

$$w_i = \frac{z_i}{e(X_i)} + \frac{1-z_i}{1-e(X_i)} \quad (1.10)$$

to estimate ATE as $\widehat{\text{ATE}} = \hat{\beta}_1$ (Robins et al., 2000); or with weights as

$$w_i = z_i + \frac{(1-z_i) e(X_i)}{1-e(X_i)} \quad (1.11)$$

to estimate ATT as $\widehat{\text{ATT}} = \hat{\beta}_1$ (Hirano, Imbens, & Ridder, 2003; Morgan & Todd, 2008).

### Outcome Analysis on the Entire Original Data with Propensity Score Adjustment

Lastly, an ATE also can be estimated as $\widehat{\text{ATE}} = \hat{\beta}_1$ by simply running the following regression with propensity score adjustment on the entire original data:

$$r_i = \beta_0 + \beta_1 z_i + \beta_2 e(X_i) + \beta_3 z_i \times e(X_i) + \varepsilon_i \quad (1.12)$$

Note that various methods of outcome analysis after matching or related method as described above are parametric and suitable for continuous outcomes. For categorical outcomes, some nonparametric methods can be used based on specific outcomes (Rosenbaum, 2010). See also Austin (2007) and Kurth et al. (2006) for odds ratios, Austin (2010) for proportions, and Austin and Schuster (2014) for survival outcomes.

## ISSUES IN PROPENSITY SCORE ANALYSIS

Since Rosenbaum and Rubin (1983b) theorized propensity score analysis, the past 30 years have witnessed a methodological development of propensity score analysis that has almost reached its maturity. Propensity score analysis has been applied to many different research fields such as medicine, health, economy, and education. However, both methodological and practical challenges persist for the use of propensity score analysis. These include how to assess the robustness of propensity score analysis to avoid violation of balance assumptions, under what conditions propensity score matching is efficient, how to implement propensity score analysis effectively on complex data, and what are relevant considerations after implementing propensity score analysis. These issues are described in the following subsections and discussed in detail in later chapters in this book.

### Issues in Propensity Score Estimation

How to select covariates is a natural question in building propensity score estimation models. Intuitively, one would include as many observed covariates as possible in a propensity score model to predict the probability of a unit being assigned to the treatment group. The danger of this approach is that some covariates may be influenced by the treatment, and therefore, the ignorability assumption is violated. Also, some covariates may not have any association with the outcome, and including such covariates will increase the variance of the estimated treatment effect while selection bias is not reduced (Brookhart et al., 2006). In addition, some researchers have recommended that higher-order moments of covariates and interactions between covariates should be examined in propensity score models (Austin, 2011; Imai et al., 2008; Morgan & Todd, 2008). The drawback of these models is, however, that they rely heavily on functional form assumptions (Steiner & Cook, 2013). In practice, Rubin (2001) recommended that covariate selection should be done based on theory and prior research without using the observed outcomes. Another caveat for propensity score estimation is that model fit or significance of covariates is not of interest because the concern is not with the parameter estimates of the model, but rather with the resulting balance of the covariates (Austin, 2011; Brookhart et al., 2006; Rubin, 2004; Setoguchi, Schneeweiss, Brookhart, Glynn, & Cook, 2008; Stuart, 2010).

If the number of covariates is large and the propensity score functional form appears to be complex, some recommend using generalized boosted models, a nonparametric, data-adaptive approach, to estimate propensity scores (Lee, Lessler, & Stuart, 2010; McCaffrey, Ridgeway, & Morral, 2004; Ridgeway & McCaffrey, 2007; Setoguchi et al., 2008). Chapter 3 presents a more detailed discussion about the generalized boosted models for estimating propensity scores.

Another concern about propensity score estimation is that one can only account for observed covariates in propensity score models. Sensitivity analysis that assesses the potential impact of unobserved confounders on the treatment effect is a useful alternative and should always complement propensity score analysis (Steiner & Cook, 2013). The literature has provided some information about sensitivity analysis of unobserved covariates in propensity score analysis (e.g., McCandless, Gustafson, & Levy, 2007; Rosenbaum, 1987; Rosenbaum & Rubin, 1983a). Chapters 12, 13, and 14 provide more discussions of the robustness of propensity score analysis results against hidden bias due to missing data or unobserved covariates in observational studies.

## Issues in Propensity Score Matching

Propensity score matching is the core of propensity score analysis, and the efficiency of propensity score matching depends on whether the treatment and control groups have sufficient overlap or common support in propensity scores. Matching with or without replacement is another dilemma in propensity score matching. Matching without replacement might not produce quality balance in covariates for small samples, whereas matching with replacement may result in duplicated control units, which violates the basic statistical assumption of independent observations, although the choice of matching with or without replacement usually has a minor effect on the treatment effect's bias (Ho et al., 2007, 2011; Steiner & Cook, 2013; Stuart, 2010). Chapter 4 provides a detailed discussion of issues related to common support and matching with or without replacement.

How to evaluate matching quality is another issue in propensity score matching. The literature has proposed some statistical and graphical criteria to evaluate matching quality, but these criteria only focus on the first and second moment of each covariate's distribution (Steiner & Cook, 2013). Chapter 5 presents a detailed discussion of this topic.

## Issues in Outcome Analysis after Matching or Related Method

The performance of outcome analysis after matching depends on the data condition and quality as well as on specific aspects of the performance.

In terms of selection bias reduction, propensity score matching is usually better than subclassification, propensity score weighting, and propensity score adjustment (Austin, 2009). Lunceford and Davidian (2004) also asserted that propensity score weighting tends to produce less bias in estimates of treatment effects than does subclassification. However, propensity score matching plus regression with controlling for covariates in the outcome analysis will produce robust estimates of treatment effects regardless of the choice of propensity score matching methods (Schafer & Kang, 2008; Shadish, Clark, & Steiner, 2008). Work by Austin (2009, 2011), Austin and Mamdani (2006), Kurth et al. (2006), and Lunceford and Davidian (2004) provides more discussions of the performance of outcome analysis using propensity scores. Chapter 6 provides a comparative review on and a case study of propensity score methods, including matching, subclassification, weighting, and adjustment with propensity scores; and Chapters 7 and 8 present additional discussions on double robust and other strategies for outcome analysis using propensity scores.

### Issues in Propensity Score Analysis on Complex Data

Propensity score analysis was originally developed on cross-sectional data, which is common in most research fields. As research phenomena have become multifaceted and multidimensional, corresponding research data have become more and more complicated, including longitudinal data, multilevel data, and complex survey samples. The complexity of research data poses methodological challenges to the development and use of propensity score analysis. Part IV is devoted solely to addressing such issues in propensity score analysis on complex data. Specifically, Chapter 9 discusses longitudinal data, Chapter 10 multilevel data, and Chapter 11 survey samples.

## CONCLUSION

This chapter provides an overview of propensity score analysis along with a description of some current issues with propensity score analysis. Readers are encouraged to find specific topics in the rest of this book that may be more relevant and critical to their own research situations. We also hope this book provides a springboard for both methodological and practical researchers to further discuss and advance propensity score methods for the design and analysis of observational studies for causal inferences in the social, behavioral, and health sciences.

## REFERENCES

Agresti, A. (2013). *Categorical data analysis* (3rd ed.). Hoboken, NJ: Wiley.
Austin, P. C. (2007). The performance of different propensity score methods for estimating marginal odds ratios. *Statistics in Medicine, 26*(16), 3078–3094.
Austin, P. C. (2009). Type I error rates, coverage of confidence intervals, and variance estimation in propensity-score matched analyses. *International Journal of Biostatistics, 5*(1), 1557–4679.
Austin, P. C. (2010). The performance of different propensity score methods for estimating differences in proportions (risk differences or absolute risk reductions) in observational studies. *Statistics in Medicine, 29*(20), 2137–2148.
Austin, P. C. (2011). An introduction to propensity score methods for reducing the effects of confounding in observational studies. *Multivariate Behavioral Research, 46*(3), 399–424.
Austin, P. C., & Mamdani, M. M. (2006). A comparison of propensity score methods: A case-study estimating the effectiveness of post-AMI statin use. *Statistics in Medicine, 25*(12), 2084–2106.
Austin, P. C., & Schuster, T. (2014). The performance of different propensity score methods for estimating absolute effects of treatments on survival outcomes: A simulation study. *Statistical Methods in Medical Research*.
Brookhart, M. A., Schneeweiss, S., Rothman, K. J., Glynn, R. J., Avorn, J., & Stürmer, T. (2006). Variable selection for propensity score models. *American Journal of Epidemiology, 163*(12), 1149–1156.
Caliendo, M., & Kopeinig, S. (2008). Some practical guidance for the implementation of propensity score matching. *Journal of Economic Surveys, 22*(1), 31–72.
Cochran, W. G. (1965). The planning of observational studies of human populations. *Journal of the Royal Statistical Society, Series A, 128*(2), 234–266.
Cochran, W. G., & Rubin, D. B. (1973). Controlling bias in observational studies: A review. *Sankhyā: The Indian Journal of Statistics, Series A, 35*(4), 417–446.
Cox, D. R. (1958). *The planning of experiments*. New York: Wiley.
Dehejia, R. H., & Wahba, S. (2002). Propensity score matching methods for nonexperimental causal studies. *Review of Economics and Statistics, 84*, 151–161.
Diamond, A., & Sekhon, J. S. (2013). Genetic matching for estimating causal effects: A general multivariate matching method for achieving balance in observational studies. *Review of Economics and Statistics, 95*(3), 932–945.
Gu, X. S., & Rosenbaum, P. R. (1993). Comparison of multivariate matching methods: Structures, distances, and algorithms. *Journal of Computational and Graphical Statistics, 2*(4), 405–420.
Guo, S., Barth, R. P., & Gibbons, C. (2006). Propensity score matching strategies for evaluating substance abuse services for child welfare clients. *Children and Youth Services Review, 28*(4), 357–383.
Hansen, B. B. (2004). Full matching in an observational study of coaching for the SAT. *Journal of the American Statistical Association, 99*(467), 609–618.
Heckman, J. J., Ichimura, H., & Todd, P. E. (1997). Matching as an econometric

evaluation estimator: Evidence from evaluating a job training programme. *Review of Economic Studies, 64*(4), 605–654.

Heckman, J. J., & Robb, R., Jr. (1985). Alternative methods for evaluating the impact of interventions: An overview. *Journal of Econometrics, 30*(1–2), 239–267.

Hirano, K., Imbens, G. W., & Ridder, G. (2003). Efficient estimation of average treatment effects using the estimated propensity score. *Econometrica, 71*(4), 1161–1189.

Ho, D. E., Imai, K., King, G., & Stuart, E. A. (2007). Matching as nonparametric preprocessing for reducing model dependence in parametric causal inference. *Political Analysis, 15*, 199–236.

Ho, D. E., Imai, K., King, G., & Stuart, E. A. (2011). MatchIt: Nonparametric preprocessing for parametric causal inference. *Journal of Statistical Software, 42*(8), 1–28.

Holland, P. W. (1986). Statistics and causal inference. *Journal of the American Statistical Association, 81*(396), 945–960.

Hong, G., & Raudenbush, S. W. (2006). Evaluating kindergarten retention policy: A case study of causal inference for multilevel observational data. *Journal of the American Statistical Association, 101*(475), 901–910.

Horvitz, D. G., & Thompson, D. J. (1952). A generalization of sampling without replacement from a finite universe. *Journal of the American Statistical Association, 47*(260), 663–685.

Hudgens, M. G., & Halloran, M. E. (2008). Toward causal inference with interference. *Journal of the American Statistical Association, 103*(482), 832–842.

Imai, K., King, G., & Stuart, E. A. (2008). Misunderstandings between experimentalists and observationalists about causal inference. *Journal of the Royal Statistical Society, Series A, 171*(2), 481–502.

Imbens, G. W. (2004). Nonparametric estimation of average treatment effects under exogeneity: A review. *Review of Economics and Statistics, 86*(1), 4–29.

Kurth, T., Walker, A. M., Glynn, R. J., Chan, K. A., Gaziano, J. M., Berger, K., et al. (2006). Results of multivariable logistic regression, propensity matching, propensity adjustment, and propensity-based weighting under conditions of nonuniform effect. *American Journal of Epidemiology, 163*(3), 262–270.

Lee, B. K., Lessler, J., & Stuart, E. A. (2010). Improving propensity score weighting using machine learning. *Statistics in Medicine, 29*(3), 337–346.

Lunceford, J. K., & Davidian, M. (2004). Stratification and weighting via the propensity score in estimation of causal treatment effects: A comparative study. *Statistics in Medicine, 23*(19), 2937–2960.

McCaffrey, D. F., Ridgeway, G., & Morral, A. R. (2004). Propensity score estimation with boosted regression for evaluating causal effects in observational studies. *Psychological Methods, 9*(4), 403–425.

McCandless, L. C., Gustafson, P., & Levy, A. (2007). Bayesian sensitivity analysis for unmeasured confounding in observational studies. *Statistics in Medicine, 26*(11), 2331–2347.

Morgan, S. L., & Todd, J. J. (2008). A diagnostic routine for the detection of consequential heterogeneity of causal effects. *Sociological Methodology, 38*(1), 231–281.

Ridgeway, G., & McCaffrey, D. F. (2007). Comment: Demystifying double robustness: A comparison of alternative strategies for estimating a population mean from incomplete data. *Statistical Science, 22*(4), 540–581.

Robins, J. M., Hernán, M. Á., & Brumback, B. (2000). Marginal structural models and causal inference in epidemiology. *Epidemiology, 11*(5), 550–560.

Rosenbaum, P. R. (1987). Sensitivity analysis for certain permutation inferences in matched observational studies. *Biometrika, 74*(1), 13–26.

Rosenbaum, P. R. (1989). Optimal matching for observational studies. *Journal of the American Statistical Association, 84*(408), 1024–1032.

Rosenbaum, P. R. (1991). A characterization of optimal designs for observational studies. *Journal of the Royal Statistical Society, 53*(3), 597–610.

Rosenbaum, P. R. (2010). *Observational studies* (2nd ed.). New York: Springer-Verlag.

Rosenbaum, P. R., & Rubin, D. B. (1983a). Assessing sensitivity to an unobserved binary covariate in an observational study with binary outcome. *Journal of the Royal Statistical Society, Series B (Methodological), 45*(2), 212–218.

Rosenbaum, P. R., & Rubin, D. B. (1983b). The central role of the propensity score in observational studies for causal effects. *Biometrika, 70*(1), 41–55.

Rosenbaum, P. R., & Rubin, D. B. (1984). Reducing bias in observational studies using subclassification on the propensity score. *Journal of the American Statistical Association, 79*(387), 516–524.

Rosenbaum, P. R., & Rubin, D. B. (1985). Constructing a control group using multivariate matched sampling methods that incorporate the propensity score. *American Statistician, 39*(1), 33–38.

Rubin, D. B. (1974). Estimating causal effects of treatments in randomized and nonrandomized studies. *Journal of Educational Psychology, 66*(5), 688–701.

Rubin, D. B. (1977). Assignment to treatment group on the basis of a covariate. *Journal of Educational and Behavioral Statistics, 2*(1), 1–26.

Rubin, D. B. (1980). Randomization analysis of experimental data: The Fisher randomization test comment. *Journal of the American Statistical Association, 75*(371), 591–593.

Rubin, D. B. (1986). Statistics and causal inference: Comment: Which ifs have causal answers. *Journal of the American Statistical Association, 81*(396), 961–962.

Rubin, D. B. (2001). Using propensity scores to help design observational studies: Application to the tobacco litigation. *Health Services and Outcomes Research Methodology, 2*(3–4), 169–188.

Rubin, D. B. (2004). On principles for modeling propensity scores in medical research. *Pharmacoepidemiology and Drug Safety, 13*(12), 855–857.

Rubin, D. B., & Thomas, N. (2000). Combining propensity score matching with additional adjustments for prognostic covariates. *Journal of the American Statistical Association, 95*(450), 573–585.

Schafer, J. L., & Kang, J. (2008). Average causal effects from nonrandomized studies: A practical guide and simulated example. *Psychological Methods, 13*(4), 279–313.

Setoguchi, S., Schneeweiss, S., Brookhart, M. A., Glynn, R. J., & Cook, E. F. (2008). Evaluating uses of data mining techniques in propensity score estimation: A simulation study. *Pharmacoepidemiology Drug Safety, 17*(6), 546–555.

Shadish, W. R., Clark, M. H., & Steiner, P. M. (2008). Can nonrandomized experiments yield accurate answers?: A randomized experiment comparing random and nonrandom assignments. *Journal of the American Statistical Association, 103*(484), 1334–1344.

Sobel, M. E. (1996). An introduction to causal inference. *Sociological Methods and Research, 24*(3), 353–379.

Sobel, M. E. (2006). What do randomized studies of housing mobility demonstrate?: Causal inference in the face of interference. *Journal of the American Statistical Association, 101*(476), 1398–1407.

Steiner, P. M., & Cook, D. (2013). Matching and propensity scores. In T. D. Little (Ed.), *The Oxford handbook of quantitative methods* (Vol. 1, pp. 237–259). New York: Oxford University Press.

Stuart, E. A. (2010). Matching methods for causal inference: A review and a look forward. *Statistical Science, 25*(1), 1–21.

Winship, C., & Morgan, S. L. (1999). The estimation of causal effects from observational data. *Annual Review of Sociology, 25*, 659–706.

# CHAPTER 2

# Overview of Implementing Propensity Score Analyses in Statistical Software

## Megan Schuler

Although some basic propensity score analyses can be implemented by writing a limited amount of code, many common statistical packages, including R, SAS, and STATA, now have a variety of robust propensity score packages that offer the ability to implement more advanced techniques (e.g., full matching, kernel matching, and subclassification). Additionally, many feature built-in balance diagnostic functions to examine the performance of the propensity score procedure. This chapter provides an overview of the capabilities of existing software packages with respect to propensity score estimation, analysis (including matching, weighting, and subclassification), and balance diagnostics. Sample syntax is provided for each package discussed.

## ESTIMATING THE PROPENSITY SCORE

We first review methods to estimate the propensity score. The propensity score model estimates the probability of treatment assignment based on observed pre-treatment covariates. Propensity score models are often estimated using parametric modeling, particularly logistic regression, although nonparametric methods such as regression trees and boosted modeling may provide better results in some cases (Lee, Lessler, & Stuart, 2009; McCaffrey, Ridgeway, & Morral, 2004; Setoguchi, Schneeweiss,

Brookhart, Glynn, & Cook, 2008). See Chapters 1 and 3 in this book for detailed discussions of propensity score estimation.

We now present basic sample code for estimating the propensity score using logistic regression in R, SAS, and STATA. For simplicity, the sample syntax presented is in reference to a dataset "mydata" with a binary treatment indicator ("treat"), a continuous outcome ("cont_out"), a binary outcome ("bin_out"), five baseline covariates ("x1" – "x5") and an ID variable ("id").

### Estimating the propensity score in R with logistic regression

```
R> <ps.out <- glm(treat~x1+x2+x3+x4+x5, data=mydata,
    family=binomial)
R> mydata$pscore <- predict(ps.out, type="response")
```

### Estimating the propensity score in SAS with logistic regression

```
SAS> proc logistic data=mydata descending;
    model treat=x1 x2 x3 x4 x5;
    output out=mydata_ps prob=pscore;
    run;
```

### Estimating the propensity score in STATA with logistic regression

```
STATA> logistic treat x1 x2 x3 x4 x5
STATA> predict pscore
```

## MATCHING METHODS

In brief, matching methods create a subset of the original sample in which treated individuals are matched to control individuals who are similar with respect to specified covariates. The final analysis is then conducted among the matched subset. Since controls are generally matched to the treated individuals, the typical estimand for matching is the average treatment effect for the treated (ATT). See Chapters 1 and 4 in this book for discussions of various matching methods and their caveats. There are many different matching algorithms; a sample syntax is provided below for some of the most common methods.

The *MatchIt* package for R (Ho, Imai, King, & Stuart, 2011) is one of the most comprehensive matching packages available and can implement a wide variety of matching methods including nearest neighbor, optimal, full, exact, and coarsened exact matching, as well as propensity score subclassification. There are several matching macros for SAS, including the %GMATCH and %VMATCH macros maintained by the Mayo Clinic (Kosanke & Bergstralh, 2004a, 2004b) and the %PSMatching macro (Coca-Perraillon, 2007). In STATA, matching can be implemented using the *psmatch2* package (Leuven & Sianesi, 2012) or the *teffects* command available in STATA 13 (which is an expansion of *psmatch2*).

## *k*:1 Nearest Neighbor Matching

Perhaps the most common and conceptually straightforward matching approach is $k$:1 nearest neighbor matching, alternatively known as $k$:1 local optimal or $k$:1 greedy matching (Rubin, 1973). Nearest neighbor matching is a local (i.e., "greedy") algorithm that optimizes matching individual by individual, unlike global matching algorithms (discussed later), which optimize matching for the sample as a whole. Matches are determined by finding control individuals with the smallest distance (with respect to the metric of interest) from the given treated individual. In the context of propensity score matching, a commonly used metric is the absolute difference in the propensity score. Ties (i.e., when two or more control individuals are the same distance from the treated individual) are handled differently in different packages—a matched control may be chosen by random draw among all tied individuals, or all tied individuals may be used as matched controls.

### Nearest Neighbor Matching in R with *MatchIt*

In *MatchIt*, the default matching method is 1:1 nearest neighbor matching without replacement, with matching based on the absolute difference of the propensity scores. By default, propensity scores are estimated using logistic regression (i.e., `distance="logit"`), although other parametric options are available such as probit regression (`distance="probit"`). Alternatively, the metric can be changed to Mahalanobis distance with `distance="mahalanobis"`. The matching ratio can be increased to $k$:1 with `ratio=k`. By default, individuals are ranked by propensity score values and matching starts with largest first; random ordering can be specified with `m.order="random"`. The `caliper=c` option specifies a caliper of $c$ units in terms of standard deviations of the given distance metric. Variables for exact matching are specified as `exact=c("x1","x2")`; variables for Mahalanobis matching are specified as `mahvars=c("x1","x2")`.

The matched dataset can be obtained with the `match.data()` command; this dataset includes a variable called weights which should be used

# Implementing Propensity Score Analyses in Statistical Software

as a frequency weight in any analysis when matching with replacement. More details and examples are provided in the *MatchIt* documentation (Ho et al., 2011).

## Examples of *k*:1 matching without replacement

```
# Install MatchIt package prior to first use
R> install.packages("MatchIt")
# Call MatchIt library in every R session
R> library(MatchIt)
# 1:1 matching
R> m.out <- matchit(treat~x1+x2+x3+x4+x5, data=mydata)
# 2:1 matching, with caliper of 0.15 PS standard deviations
R> m.out <- matchit(treat~x1+x2+x3+x4+x5, data=mydata,
   method= "nearest", ratio=2, caliper=0.15)
# 2:1 matching, random sorting
R> m.out <- matchit(treat~x1+x2+x3+x4+x5, data=mydata,
   method= "nearest", ratio=2, m.order="random")
# 1:1 matching, Mahalanobis metric
R> m.out <- matchit(treat~x1+x2+x3+x4+x5, data=mydata,
   method="nearest", distance=mahalanobis)
```

## Examples of *k*:1 matching with replacement

```
# 2:1 matching with replacement
R> m.out <- matchit(treat~x1+x2+x3+x4+x5, data=mydata,
   method= "nearest", ratio=2, replace=T)
# 3:1 matching with replacement, probit regression,
   with caliper
R> m.out <- matchit(treat~x1+x2+x3+x4+x5, data=mydata,
   method= "nearest", ratio=3, distance="probit", caliper=0.20,
   replace=T)
```

## Combining nearest neighbor with Mahalanobis or exact matching

```
# 1:1 nearest neighbor matching, Mahalanobis matching on x1
   and x2
R> m.out <- matchit(treat~x1+x2+x3+x4+x5, data=mydata,
   method="nearest", mahvars=c("x1","x2"), caliper=0.25)
# 1:1 nearest neighbor matching, exact matching on x1 and x2
R> m.out <- matchit(treat~x1+x2+x3+x4+x5, data=mydata,
   method="nearest", exact=c("x1","x2"))
```

## Example of estimating treatment effect after matching

```
# Obtain matched dataset from MatchIt output
R> m.mydata <- match.data(m.out)
# Matched without replacement: conduct t-test
```

```
R> t.test(m.mydata$cont_out[m.mydata$treat==1],
   m.mydata$cont_out[m.mydata$treat==0])
# Alternatively, regression model
R> lm(cont_out~treat, data=m.mydata)
# Regression model including covariates
R> glm(bin_out~treat+x1+x2+x3+x4+x5, data=m.mydata,
   family=binomial)
# Matched with replacement, use frequency weights
R> glm(bin_out~treat+x1+x2+x3+x4+x5, data=m.mydata,
   weights=weights, family=binomial)
```

### Nearest Neighbor Matching in SAS with %GMATCH Macro

The %GMATCH macro performs $k$:1 nearest neighbor matching without replacement, with 1:1 matching as the default. The propensity score must be estimated prior to running the macro, such that the dataset passed to the macro includes the variable to match on (typically the propensity score or the logit of the propensity score), specified by the mvars option. The distance metric is defined as the absolute difference between the paired treated and control individuals on the matching variable. The number of controls matched to each treated individual is specified by ncontls=k. %GMATCH does not have an option to match with replacement. The dmaxk option specifies a caliper—the input is in absolute units of the matching variable. It is recommended that the treated and control groups are both randomly sorted prior to matching; the random seed for sorting can be specified by the seedca option for the treated group and seedco for the control group. %GMATCH returns a dataset of the matched sample. See Faries, Leon, Maria Haro, and Obenchain (2010) for a detailed example.

### Examples of $k$:1 matching without replacement

```
/* Include %GMATCH
SAS> %include 'gmatch.sas';
/* 1:1 nearest neighbor matching, matching on propensity score
SAS> %gmatch(data=mydata_ps, group=treat, id=id,
     mvars=pscore, seedca=111222, seedco=111333, out=matched);
/* 2:1 matching, matching on PS, caliper=0.10 units
SAS> %gmatch(data=mydata_ps, group=treat, id=id;
     mvars=pscore, dmaxk=0.10, ncontls=2, seedca=111222,
     seedco=111333, out=matched);
```

### Example of caliper matching

```
/* Want to specify caliper in terms of SD of PS logit
/* Calculate standard deviation of logit of propensity score
```

*Implementing Propensity Score Analyses in Statistical Software*

```
SAS> proc means std data=mydata_ps;
     var logit_ps;
     output out=std_ps (keep=std) std=std;
     run;
/* Create new variable that is 0.20 SD of logit of PS
SAS> data std_ps; set std_ps;
     std=0.2*std;
     run;
/*Create macro variable that specifies caliper size
     for matching
SAS> data _null_;
     set std_ps;
     call symput('stdcal',std);
     run;
/* 2:1 caliper matching, caliper=0.20 SD of logit of PS
SAS> %gmatch(data=mydata_ps, group=treat, id=id,
     mvars=logit_ps, dmaxk=&stdcal, ncontls=2, seedca=111222,
     seedco=111333, out=matched);
```

## Nearest Neighbor Matching in SAS with %PSMatching Macro

The %PSMatching macro performs nearest neighbor matching and caliper matching, and allows both matching without replacement and matching with replacement. $k$:1 nearest neighbor matching is performed by specifying method=nn and numberofcontrols=k. Caliper matching is performed by specifying method=caliper and caliper=c. The propensity score must be estimated prior to running the macro, such that the dataset passed to the macro already includes the propensity score. These data must be passed to the macro as two separate datasets, one for the controls and one for the treated. The treated and control datasets are randomly sorted prior to matching. The macro returns a dataset where each row corresponds to a matched pair and the variables are pair number, control individual's ID "IdSelectedControl," control propensity score "PScoreControl," treated individual's ID "MatchedToTreatID" and treated propensity score "PScoreTreat." More details are given in Coca-Perraillon (2007).

### Examples of $k$:1 matching, with and without replacement

```
/* Include %PSMatching macro
SAS> %include 'PSMatching.sas';
/* Have previously estimated propensity score "pscore"
/* Separate datasets for treated and control, only contain ID
and propensity score (or alternatively logit of PS)
SAS> data mydataC mydataT;
     set mydata_ps;
```

```
          if treat=0 then do;
            idC=id; pscoreC=pscore; output mydataC;
          end;
          if treat=1 then do;
            idT=id; pscoreT=pscore; output mydataT;
          end;
     /* 1:1 nearest neighbor matching without replacement
SAS>    %PSMatching(datatreatment=mydataT, datacontrol= mydataC,
          method=nn, numberofcontrols=1, replacement=no,
          out=matches);
     /* 2:1 caliper matching with replacement, 0.10 caliper
SAS>    %PSMatching(datatreatment= mydataT, datacontrol= mydataC,
          method=caliper, caliper=0.10, numberofcontrols=2,
          replacement=yes, out=matches);
```

## Nearest Neighbor Matching in STATA with *psmatch2*

The *psmatch2* package in STATA performs k:1 matching. Matching with replacement is the default; matching without replacement is only available for 1:1 matching and can be specified with the noreplace option. By default, matching is based on the propensity score estimated by probit regression; other options include logistic regression of the propensity score and Mahalanobis matching. Matching is preformed based on the order of individuals in the given dataset, so random sorting or sorting based on propensity score magnitude is recommended.

Depending on the treatment effect of interest and whether one would like to adjust for additional covariates in the final analysis, one can obtain treatment effect estimates from *psmatch2* directly or estimate separately based on the matching results (reflected in the generated variable _weight). See documentation for details on the treatment effect estimates provided in *psmatch2*.

### Examples of k:1 matching, with and without replacement

```
// Install psmatch2.ado file
STATA> findit psmatch2
// Sort individuals randomly before matching
// Set random seed prior to psmatch2 to ensure replication
STATA> set seed 1234
STATA> generate sort_id = uniform()
STATA> sort sort_id
// 1:1 matching with replacement, estimate PS with
        logistic regression
```

```
STATA> psmatch2 treat x1 x2 x3 x4 x5, logit
// 2:1 matching without replacement
STATA> psmatch2 treat x1 x2 x3 x4 x5, logit noreplace n(2)
// 2:1 matching with replacement and caliper,
PS previously estimated
STATA> psmatch2 treat, pscore(pscore) n(2) cal(0.20)
// 1:1 matching Mahalanobis metric, with caliper
STATA> psmatch2 treat, mahal(x1 x2 x3 x4 x5) cal(0.10)
```

## Example of estimating treatment effect after matching

```
// ATT (default estimand) for both outcome variables
STATA> psmatch2 treat x1 x2 x3 x4 x5, outcome(cont_out bin_out)
       logit
// Regression approach: Equivalent to ATT estimates
from psmatch2
// Note: if matched without replacement, _weight=1 for all
STATA> psmatch2 treat x1 x2 x3 x4 x5, logit
STATA> regress cont_out treat [iweight=_weight] if _weight!=.
// Regression including covariates
STATA> regress cont_out treat x1 x2 x3 x4 x5 [iweight=_weight]
       if _weight!=.
```

## Nearest Neighbor Matching in STATA 13 with *teffects*

Nearest neighbor matching in *teffects* is performed using the psmatch command and is similar to that in *psmatch2*, with some important differences. *teffects* only allows nearest neighbor matching with replacement, and the treatment effect standard errors are calculated differently from *psmatch2* (details in Abadie & Imbens, 2012; STATA 13 documentation). Logistic regression for propensity score estimation is default in *teffects* (rather than probit), and the default treatment effect estimated also differs (*teffects*'s atet option estimates the ATT). Mahalanobis matching can also be performed in *teffects* using the nnmatch command.

## Examples of nearest neighbor matching and Mahalanobis matching

```
// 2:1 matching with replacement, ATT effect
STATA> teffects psmatch (cont_out)(treat x1 x2 x3 x4 x5),
       nn(2) atet
// 1:1 matching, Mahalanobis metric, ATT effect
STATA> teffects nnmatch (cont_out x1 x2 x3 x4 x5) (treat),
       atet
```

## More Advanced Matching Methods

We now discuss some of the more recent alternatives to nearest neighbor matching, including coarsened exact matching, radius matching, kernel matching, and optimal matching. See Chapter 1 for an overview of the advanced matching methods, except for coarsened exact matching that is briefly described below.

### Coarsened Exact Matching

Coarsened exact matching (CEM) provides a feasible alternative to exact matching for continuous covariates or categorical covariates with many categories. This method temporarily coarsens (i.e., discretizes) covariates and then performs exact matching within covariate strata. Individuals in strata that do not successfully match at least one treated with at least one control individual are not included in the matched set. After matching, the coarsened versions of the variables are discarded, and the final analysis proceeds with the original variables (Blackwell, Iacus, King, & Porro, 2009). CEM bounds the maximum imbalance between groups as a function of the coarsening—as the bins become smaller, matched individuals become more similar. CEM is a variable-ratio matching approach, so weights must be used in the final analysis to account for different strata sizes. Alternatively, one may constrain CEM such that all strata have the same number of treated and control individuals.

*Coarsened Exact Matching in R with MatchIt.* CEM can be performed in *MatchIt* by specifying `method="cem"`; *MatchIt* calls the *cem* package. Variables will be coarsened automatically with CEM's binning algorithm; alternatively, the user can specify cutpoints for particular variables. See Iacus, King, and Porro (2009) for more details of CEM, including specifying cutpoints, restricting to $k$-to-$k$ matching, and estimating treatment effects.

### Examples of coarsened exact matching

```
# CEM with automatic binning
R> m.out <- matchit(treat~x1+x2+x3+x4+x5, data=mydata,
    method="cem")
# Obtain matched dataset from selected MatchIt output
R> m.mydata <- match.data(m.out)
# Estimate treatment effects; CEM weight is frequency weight
R> lm(cont_out~treat+x1+x2+x3+x4+x5, data=m.mydata,
    weights=weights)
```

# Implementing Propensity Score Analyses in Statistical Software

Coarsened Exact Matching in STATA. CEM can be implemented in STATA with the user-contributed package *cem*. This package was written by the same authors as the R *cem* package and thus implements the same algorithm. See more details in Blackwell, Iacus, King, and Porro (2009).

## Examples of coarsened exact matching

```
/* Install cem package
STATA> findit cem
/* CEM with automatic binning
STATA> cem x1 x2 x3 x4 x5, treatment(treat)
/* CEM with user-specified cutpoints for x3
STATA> cem x1 x2 x3 (0 1.5 4 7 9 14) x4 x5, treatment(treat)
/* Estimate treatment effects (using weights)
STATA> regress cont_out treat x1 x2 x3 x4 x5
       [iweight=cem_weights]
/* Constrain strata to have same number of treated and
       controls
STATA> cem x1 x2 x3 x4 x5, treatment(treat) k2k
/* Estimate treatment effects (no weighting)
STATA> regress cont_out treat x1 x2 x3 x4 x5
```

## Radius Matching

Radius matching matches a treated individual to all controls within the specified radius and thus is essentially a variable-ratio form of caliper matching (Dehejia & Wahba, 2002; Ming & Rosenbaum, 2000, 2001). This approach can offer greater precision relative to *k*:1 caliper matching when some treated individuals have many close controls.

Radius Matching in SAS with the %PSMatching Macro. Radius matching is performed by specifying `method=radius` and `caliper=c`. The propensity score must be estimated prior to running the macro, such that the dataset passed to the macro already includes the propensity score.

```
/* Radius matching
SAS> %PSMatching(datatreatment= mydataT, datacontrol= mydataC,
    method=radius, caliper=0.20, replacement=no,
    out=matches);
```

*Radius matching in STATA with* psmatch2. Radius matching is performed using the `radius` option and `caliper(c)`.

```
// Radius matching
STATA> psmatch2 treat x1 x2 x3 x4 x5, logit radius
       caliper(0.10)
```

## Kernel Matching

Kernel matching matches each treated individual to a weighted average of all the controls. Weights are proportional to the distance between a given control and the treated individual, such that closer controls receive larger weights.

*Kernel matching in STATA with psmatch2.* Kernel matching can be performed with the *psmatch2* package. There are several options for the choice of kernel (default is Epanechnikov kernel) and the bandwidth can be varied with the bwidth option. Increasing the bandwidth improves the smoothness of the density function, which may increase bias and yet may decrease variance.

```
Examples of kernel matching

// Kernel matching, PS estimated with logistic regression
STATA> psmatch2 treat x1 x2 x3 x4 x5, kernel logit
// Kernel matching, bandwidth=0.10
STATA> psmatch2 treat x1 x2 x3 x4 x5, kernel logit bwidth(0.10)
// Estimate ATT for outcome variable(s)
STATA> psmatch2 treat x1 x2 x3 x4 x5, kernel outcome(cont_out)
```

## Optimal Matching

Unlike greedy nearest neighbor matching, optimal matching seeks to maximize balance across all individuals by considering a global distance measure (Rosenbaum, 2002). Optimal matching is preferred when well-matched pairs, rather than well-matched groups, are of interest (Stuart, 2010).

*Optimal Matching in R with MatchIt.* Optimal $k$:1 matching in *MatchIt* calls the package *optmatch* (Hansen & Klopfer, 2006).

### Examples of optimal matching
```
# Optimal matching with a 2:1 ratio
R> m.out<-matchit(treat~x1+x2+x3+x4+x5,data=mydata,
   method="optimal", ratio=2)
```

```
# Optimal matching with a variable ratio
R> m.out<-matchit(treat~x1+x2+x3+x4+x5,data=mydata,
    method="optimal")
# Obtain matched dataset from selected MatchIt output
R> m.mydata <- match.data(m.out)
# Estimate treatment effects (using weights)
R> lm(cont_out~treat+x1+x2+x3+x4+x5, data=m.mydata,
    weights=weights)
```

Optimal Matching in SAS with %VMATCH Macro. The %VMATCH macro performs optimal matching with a variable matching ratio by default; a minimum and maximum number of controls matched to each treated individuals can be specified. The input to this macro must be in the form of a treated-control distance matrix, in which the value in the ith row and the jth column represents the distance between the ith treated individual and the jth control individual. This distance matrix can be calculated with the %DIST macro.

### Examples of optimal matching

```
/* Include %DIST and %VMATCH macro
SAS> %include 'dist.sas';
SAS> %include 'vmatch.sas';
/* If have already calculated distance matrix, can run vmatch
SAS> %vmatch(dist=mydata_dist, idca=id, a=2, b=2,
    lilm=num_of_control, n=num_of_treat, firstco=C_first,lastco=
    C_last);
/* Can run %VMATCH through %DIST macro
/* Does 1:1 optimal matching
SAS> %dist(data=mydata, group=treat, id=id, mvars=pscore,
    wts=1, vmatch=Y, a=1, b=1, lilm= num_of_control, dmax=0.1,
    outm=mp1_b, summatch=n, mergeout=mpropen);
/* Optimal matching; each treated matched with 1-3 controls
SAS> %dist(data=mydata, group=treat, id=id, mvars=pscore,
    wts=1, vmatch=Y, a=1, b=3, lilm= num_of_control, dmax=0.1,
    outm=mp1_b, summatch=n, mergeout=mpropen);
```

## PROPENSITY SCORE WEIGHTING

Propensity score weighting may also be used to achieve covariate balance between treated and control groups (Hirano & Imbens, 2001; Rosenbaum, 1987). This method uses the estimated propensity score to create weights for each individual, based on their treatment group. The form of the weights is dependent on whether the ATE or ATT estimand is of interest. See Chapters 1 and 7 for more discussions of propensity score weighting schemes. ATE and ATT estimands can be obtained parametrically using logistic regression with propensity score weighting in R, SAS, or STATA.

## ATE and ATT propensity score weighting with logistic regression in R

```
# Estimate the propensity score with logistic regression
R> ps.logit <- glm(treat~x1+x2+x3+x4+x5, data=mydata,
   family=binomial)
R> mydata$pscore <- predict(ps.logit, type="response")
# Calculate ATE propensity score weights (IPTW)
R> mydata$w.ate<-ifelse(mydata$treat==1,1/mydata$pscore,1/(1-
   mydata$pscore))
# Calculate ATT propensity score weights
R> mydata$w.att<-ifelse(mydata$treat==1,1,mydata$pscore/(1-
   mydata$pscore))
# Use ATE weights as probability weights in final analysis
R> library(survey)
R> design.ate <- svydesign(ids=~1,weights=~w.ate,data=mydata)
R> svyglm(cont_out~treat+x1+x2+x3+x4+x5, design=design.ate)
# Use ATT weights as probability weights in final analysis
R> design.att <- svydesign(ids=~1,weights=~w.att,data=mydata)
R> svyglm(cont_out~treat+x1+x2+x3+x4+x5, design=design.att)
```

## ATE and ATT propensity score weighting with logistic regression in SAS

```
/* Estimate the propensity score with logistic regression
SAS> proc logistic data=mydata descending;
    model treat = x1 x2 x3 x4 x5;
    output out=mydata_ps prob=pscore;
    run;
/* Calculate ATE and ATT propensity score weights
SAS> data mydata_ps.w;
    set mydata_ps;
    w_ate= treat/pscore + (1-treat)/(1-pscore);
    w_att= treat + (1-treat)*(pscore/(1-pscore));
    run;
/* Use ATE weights as probability weights in final analysis
SAS> proc genmod data=mydata_ps.w,
    class id;
    model cont_out = treat x1 x2 x3 x4 x5 / error=B;
    weight w_ate;
    run;
```

## ATE and ATT propensity score weighting with logistic regression in STATA

```
// Estimate the propensity score with logistic
    regression
STATA> logistic treat x1 x2 x3 x4 x5
STATA> predict pscore
// Calculate ATE propensity score weights (IPTW)
STATA> g w_ate = treat/pscore + (1-treat)/(1-pscore)
// Use ATE weights as probability weights in final analysis
STATA> svyset [pw=w_ate]
STATA> svy: regress cont_out treat x1 x2 x3 x4 x5
// Calculate ATT propensity score weights
STATA> g w_att = treat + (1-treat)*(pscore/(1-pscore))
STATA> svyset [pw=w_att]
// Use ATT weights as probability weights in final analysis
STATA> svyset [pw=w_att]
STATA> svy: regress cont_out treat x1 x2 x3 x4 x5
```

The toolkit for weighting and analysis of nonequivalent groups (*twang*) package in *R* creates propensity score weights generated by nonparametric generalized boosted modeling (Ridgeway, McCaffrey, & Morral, 2013). *twang* is notable since it is one of the few propensity score packages that estimates the propensity score nonparametrically, using generalized boosted modeling (GBM), which has been shown to outperform parametric methods for estimating the propensity score under certain conditions (Lee et al., 2009; McCaffrey et al., 2004; Setoguchi et al., 2008).[1] Additionally, *twang* is one of the few propensity score programs that implements propensity score weighting, rather than matching; either ATE or ATT weighting can be specified. Additionally, *twang* has a comprehensive suite of balance diagnostics. *twang* is discussed in greater depth in Chapter 3.

## ATE and ATT propensity score weighting with GBM

```
# Set random seed in order to ensure duplication of results
R> set.seed(1234)
# Run propensity score model, calculating ATT weights
R> mydata_ps1 <- ps(treat~x1+x2+x3+x4+x5, data=mydata,
    estimand= "ATT", verbose=FALSE)
# Save ATT weight as variable to original dataset
R> mydata$w.att <- get.weights(mydata_ps1,stop.method=
    "ks.mean")
# Use ATT weights as probability weights in final analysis
R> library(survey)
R> design.att <- svydesign(ids=~1,weights=~w.att,data=mydata)
```

```
# Run propensity score model, calculating ATE weights
R> mydata_ps2 <- ps(treat~x1+x2+x3+x4+x5, data=mydata,
     estimand= "ATE", verbose=FALSE)
# Save ATE weight as variable to original dataset
R> mydata$w.ate <- get.weights(mydata_ps2,stop.method=
     "ks.mean")
```

## PROPENSITY SCORE SUBCLASSIFICATION

### Subclassification

Subclassification creates subgroups (i.e., subclasses) of individuals who have similar propensity scores, for example, by grouping individuals based on the propensity score quintile (Rosenbaum & Rubin, 1984). See Chapter 1 for a brief description of subclassification.

### Subclassifcation in R Using *MatchIt*

Subclassification can be performed in *MatchIt* by specifying method="subclass". The number of subclasses is controlled with the subclass=k option; the default is six. *MatchIt* returns a dataset with a subclass indicator variable "subclass".

### Generating subclasses based on propensity score

```
# Subclassification with 5 subclasses
R> m.out <- matchit(treat~x1+x2+x3+x4+x5, data=mydata,
     method="subclass", subclass=5)
```

### Examples of calculating subclass-specific effects

```
# Get matched data, subclass indicator variable is "subclass"
R> data.sub <- match.data(m.out)
# Subclass-specific t-test for given subclass
R> t.test(cont_out~treat, data=data.sub, subset=subclass==1)
# Equivalent to subclass-specific t-test for all subclasses
R> lm(re78~as.factor(I(subclass)) + as.factor
     (I(subclass*treat)) -1, data=data.sub)
```

### Example of ATE estimate (combining subclass-specific estimate)

```
# define N = total number of people
R> N <- dim(data.sub)[1]
# Initialize vectors for subclass-specific effects
   ("sub.effect"), and sample size("sub.N")
```

```
R> sub.effect <- rep(NA, max(data.sub$subclass))
R> sub.var <- rep(NA, max(data.sub$subclass))
R> sub.N <- rep(NA, max(data.sub$subclass))
# Run linear regression model within each subclass
R> for(s in 1:max(data.sub$subclass)){
    tmp <- lm(cont_out ~ treat, data=data.sub,
        subset=subclass==s)
    sub.effect[s] <- tmp$coef[2]
    sub.var[s] <- summary(tmp)$coef[2,2]^2
    sub.N[s] <- sum(data.sub$subclass==s) }
# Calculate overall ATE effect
R> ATE.effect <- sum((sub.N/N)*sub.effect)
R> ATE.stderror <- sqrt(sum((sub.N/N)^2*sub.var))
```

## Subclassification in SAS

Subclassification can be performed in SAS by first estimating the propensity score, ranking individuals based on propensity score, and creating subclasses of individuals based on $q$-quantiles (e.g., quintiles in order to form five subclasses). Once subclasses are formed, subclass-specific effects can be estimated. Overall effects can be estimated by creating weights and generating the weighted average of subclass-specific effects. Faries et al. (2010) provide a detailed example, including macros for balance diagnostics across subgroups. Lanehart et al. (2012) discusses an alternate method of calculating an overall treatment effect via precision weighting of the subclass-specific effects (as shown in the sample code below). Note that this approach assumes that treatment effects are constant across subclasses.

### Creating 5 propensity score subclasses

```
/* After generating propensity scores, create quintiles
SAS> proc rank data = mydata_ps groups=5 out= ps_strataranks;
    var pscore;
    ranks ps_quint;
    run;
/* Sort data by quintiles
SAS> proc sort data = ps_strataranks;
    by ps_quint;
```

### Estimating subclass-specific and overall effect estimates

```
/* Binary outcome: Mantel-Haenszel stratified analysis
SAS> proc freq data= ps_strataranks;
    table ps_quint*treat*bin_out / nocol cmh;
run;
```

```
/* Continuous outcome: can combine subclass-specific t-tests
SAS> proc ttest data=ps_strataranks;
   by ps_quint;
   class treat;
   var cont_out;
   ods output statistics = strata_out;
/* Calculate weights (weight is inverse of square of SE
   of group difference); weight group differences
SAS> data weights;
   set strata_out;
   if class = 'Diff (1-2)';
   wt_i = 1/(StdErr**2);
   wt_diff = wt_i*Mean;
/* Sum weighted means
SAS> proc means noprint data = weights;
   var wt_i wt_diff;
   output out = total sum = sum_wt sum_diff;
/* Calculate and output overall treatment difference, SE
SAS> data overall;
   set total;
   diff_mean = sum_diff/sum_wt;
   diff_SE = SQRT(1/sum_wt);
SAS> proc print data = overall;
   run;
```

## Subclassification in STATA

As in SAS, subclassification can be performed in STATA by first estimating the propensity score, ranking individuals based on the propensity score, and creating subclasses of individuals based on $q$-quantiles. In this example, we combine subclass-specific effects using a Mantel–Haenszel approach for the binary outcome and a Van Elteren approach for the continuous outcome, both of which assume treatment effects are constant across subclasses.

### Creating 5 propensity score subclasses

```
// After generating propensity score, can create quintiles
STATA> xtile pscore_5 = pscore, nq(5)
```

### Estimating subclass-specific and overall effect estimates

```
// Binary outcome: Mantel-Haenszel stratified analysis
STATA> cc out_bin treat, by(pscore_5) bd
// Continuous outcome: Van Elteren test (Stratified Wilcoxon
     rank sum)
STATA> vanelteren out_cont, by(treat) strata(pscore_5)
```

## Full Matching

Full matching is a type of subclassification that forms subclasses comprised of one treated individual and one or more controls (Ho et al., 2011; Rosenbaum, 2002). See Chapter 1 for a description of full matching.

### Full Matching in R Using *MatchIt*

Full matching is implemented in *MatchIt* by specifying method = "full". Full matching, like optimal matching, uses the *optmatch* package (Hansen & Klopfer, 2006).

### Examples of full matching

```
R> m.out <- matchit(treat~x1+x2+x3+x4+x5, data=mydata,
     method="full")
# Constrained full matching: 2-5 controls per
     treated individual
R> m.out <- matchit(treat~x1+x2+x3+x4+x5, data=mydata,
     method="full", min.controls=2, max.controls=5)
# Obtain matched dataset from selected MatchIt output
R> matched.mydata <- match.data(m.out)
# Outcome regression, use frequency weights
R> lm(cont_out~treat+x1+x2+x3+x4+x5, data=matched.mydata,
     weights=weights)
```

## BALANCE DIAGNOSTICS

Assessing covariate balance when using propensity score methods is fundamental, since achieving good balance between groups indicates that the propensity score was adequate modeled and utilized. See Chapters 1 and 5 for detailed discussions of balance diagnostics.

### Balance Diagnostics Using R

A major advantage of robust propensity score packages, such as *MatchIt* and *twang*, is that they offer an extensive array of built-in diagnostic features.

### Diagnostic Methods in R Using *MatchIt*

Running the summary command on the output object from *MatchIt* returns a comprehensive balance table, showing covariate balance before and after matching, as well as a sample size summary. Specifying standardize=T in the summary command returns standardized mean difference (SMD) statistics for each covariate in the propensity score model. *MatchIt* provides numerous diagnostic plots (see Figure 2.1), including an effect size plot, which shows the SMDs for each covariate before and after matching. *MatchIt* also can generate a jitter plot showing the propensity score distributions across unmatched treated, matched treated, unmatched control, and matched control individuals; this plot helps assess whether there is sufficient propensity score overlap between the treated and control groups. *MatchIt* also provides histograms of the propensity score in the original treated, matched treated, original control, and matched control groups.

```
# 1:1 matching
R> m.out <- matchit(treat~x1+x2+x3+x4+x5, data=mydata)
# Print balance table
R> summary(m.out, standardize=T)
# Plot of absolute SMD for all covariates, before and after
    matching
R> plot(summary(m.out, standardize=T), interactive=F)
# Jitter plot of propensity scores
R> plot(m.out, type = "jitter", interactive = F)
# Propensity score histogram plot
R> plot(m.out, type = "hist")
```

### Diagnostic Methods in R Using *twang*

*twang* provides a comprehensive balance table showing covariate balance before and after propensity score weighting; this table includes standardized mean difference statistics for each covariate in the propensity score model.

```
# Run propensity score model, calculating ATT weights
# Print balance table
R> bal.table(mydata_ps)
```

One important factor to check is the effective sample size after weighting. If this is significantly smaller than the original sample size, then it indicates that many individuals are being downweighted toward 0 and thus are not providing meaningful matches.

```
# Provides quick summary of balance, effective sample size
R> summary(mydata_ps)
```

*twang* also provides many useful diagnostic graphics (see Figure 2.2). One option is a side-by-side box plot of the propensity scores in the

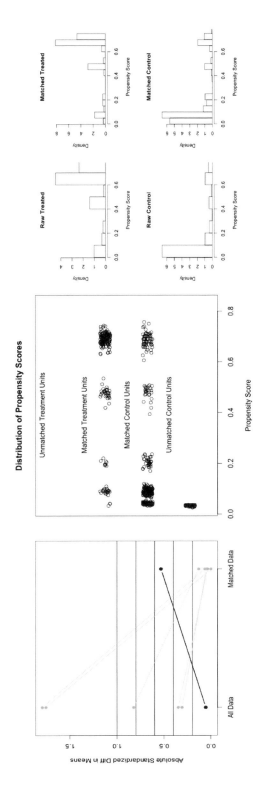

**FIGURE 2.1.** Effect size plot (left), propensity score jitter plot (middle), and propensity score histogram (right) from the *MatchIt* package.

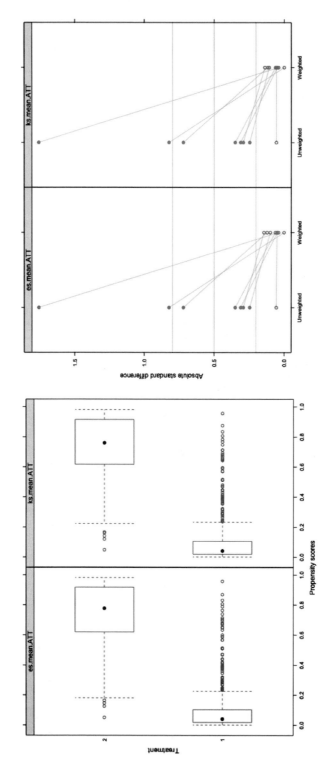

**FIGURE 2.2.** Box plot of propensity scores (left) and effect size plot (right) from the *twang* package.

treatment and control groups, so as to assess overlap (common support). Additionally, *twang* provides an effect size plot, showing the absolute SMDs in each covariate before and after weighting.

```
# Boxplot of Propensity Scores
R> plot(t mydata_ps, plots="boxplot")
# Effect Size plots
R> plot(mydata_ps, plots="es")
```

Assessing propensity score weights for extreme outliers is also an important step. Extreme weights increase the variance of the treatment estimate and may give undue influence to individuals with large weights. Weight trimming is often performed in the case of extreme weights (e.g., replace large weights with value of 90th percentile weight) (Robins, Hernan, & Brumback, 2000).

```
# Check distribution of weights within each treatment group
R> summary(mydata$w.att[mydata$treat==1])
R> summary(mydata$w.att[mydata$treat==0])
```

## Balance Diagnostics Using SAS and STATA

### Diagnostic Methods in SAS

Please see Faries et al. (2010) for a detailed discussion of assessing covariate balance in the context of matching, subclassification, and weighting—several diagnostic macros are provided as well as sample code. Sample code for assessing propensity score overlap between treatment groups is presented below.

### Example code for checking propensity score overlap

```
/* Sort data by treatment groups
SAS> proc sort data = mydata_ps;
by treat;
/* Boxplot of PS by treatment group
SAS> proc boxplot data= mydata_ps;
    symbol width = 2;
    plot pscore*treat;
    run;
/* Stacked histogram of PS by treatment group
SAS> ODS graphics on;
    proc univariate noprint data= mydata_ps;
    var pscore;
    class treat;
```

```
histogram pscore / nrows=2 ;
run;
ODS graphics off;
```

### Diagnostic Measures in STATA Using *psmatch2*

After performing matching with *psmatch2*, diagnostics can be assessed with several built-in commands. The pstest command prints a balance table comparing the treated and control groups; specifying the both option shows balance before and after matching. Pstest reports standardized % bias, which is similar to standardized mean difference. Specifying the graph option generates a plot of the standardized % bias for each covariate (see Figure 2.3).

```
// Balance table and plot
STATA> pstest x1 x2 x3 x4 x5, both graph
```

Additionally, the psgraph command generates a plot comparing histograms of the propensity score in the treated and control group.

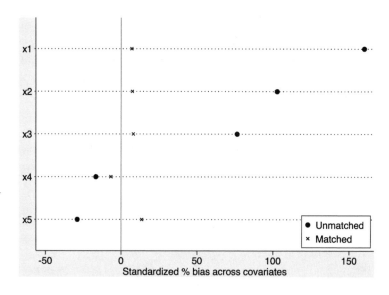

**FIGURE 2.3.** Plot of standardized percent bias before and after matching from the *psmatch2* package.

## CONCLUSION

If propensity score matching or subclassification is of interest, *MatchIt* is recommended since it offers the most extensive capabilities. *MatchIt* also provides comprehensive balance statistics and diagnostic plots that greatly facilitate assessing propensity score performance. *MatchIt* is straightforward to use and has extensive documentation and sample code (see Ho et al., 2011). STATA also offers numerous matching options, including nearest neighbor, Mahalanobis, radius, kernel, and coarsened exact matching. In general, matching programs in STATA are straightforward to use and well documented. Balance statistics and diagnostic plots are available, but not as comprehensive as in *MatchIt* or *twang*. One drawback in STATA is that $k$:1 matching without replacement is not available. SAS also offers a broad array of matching options, including optimal matching. There are macros available to facilitate balance checking and diagnostics; these tend to be separate from the macros that perform the matching. In general, propensity score analysis in SAS requires a bit more coding for the analyst compared to other software packages. Faries et al. (2010) is recommended as a comprehensive tutorial to propensity score analysis in SAS.

The *twang* package is recommended if propensity score weighting is of interest. *twang* offers the advantage of nonparametric estimation for the propensity score which has been shown to improve performance in some cases. *twang* implements either ATE or ATT weighting, provides extensive balance diagnostics, and is well documented with extensive sample code.

## RECOMMENDED RESOURCES

### General

Caliendo, M., & Kopeinig, S. (2008). Some practical guidance for the implementation of propensity score matching. *Journal of Economic Surveys, 22*, 31–72.

Stuart, E. A. (2010). Matching methods for causal inference: A review and a look forward. *Statistical Science, 25*, 1–21.

Elizabeth Stuart's propensity score software webpage
*www.biostat.jhsph.edu/~estuart/propensityscoresoftware.html*

Gives an overview of many software packages and macros for R, SAS, STATA and SPSS, as well as software for assessing sensitivity to unmeasured confounders.

## For R

*MatchIt* documentation
http://cran.r-project.org/web/packages/MatchIt/MatchIt.pdf
More details on the *MatchIt* package.

*twang* documentation
http://cran.r-project.org/web/packages/twang/twang.pdf
More details on the *twang* package.

*twang* tutorial
http://cran.r-project.org/web/packages/twang/vignettes/twang.pdf
Provides step-by-step example of using propensity score weighting on the well-known Lalonde data.

http://sekhon.berkeley.edu/matching
More information on the *Matching* package in R, based on a genetic search algorithm.

## For SAS

SAS macros are available through the Mayo Clinic and at www.math.smith.edu/sasr/examples.php

Faries, D. E., Leon, A. C., Maria Haro, J., & Obenchain, R. L. (2010). *Analysis of observational health care data using SAS*. Cary, NC: SAS Institute.

## For STATA

*psmatch2* documentation
http://repec.org/bocode/p/psmatch2.html

*teffects* documentation
www.stata.com/manuals13/te.pdf

Comparison of *teffects* and *psmatch2*
www.ssc.wisc.edu/sscc/pubs/stata_psmatch.htm

## NOTE

1. Note that *twang* performs propensity score weighting only. It is possible to input propensity scores estimated by *twang* into *MatchIt* in order to perform propensity score matching and subclassification based on nonparametric propensity scores.

## REFERENCES

Abadie, A., & Imbens, G. W. (2011). Bias-corrected matching estimators for average treatment effects. *Journal of Business and Economic Statistics, 29,* 1–11.

Abadie, A., & Imbens, G. W. (2012). *Matching on the estimated propensity score.* Cambridge, MA: Harvard University and the National Bureau of Economic Research. Available at *www.hks.harvard.edu/fs/aabadie/pscore.pdf.*

Blackwell, M., Iacus, S., King, G., & Porro, G. (2009). CEM: Coarsened exact matching in Stata. *Stata Journal, 9,* 524–546.

Brookhart, M. A., Schneeweiss, S., Rothman, K. J., Glynn, R. J., Avorn, J., & Sturmer, T. (2006). Variable selection for propensity score models. *American Journal of Epidemiology, 163,* 1149–1156.

Coca-Perraillon, M. (2007). Local and global optimal propensity score matching. In SAS *Global Forum 2007,* Paper 185–2007.

Dehejia, R. H., & Wahba, S. (2002). Propensity score matching methods for nonexperimental causal studies. *Review of Economics and Statistics, 84*(1), 151–161.

Faries, D. E., Leon, A. C., Maria Haro, J., & Obenchain, R. L. (2010). *Analysis of observational health care data using SAS.* Cary, NC: SAS Institute.

Hansen, B. B., & Klopfer, S. O. (2006). Optimal full matching and related designs via network flows. *Journal of Computational and Graphical Statistics, 15,* 609–627.

Hirano, K., & Imbens, G. (2001). Estimation of causal effects using propensity score weighting: An application to data on right heart catheterization. *Health Services and Outcomes Research Methodology, 2,* 259–278.

Ho, D., Imai, K., King, G., & Stuart, E. A. (2011). MatchIt: Nonparametric preprocessing for parametric causal inference. *Journal of Statistical Software, 42,* 1–44.

Iacus, S., King, G., & Porro, G. (2009). CEM: Software for Coarsened Exact Matching. *Journal of Statistical Software, 30,* 1–27.

Kosanke, J., & Bergstralh, E. (2004a). gmatch: Match 1 or more controls to cases using the GREEDY algorithm. Available at *http://mayoresearch.mayo.edu/mayo/research/biostat/upload/gmatch.sas.*

Kosanke, J., & Bergstralh, E. (2004b). Match cases to controls using variable optimal matching. Available at *http://mayoresearch.mayo.edu/mayo/research/biostat/upload/vmatch.sas.*

Lanehart, R. E., Rodriguez de Gil, P., Kim, E. S., Bellara, A. P., Kromrey, J. D., & Lee, R. S. (2012). Propensity score analysis and assessment of propensity score approaches using SAS procedures. In *SAS Global Forum,* Paper 314–2012.

Lee, B., Lessler, J., & Stuart, E. A. (2009). Improving propensity score weighting using machine learning. *Statistics in Medicine, 29,* 337–346.

Leuven, E., & Sianesi, B. (2012). PSMATCH2: Stata module to perform full Mahalanobis and propensity score matching, common support graphing, and covariate imbalance testing. Available at *http://ideas.repec.org/c/boc/bocode/s432001.html.*

McCaffrey, D. F., Ridgeway, G., & Morral, A. R. (2004). Propensity score estimation with boosted regression for evaluating causal effects in observational studies. *Psychological Methods, 9*, 403–425.

Ming, K., & Rosenbaum, P. R. (2000). Substantial gains in bias reduction from matching with a variable number of controls. *Biometrics, 56*, 118–124.

Ming, K., & Rosenbaum, P. R. (2001). A note on optimal matching with variable controls using the assignment algorithm. *Journal of Computational and Graphical Statistics, 10*(3), 455–463.

Morgan, S. L., & Todd, J. L. (2008). A diagnostic routine for the detection of consequential heterogeneity of causal effects. *Sociological Methodology, 38*, 231–281.

Ridgeway, G., McCaffrey, D., & Morral, A. (2013). *Twang*: Toolkit for weighting and analysis of nonequivalent groups. Software for using matching methods in R. Available at *http://cran.r-project.org/web/packages/twang/index.html*.

Robins, J. M., Hernan, M. A., & Brumback, B. (2000). Marginal structural models and causal inference in epidemiology. *Epidemiology, 11*, 550–560.

Rosenbaum, P. R. (1987). Model-based direct adjustment. *Journal of the American Statistical Association, 82*, 387–394.

Rosenbaum, P. R. (2002). *Observational studies* (2nd ed.). New York: Springer.

Rosenbaum, P. R., & Rubin, D. B. (1983). The central role of the propensity score in observational studies for causal effects. *Biometrika, 70*, 41–55.

Rosenbaum, P. R., & Rubin, D. B. (1984). Reducing bias in observational studies using subclassification on the propensity score. *Journal of the American Statistical Association, 79*, 516–524.

Rosenbaum, P. R., & Rubin, D. B. (1985). Constructing a control group using multivariate matched sampling methods that incorporate the propensity score. *American Statistician, 39*, 33–38.

Rubin, D. B. (1973). Matching to remove bias in observational studies. *Biometrics, 29*, 159–184.

Sekhon, J. S. (2011). Multivariate and propensity score matching software with automated balance optimization: The Matching package for R. *Journal of Statistical Software, 42*(7), 1–52.

Setoguchi, S., Schneeweiss, S., Brookhart, M. A., Glynn, R. J., & Cook, E. F. (2008). Evaluating uses of data mining techniques in propensity score estimation: A simulation study. *Pharmacoepidemiology and Drug Safety, 17*, 546–555.

Stuart, E. A. (2010). Matching methods for causal inference: A review and a look forward. *Statistical Science, 25*, 1–21.

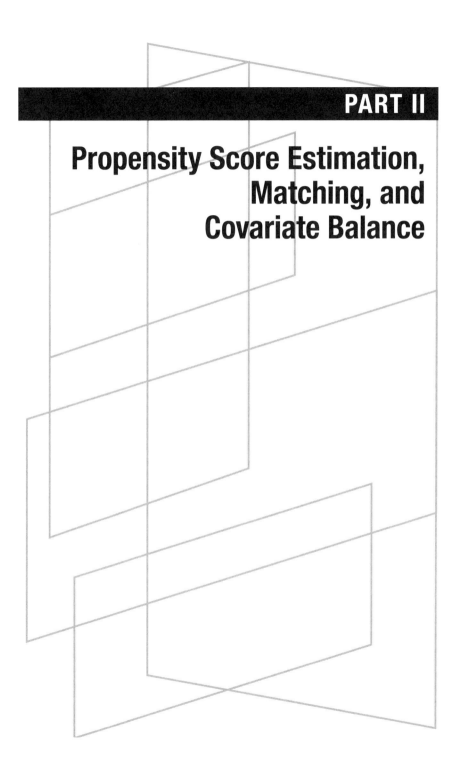

# PART II

# Propensity Score Estimation, Matching, and Covariate Balance

# CHAPTER 3

# Propensity Score Estimation with Boosted Regression

**Lane F. Burgette
Daniel F. McCaffrey
Beth Ann Griffin**

The theory of propensity score analysis is elegant. Provided strong ignorability holds, the single propensity score is all that is required to control for pretreatment differences between two treatment groups or a treatment and a control group. In practice, however, propensity score analysis involves a number of key steps, each with its own set of complexities. This chapter describes the propensity score estimation step of a propensity score analysis and provides an illustrative example of how to estimate propensity scores using generalized boosted models (Hastie, Tibshirani, & Friedman, 2009).

In observational studies, propensity scores are almost always unknown and therefore must be estimated from the observed data at hand. If estimated incorrectly, propensity scores can add bias and unnecessary variance to treatment effect estimates. Researchers and analysts must work carefully to obtain stable propensity scores with good balancing properties. In doing so, they face a variety of critical issues.

Several years ago, after spending considerable time building a propensity score model using methods that were then state of the art (Dehejia & Wahba, 1999; Rosenbaum & Rubin, 1985) only to remain unsatisfied with the results, we turned to a novel statistical method at that time—generalized boosted modeling (GBM; Ridgeway, 1999) to estimate propensity scores. GBM developed in the intersection of machine learning and statistics and seemed to be ideal for estimating propensity scores. Specifically, GBM predicted dichotomous outcomes (such as treatment assignment) more accurately than other available methods (such as logistic regression, Schonlau, 2005, or regression trees, Friedman, Hastie, & Tibshirani, 2000) and did so with an automated algorithm that selected which predictor variables were to be included in the model, the necessary interaction terms, and the most appropriate functional relationships between the predictor variables and the outcome of interest. We applied GBM to our data and found that propensity scores estimated from GBM succeeded in balancing the covariate distributions between the treatment and weighted control groups. Since that time many authors have used GBM in propensity score analysis and refined the tuning of GBM for propensity score estimation so that it selects a set of propensity scores with optimal balancing properties.

This chapter contains an overview of GBM and a discussion of the current approaches to GBM for propensity score analysis. The chapter also contains a detailed application of GBM to estimate the effects of different adolescent substance abuse treatment programs as an empirical example.

## GENERALIZED BOOSTED MODELING

The generalized boosted model is one of a class of boosting methods developed in the late 1990s and early years of the 21st century. Boosting combines many weak predictor models or classifiers to create a single powerful predictor or classifier (Hastie, Tibshirani, & Friedman, 2009, Chapter 10). Each individual weak predictor model is a poor approximation to the function of interest, but together they can approximate a smooth function just like a sequence of line segments can approximate a smooth curve. Some of the alternative boosting methods include AdaBoost (Freund & Schapire, 1997), LogitBoost (Friedman et al., 2000), and the gradient boosting machine (Friedman, 2001). Boosting has been shown to outperform alternative methods in terms of prediction error (Friedman, 2001; Madigan & Ridgeway, 2004) and is considered by some experts to be the best classifier (Breiman, 1998). It is particularly effective when the model involves a large set of covariates (Bühlmann & Yu, 2003).

The original applications of boosting used simple classification rules as the weak predictors, but GBM and other later applications use very simple regression trees as weak predictors. The use of regression trees in GBM makes it a particularly valuable predictor of dichotomous variables because they handle mixed covariate data types (continuous, discrete, or semicontinuous), including variables with missing values; they are computationally speedy; they automatically accommodate nonlinear and interactive effects; the fitted values are invariant to strictly monotonic transformations of the explanatory variables; and covariates that never result in the best split are never used. Each of these characteristics is especially desirable in the context of propensity score estimation.

To provide more details, regression tree models partition the values of the covariates into disjoint sets and then assign a constant value to each set in order to model the outcome. The fitted values for the outcome are allowed to vary across partitions. While each individual partition is very simple—every split is binary and depends on a single covariate—the process can segment the data in complex ways and therefore may describe complex relationships between the covariates and the outcome of interest. Breiman, Friedman, Olshen, and Stone (1984) provide details fitting regression trees and their properties.

By applying boosting to regression trees, GBM retains the attractive features of trees, but by combining many simple trees it yields smoother fits (see Figure 3.1) and better predictions than trees (Friedman et al., 2000; Friedman, 2001). Like all boosting methods, GBM uses what is

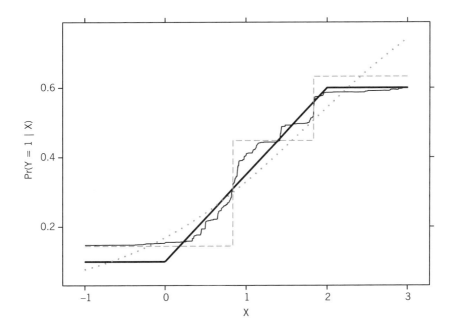

**FIGURE 3.1.** Comparison of fitted values from different models. The figure plots the fit from GBM (solid, thin curve), tree (dashed curve), and logistic (dotted curve) regression models, along with a true data-generating model (thick, solid curve).

known as a "forward stagewise additive algorithm" to develop the propensity score model (Hastie et al., 2009). This means that, at each step of the algorithm used to build a GBM, a new simple regression tree is added to the model from the previous steps without changing any of the previous regression tree fits. GBM models the log-odds of treatment assignment, $g(\mathbf{x}) = \log\{e(\mathbf{x})/[1 - e(\mathbf{x})]\}$, where for a vector of covariates $\mathbf{x}$ and a treatment assignment indicator $z$, $e(\mathbf{x}) = \Pr(z = 1|\mathbf{x})$ and $e(\mathbf{x}) = 1/\{1 - \exp[-g(\mathbf{x})]\}$. The algorithm initially sets the estimate of the propensity score function $\hat{g}(\mathbf{x})$ to the sample log odds of receiving treatment, $\log[\bar{z}/(1 - \bar{z})]$, where $\bar{z}$ is the average treatment assignment indicator for the entire sample. The next step of the algorithm fits a simple regression tree, $h_2(\mathbf{x})$, to the residuals from the current estimate of the propensity score. The current estimate of the propensity score equals $1/\{1 + \exp[-\hat{g}_1(\mathbf{x})]\}$, so the residuals are $r_i = z_i - 1/\{1 + \exp[-\hat{g}_1(\mathbf{x})]\}$, and $h_2(\mathbf{x})$ is the best fitting regression tree function of the covariates for these residuals. The model is updated to $\hat{g}_2(\mathbf{x}) = \hat{g}_1(\mathbf{x}) + \lambda h_2(\mathbf{x})$, and the parameter $\lambda$ is a shrinkage factor that is less than one that helps make the fitted model smoother and improves the accuracy of the prediction. The algorithm now repeats. Residuals are calculated using the new model, and a new simple regression tree is fit to these residuals.[1] The algorithm continues until it reaches the maximum number of iterations that we specify.

The number of iterations determines the model's complexity and must be determined from the data. With each iteration of the algorithm, a GBM becomes more complex, fitting additional features of the data. With too few iterations, a GBM does not capture important features of the data. With too many iterations, it overfits the data. Analysts typically use external fit indices such as cross-validation prediction error (Hastie et al., 2009). For propensity score analysis, we use covariate balance to choose the iterations in the GBM, as described later in the chapter.

Figure 3.2 demonstrates the GBM algorithm in a simple example using data from a study on the effectiveness of adolescent substance use treatment in which receipt of treatment is modeled as a function of substance use as measured by the Substance Intensity Index (SII). For demonstration purposes, the model includes only one covariate; in practice, we would typically control for many more variables. In each panel, the horizontal axis is SII and the vertical axis is the log-odds of treatment. The short line segments at the top and bottom of the figure plot the SII values of treatment and control units (e.g., subjects), respectively. In Figure 3.2a the black line shows the value of the GBM at its initial value, the sample log-odds of treatment. The gray line is fit from a linear logistic regression model. The black lines in Figures 3.2b, c, and d show the value of the GBM

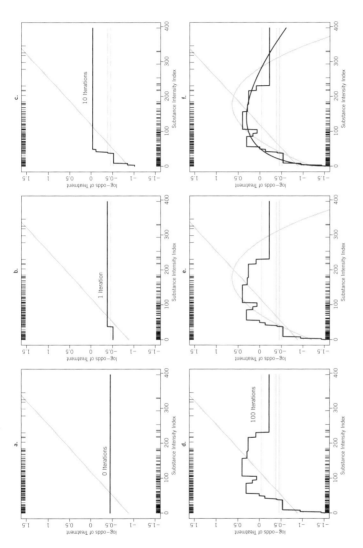

**FIGURE 3.2.** Example of the GBM fitting process. These figures illustrate GBM fits at various iterations of the fitting process and compares the fit with logistic regression. The black line in panels a–d is for the current GBM fit and the straight gray line is from logistic regression; other gray lines are other GBM fits to Substance Intensity Index (SII). The short line segments at the top and bottom of each panel show the values of the treatment and control units. Panels a, b, c, and d plot GBM fits at after 0, 1, 10, and 100 iterations, respectively. Panel e adds a logistic regression fit with a quadratic term (solid gray curve) to SII, and panel f adds predictions from GBM (black line) and logistic regression (with quadratic term, black curve) fits to the square root of SII. The gray line for the GBM fit to SII is hidden by the black line for the GBM fit to the square root of SII because GBM is invariant to monotonic transformations of the covariates.

after 1, 10, and 100 iterations. After 1 iteration there is one split indicating that youth with very low values of the SII have a lower probability (lower log-odds) of receiving treatment, which is consistent with our expectation since these youth would have less need for treatment. By 100 iterations, the GBM is a somewhat smooth function that reaches its maximum at value of 106 for the SII and then turns down slightly. Figure 3.2e shows the same figure with the curve from a logistic regression model with quadratic term. The logistic regression fit is no longer monotonically increasing, but the fit is poor, especially for cases with a high value of the index. Figure 3.2f adds fits from a GBM and a logistic regression model fit to the square root of the SII. The logistic regression model included linear and quadratic terms in the square root of the index. Now the logistic and GBM models are well aligned, and the logistic model fits the data much better. However, the logistic regression fit required knowing the best transformation of SII. The GBM fit is the same using the raw or transformed index because, as noted earlier, GBM is invariant to monotone transformations of the covariates.

The example also demonstrates another advantageous feature of GBM: the estimates flatten out at the extreme values of the covariate where the data are sparse. This feature helps GBM avoid propensity scores that come spuriously close to zero or one, which can greatly stabilize propensity score weighted estimators. As shown in the example, logistic regression is more likely to produce extreme propensity score values.

## TREATMENT EFFECT ESTIMANDS USED IN PROPENSITY SCORE ANALYSIS

In this section, we use the potential outcomes framework to define treatment effects that tend to be of primary interest in most studies using propensity score analysis and present a general approach to their estimation via weighted means. As discussed in Chapter 1, propensity scores can be used for matching, subclassification (or stratification), or weighting. Propensity scores estimated via GBM can be used for any of those purposes, though in this chapter we focus on using GBM to estimate propensity score weights. There is evidence that using GBM to estimate propensity scores works particularly well when applied to weighting (Harder, Stuart, & Anthony, 2010; Lee, Lessler, & Stuart, 2010). Also, the Toolkit for Weighting and Analysis of Nonequivalent Groups (*twang*) package (Ridgeway, McCaffrey, Morral, Burgette, & Griffin, 2012) in the R environment (R Development Core Team, 2008), which we have developed to model propensity scores using GBM, assumes propensity score analysis using weighting.

The two estimands we consider are the average treatment effect on the population (ATE) and the average effect of treatment on the treated (ATT; Wooldridge, 2002). We let $r_1$ and $r_0$ equal the potential outcomes for treatment and control, respectively, then ATE = $E(r_1) - E(r_0)$, where the expectation is over the entire population or sample. Under the standard ignorability assumptions, a consistent weighted estimator is

$$\widehat{\text{ATT}} = \frac{\sum_{i=1}^{N} r_i z_i / e(\mathbf{x}_i)}{\sum_{i=1}^{N} z_i / e(\mathbf{x}_i)} - \frac{\sum_{i=1}^{N} r_i (1-z_i)/[1-e(\mathbf{x}_i)]}{\sum_{i=1}^{N} (1-z_i)/[1-e(\mathbf{x}_i)]}$$

(Imbens, 2004). In contrast, ATT = $E(r_1 \mid z = 1) - E(r_0 \mid z = 1)$, the average effect of treatment for units like those who received treatment. Again, under the standard ignorability assumptions, a consistent weighted estimator for the ATT is

$$\widehat{\text{ATT}} = \frac{\sum_{i=1}^{N} r_i z_i}{\sum_{i=1}^{N} z_i} - \frac{\sum_{i=1}^{N} r_i (1-z_i)e(\mathbf{x}_i)/[1-e(\mathbf{x}_i)]}{\sum_{i=1}^{N} (1-z_i)e(\mathbf{x}_i)/[1-e(\mathbf{x}_i)]}$$

(Imbens, 2004). For both ATE and ATT, in practice, the estimated propensity scores replace the unknown values.

## USING GBM TO ESTIMATE PROPENSITY SCORES

The first step to modeling the propensity scores is selecting which covariates to use. The choice is clearly substantive, but some general rules apply. Omitting pretreatment variables that predict outcome and treatment assignment will lead to bias (Drake, 1993), so including all available pretreatment variables that are thought to do both is desirable. Since the computational time increases slowly with the number of variables included in the modeling, using a large number of variables is quite feasible in GBM. Moreover, GBM can sort out variables that are not predictive of treatment status and not use them in the final model, so including many candidate variables in the GBM generally may be preferable to pre-selecting variables. However, variables that relate to the outcome only through their effect on treatment assignment should be excluded because using them in propensity score modeling can make estimation inefficient and actually increase hidden bias due to omitted variables (Brookhart et al., 2006; Meyer et al., 2011). Additionally, when the number of variables is very large relative to the sample size, GBM may not find balance. In such cases, use of expert opinion or empirical investigations to identify covariates related to the outcomes of interest may lead to better balance and treatment effect estimates.

After selecting variables for the modeling, fitting GBM to treatment assignment data requires setting two tuning parameters and choosing the number of iterations for the algorithm. The first tuning parameter is the complexity of the simple regression tree used in the boosting algorithm. Trees with more splits can fit higher degree interactions. More specifically, a tree can fit interactions of degree equal to the number of splits less one. In our experience, we typically default to four splits, which allows for three-way interactions. The other tuning parameter is the shrinkage applied at each iteration of the algorithm as described above. Small values on the order of 0.0005 result in smoother estimates, which can help reduce extraneous variability in the propensity scores. We tend to choose values of 0.001 or 0.0005 in practice. Computational time increases almost linearly with the reciprocal of the shrinkage factor, so, to improve speed, larger values might need to be chosen with large datasets and many predictors.

## Balance Metrics

Rosenbaum and Rubin (1983) show that the propensity score is a balancing score: conditional on it, the distribution of the covariates is the same for the treatment and control groups. Similarly, weighting by the propensity score also balances the distributions of covariates between the treatment and control group. Good propensity score estimates should balance the covariates between treatment groups. We use two balance measures to assess the performance of the propensity score estimates from each iteration of GBM: the standard bias (SB, also called the absolute standardized mean difference [ASMD] or standardized effect size [ES]; McCaffrey, Ridgeway, & Morral, 2004), and the Kolmogorov–Smirnov standardized bias (KS).

### Standardized Bias

For each covariate, the standardized bias equals the absolute value of the difference between the weighted mean for the treatment group and the weighted mean for the control group divided by the unweighted standard deviation of the pooled sample for ATE or divided by the unweighted standard deviation of the treatment group for ATT. More specifically, for ATE, for covariate $k$ ($k = 1, \ldots, K$), $SB_k = |\bar{x}_{k1} - \bar{x}_{k0}|/s_k$, where $\bar{x}_{kz}$ is the weighted mean of the covariate for treatment ($z = 1$) or control ($z = 0$) and $s_k$ is the standard deviation of the covariate for the pooled sample. The weights are $1/\hat{e}(\mathbf{x})$ for members of the treatment group and $1/[1 - \hat{e}(\mathbf{x})]$ for members of the control group, where $\hat{e}(\mathbf{x})$ is the GBM estimate of the propensity score. For ATT, $SB_k = |\bar{x}_{k1} - \bar{x}_{k0}|/s_{k1}$, where the weights equal 1 for members of the treatment group and $\hat{e}(\mathbf{x})/[1 - \hat{e}(\mathbf{x})]$ for members of the control group and $s_{k1}$ is the standard deviation of the covariate for the treatment group.

As noted below, tuning GBM requires a single summary statistic rather than standardized bias for each covariate. Thus, we use either the mean or the maximum across the $K$ covariates.[2] We then select as "optimal" the iteration of GBM that minimizes this overall summary statistic and use the estimated propensity scores from this "optimal" iteration in our propensity score analysis.

### KS Statistic

The KS statistic depends on the weighted empirical distribution functions for the treatment and control samples. For covariate $k$, these are defined as

$$EDF_{zk}(x) = \frac{\sum_{i=1}^{N} w_i I(z_i = z) I(x_i \leq x)}{\sum_{i=1}^{N} w_i I(z_i = z)}$$

for $z = 0$ or 1, where $I(z_i = z)$ equals 1 if this is true and 0 otherwise and similarly for $I(x_i \leq x)$. Again, for ATE the weights are $1/\hat{e}(\mathbf{x})$ and $1/[1 - \hat{e}(\mathbf{x})]$ for the treatment or the control groups, respectively, and for ATT they are 1 for treatment and $\hat{e}(\mathbf{x})/[1 - \hat{e}(\mathbf{x})]$ for control. The KS statistic for each covariate is

$$KS_k = \sup_x | EDF_{1k}(x) - EDF_{0k}(x) |$$

The KS is valuable because it compares entire distributions rather than just means. We use either the mean or the maximum of the $KS_k$ across covariates to select the optimal iteration of GBM for obtaining our estimates of the propensity scores in our propensity score analysis.

### Choosing the Number of Iterations for GBM

As discussed above, we must use the data to select the number of iterations for the GBM fit. For propensity score estimation we choose the number of iterations that gives the best balance between the treatment and control groups on the covariates according to a selected balance metric. Specifically, we run the GBM algorithm for one iteration and use the resulting fit to calculate a score on the desired balance metric. We then add a second iteration and again calculate the balance statistic. We repeat this process for a very large number of iterations calculating the balance statistic at each iteration, and then we search across the iterations to find the number that optimizes our balance metric.

This approach to choosing the number of iterations works because with few iterations there is very little variation in the propensity scores since the model has not yet recovered the features of the data that differentiate units that are common in the treatment group and those that are not. These propensity scores cannot balance the groups since they do not differentiate units. As the GBM algorithm proceeds through more iterations, the resulting models fit closer and closer to the observed treatment assignment indicators. When the number of iterations gets large, the propensity scores become nearly uniformly close to one in the treatment group and nearly uniformly zero in the control group. Such propensity scores also cannot balance the groups since all units in the treatment get roughly the same propensity score and similarly for the control group. Consequently, balance is initially poor, tends to improve as we add iterations to the GBM algorithm, reach an optimum, and then decline, so it can be used to tune the algorithm.

## Stopping Rules and Balance Assessment

We refer to the balance metrics above as "stopping rules" when fitting GBM to estimate propensity scores, and typically we work with one of four stopping rules when implementing a propensity score analysis: the mean or maximum SB or the mean or maximum KS.

Once the optimal iteration of GBM is selected based on the chosen "stopping rule" for a particular propensity score analysis, we also use the balance statistics for individual covariates and the summary statistics to judge the quality of the weighting and the potential for remaining bias. Overall, we like SB to be less than 0.20 for all variables because SB is like an effect size and values less than 0.20 are considered small (Cohen, 1998). Other authors suggest 0.25 as sufficient to reduce most bias (Cochran, 1968; Ho, Imai, King, & Stuart, 2007). Unlike standardized bias, the distribution of the KS statistic depends on the sample size, so there can be no universal objective guideline for what constitutes a large or small value. For modest to large sample sizes, we tend to consider KS statistics greater than 0.10 as indications of imbalance. The KS statistic is very useful for comparing among models because even if there are no absolute standards, the relative sizes of the KS statistics for weights from different model fits can rank the models.

Because the weights and balance statistics are specific to ATE or ATT, GBM must be tuned using either ATE or ATT specific stopping rules. Conveniently, the *twang* package in R contains functions for estimating propensity score models using GBM tuned by one or more of the balance statistics which can be specific to match the treatment effect estimand of interest.

It is possible that propensity scores that yield good balance for ATE will not do the same for ATT, and vice versa. For instance, suppose the treatment is tutoring for students who are struggling with reading. The students in the program would all have low reading scores, and the group could not be weighted to match a general population that includes students with high reading scores. Thus, it would be hard to achieve ATE balance with this treatment group and a general population control group. However, a general population control group can be weighted to match the treatment group using ATT weights by giving large weights to students with low reading scores (who are not enrolled in tutoring) and small weights to all the other students. Even in less dramatic situations, propensity scores tuned for ATT weighting might not yield balance for ATE weighting, and vice versa.

## Performance of GBM for Estimating Propensity Score Weights

Multiple studies have compared weighting with GBM-estimated propensity scores to other methods for estimating causal effects and found that it performs well relative to other methods. For example, McCaffrey et al. (2004) compared GBM with logistic regression for estimating ATT and found that GBM generated weights that better balanced covariates and yielded smaller standard errors for the treatment effects. Harder et al. (2010) tested multiple propensity score estimation methods including GBM and applied each to one-to-one matching, full-matching, stratification or subclassification, ATT weighting, and ATE weighting. This resulted in 15 methods for estimating causal effects, which they applied to a single data set. GBM worked relatively well in all the methods balancing nearly all variables, and no other model worked as consistently well. In addition, GBM with ATT weighting and logistic regression with ATE weighting were the only methods to balance all the covariates to have SB below 0.25. Lee, Lessler, and Stuart (2010, 2011) compared GBM to other methods in large simulation studies and found that GBM yielded estimated treatment effects with smaller relative bias and greater precision than the other methods. Random forests (Breiman, 2001) also performed well.

## MORE THAN TWO TREATMENT CONDITIONS

Although many studies involve just two treatments, many also involve three or more. McCaffrey et al. (2013) discuss the use of propensity score weighting and GBM to estimate the effects of two or more treatments. They focus on the estimation of pairwise effects. In a study of three treatments A, B, and C, the pairwise effects are the effect of A relative to B, A relative to C, and B relative to C. Although pairwise effects are not the only effects that might be of interest with multiple treatments, they are often of interest.

McCaffrey and colleagues (2013) consider pairwise ATE and ATT. To estimate pairwise ATE, they suggest using GBM for dichotomous outcomes repeatedly to model indicators for each treatment group. Their procedure consists of the following steps:

1. Creating a dichotomous indicator variable $z_{ji} = 1$ if observation $i = 1, \ldots, N$ received treatment $j$ and 0 otherwise.

2. Modeling $z_{ji}$ using GBM with an ATE stopping rule and the selected observed covariates.

3. Calculating the ATE weights, $w_{ji}$, from the resulting GBM fit.

4. Repeating for each treatment.

5. Estimate pairwise treatment effects as

$$\frac{\sum_{i=1}^{N} r_i z_{ji} w_{ji}}{\sum_{i=1}^{N} z_{ji} w_{ji}} - \frac{\sum_{i=1}^{N} r_i z_{ki} w_{ki}}{\sum_{i=1}^{N} z_{ki} w_{ki}}$$

where $r_i$ is an outcome of interest, $z_{ji}$ and $z_{ki}$ are indicators for the pair of treatments being compared, and $w_{ji}$ and $w_{ki}$ are the ATE for weights treatments $j$ and $k$ for observation $i$. That is to say, each estimated pairwise treatment effect is the difference in the ATE weighted means.

For pairwise ATT, McCaffrey et al. (2013) suggest for each pair of treatments to:

1. Restrict the sample to observations from the pair of treatments.
2. Use GBM for ATT for the two-group unit to estimate ATT weights.
3. Use the ATT weights to estimate the desired causal effect.

That is, we restrict the sample to two treatments and apply the two-group GBM methods described earlier in the chapter. We repeat this for all the pairwise treatment effects that are of interest.

For both ATE and ATT, we estimate weights through repeated use of the GBM for two groups. The tools developed for two groups can be used for multiple groups. However, it can be useful to have an overall assessment of balance across the multiple treatments. For pairwise comparisons, we propose the maximum of the pairwise statistics over all pairs as the summary of the balance; we consider groups to be jointly balanced when this statistic is small, for example, less than 0.20.[3]

Repeatedly applying the two-group GBM model to calculate weights provides a means of estimating weights, but it does not provide the joint probability of treatment assignment. Theoretical results on weighting assume that the joint probabilities are used, so repeated use of the two-group solution is somewhat ad hoc; however, since each experimental unit is weighted by a propensity score that is defined by the probability of having received one particular treatment, the pairwise approach seems reasonable. In addition, for $K$ treatments it requires applying GBM $K(K-1)/2$ times. If we estimate the joint probabilities in a single model, then GBM will be run only one time. Until recently, this option did not exist using the available tools in R because GBM did not estimate the joint probabilities from a multinomial distribution. However, the GBM package in R now estimates multinomial models for multiple outcome categories.

The following algorithm could be used to apply the new multinomial function to propensity score estimation. Let $z_i$ take on values 1 to $K$ where $z_i = k$ if and only if $z_{ki} = 1$ or individual $i$ received treatment $k$. Let $p_k(X_i)$ equal the conditional probability that $z_i = k$ given the observed covariate $X_i$ and $p_k(X_i)$ be the GBM estimate of this probability from a multinomial model. For ATE, the weight for an individual in treatment group $k$ is $1/p_k(X_i)$. For ATT for treatment group $k$, the weight for each individual in treatment group $k'$ is $p_k(X_i)/p_{k'}(X_i)$. For pairwise comparisons, we use the maximum over pairs of the pairwise balance statistics for the GBM stopping rule. The best stopping rule for tuning GBM and the relative advantages of using probabilities from the joint model versus repeated use of the two-group GBM approaches are an area of ongoing research since the multinomial GBM fit is a new feature of the program. In the example below we use the methods of McCaffrey et al. (2013). Future research will need to test GBM with the multinomial fit.

## APPLICATION TO A SUBSTANCE ABUSE TREATMENT EVALUATION

In this section, we provide two illustrative examples of propensity score weight estimation using GBM. In the first, we have only two treatment groups (i.e., the binary treatment unit) and in the second, we have four treatment groups (i.e., the multiple treatments unit). In both examples, interest lies in obtaining ATE weights that balance the treatment groups on a set of 23 pretreatment characteristics. Both sets of weights are fit using the *twang* package in R. We begin each example by describing how to estimate the propensity score weights using the *twang* package and then discuss how to perform diagnostics that assess how well the propensity score weights balance the groups in question.

### Case Study Data

In our illustrative examples, we use data from a recent study that examined the effectiveness of biological drug screening (BDS) alone versus three other treatment conditions on drug use outcomes among adolescent substance users. The three other treatment groups are a no-treatment condition; a group of youth who received motivational enhancement therapy/cognitive-behavioral therapy 5 (MET/CBT5) only; and a group of youth who received both MET/CBT5 and BDS (MET/CBT5 + BDS). Extensive details about the study can be found in Schuler et al. (2014). In brief, the data arose from an observational study of youth who enrolled into treatment programs funded by the Substance Abuse and Mental Health Services Administration's Center for Substance Abuse Treatment (SAMHSA's CSAT) between 1998 and 2008. By design, youth were followed up at 3, 6, and 12 months post-intake and were administered the Global Appraisal of Individual Needs (GAIN) (Dennis, Titus, White, Unsicker, & Hodgkins, 2003), a comprehensive structured clinical interview that contains eight modules assessing background and demographic characteristics; substance use; physical health; risk behaviors; mental health; and environmental, legal, and educational/vocational problem areas. In the examples below, the propensity scores estimated via GBM aim to balance the treatment groups in question on 23 pretreatment characteristics measured by the GAIN.

## The Binary Treatment Case

For this binary treatment example, we use the BDS only and no-treatment condition samples from Schuler et al. (2014). Estimating propensity score weights with GBM for binary treatments can be easily implemented in *twang*. The user simply needs to make a call to the ps() function. In our case, we issue the following command:

```
> ps.binary <- ps(bds3 ~ bcs + cei0 + cjsi0 + cvs + e10 +
  eps7p0 + ers210 + female + ias5p0 + maxce0 + mhti30 +
  pos + prmhtx + race + recov0 + s2s20 + sdsm0 + sdsy0 +
  sfs8p0 + spsm0 + spsy0 + sri70 + tas5p0, data = data.binary,
  estimand = 'ATE', stop.method = "es.max", n.trees = 5000,
  verbose = FALSE).
```

The first term in the call to ps() is the formula that contains the treatment indicator (bds3) followed by a tilde ("~") and then the covariates separated by addition signs. Next is the name of the dataset "data.binary," which is a subset of the Schuler et al. dataset, restricted to the BDS only and no-treatment groups. Setting the estimand option equal to "ATE" tells the ps() function to choose the iteration of GBM that optimizes balance with respect to ATE weights and diagnostic criterion. Here n.trees is set to 5000, and only the "es.max" stopping rule is selected to choose the optimal iteration of the GBM.

A call to plot(ps.binary, plots = 1) produces a diagnostic figure for assessing whether the specified value of n.trees allowed GBM to explore sufficiently complicated models (see Figure 3.3). It plots the balance measure for a given stopping rule (here the maximum SB) as a function of the number of iterations in the GBM algorithm, with higher iterations corresponding to more complicated fitted models. As can roughly be seen in Figure 3.4, 1,361 iterations minimize the SB, and the trend after 2,000 iterations suggests that further iterations would not improve balance in this example.

The bal.table() function from the *twang* package provides a summary of the balance. It calculates both the SB and KS statistics for each covariate before and after weighting. Figure 3.4 presents a portion of the output from this function for our binary treatment example. The top half of the figure ($unw) presents the unweighted comparison of youth in the two groups. There are imbalances in terms of race. Fifty-one percent of youth receiving BDS only (tx.mn) were white (race:1) and 11% were black (race:2), compared with 39% and 18% of those who received no treatment (ct.mn). The bottom half of Figure 3.4 ($es.max.ATE) presents R output

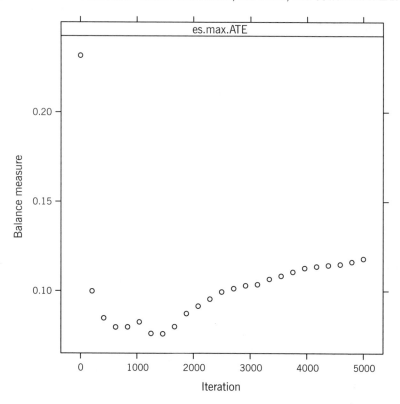

**FIGURE 3.3.** Plot generated by the plot() function in the *twang* package. Plot of the stopping rule balance measure (maximum SB) as a function of GBM iterations. The figure shows the balance statistic at each iteration of the GBM fitting algorithm for the binary treatment example. Balance is measured by the maximum SB for the 23 covariates for the ATE estimand. The *twang* package denotes this balance measure and associated stopping rule as "es.max.ATE," which is presented in the banner at the top of the plot. The best fit occurs at the minimum value at 1,361 iterations. Before that the model is underfit, and after this it is overfit, producing poorer balance of the covariates.

of balance statistics for the weighted samples. Weighting attenuates the differences found in the unweighted portion of Figure 3.4. After weighting, 49% of the BDS-only group is white and 12% is black, and the corresponding percentages are 47% and 13% for the no-treatment sample. The SB statistics for racial groups drop from over 0.20 in absolute value before weighting to about 0.04 after weighting.

Figure 3.5 shows a useful graphical summary of the SBs presented in Figure 3.4, though for the full set of pretreatment covariates rather than the truncated output of the table. Specifically, this graphic illustrates the effect of propensity score weights on the magnitude of differences between the two groups on each pretreatment covariate. These magnitudes are standardized using the ATE standardization because ATE is the estimand of interest in this example. A substantial reduction in the SB is observed for almost all the variables. The SB increases slightly after weighting for a few variables for which it was very small prior to weighting (thick lines). Closed circles indicate a statistically significant difference, many of which occur before weighting, and only a few after. Figure 3.5 was produced using the command plot (ps.binary, plots=3).

```
$unw
                tx.mn   tx.sd   ct.mn   ct.sd   std.eff.sz    stat       p      ks   ks.pval
prmhtx          0.393   0.488   0.336   0.473        0.118   2.999   0.003   0.057     0.033
prmhtx:<NA>     0.007   0.086   0.011   0.103       -0.038  -0.902   0.367   0.003     0.364
race:1          0.510   0.500   0.393   0.488        0.234  11.297   0.000   0.117     0.000
race:2          0.113   0.316   0.179   0.384       -0.210      NA      NA   0.066     0.000
race:3          0.213   0.409   0.246   0.430       -0.081      NA      NA   0.033     0.000
race:4          0.164   0.370   0.181   0.385       -0.044      NA      NA   0.016     0.000
race:<NA>       0.000   0.017   0.001   0.036       -0.064      NA      NA   0.001     0.000
$es.max.ATE
                tx.mn   tx.sd   ct.mn   ct.sd   std.eff.sz    stat       p      ks   ks.pval
prmhtx          0.386   0.487   0.350   0.477        0.074   1.702   0.089   0.036     0.489
prmhtx:<NA>     0.008   0.088   0.008   0.088       -0.001  -0.029   0.977   0.000     0.977
race:1          0.494   0.500   0.472   0.499        0.042   0.501   0.723   0.021     0.723
race:2          0.121   0.326   0.134   0.340       -0.038      NA      NA   0.013     0.723
race:3          0.218   0.413   0.223   0.416       -0.013      NA      NA   0.005     0.723
race:4          0.167   0.373   0.170   0.375       -0.008      NA      NA   0.003     0.723
race:<NA>       0.000   0.017   0.001   0.029       -0.034      NA      NA   0.001     0.723
```

FIGURE 3.4. Truncated output of bal.table() function from the *twang* package in R. Balance metrics are for BDS only and no treatment groups before and after weighting. The upper table labeled "$unw" presents balance prior to weighting. The first column presents the variable names. The covariate "prmhtx" (any mental health treatment prior to current treatment episode) is dichotomous with missing values. The row labeled "prmhtx: <NA>" gives balance for the missing data indicator variable or the proportion of missing data in the two treatment groups. The covariates "race:1" to "race:4" are race/ethnicity indicators for white, black, hispanic, and other race and "race <NA>" is the missing race indicator. The columns of balance data are: treatment mean and standard deviation ("tx.mn," "tx.sd"), control mean and standard deviation ("ct.mn," "ct.sd"), standardized group mean difference ("std.eff.sz"), the *t*-statistic ("stat") and *p*-value ("p") for testing the difference in means, the KS statistics and a *p*-value for testing it ("ks", "ks.pval"). For categorical variables with more than two levels, like race, a chi-square test is used to test for group differences with values given in the row for the first level ("race:1"). The bottom half of the figure labeled "$es.max. ATE" summarizes balance after weighting with weights from a GBM fit tuned using the maximum standardized bias (SB) stopping rule ("es.max") for the ATE estimand.

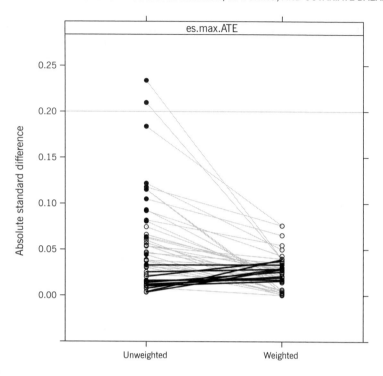

**FIGURE 3.5.** Plot generated by the plot() function in the *twang* package. Unweighted and weighted SBs for covariates in the binary treatment example. Dots on the left plot the SB for covariates prior to weighting; dots on the right plot the SB for covariates after weighting; and lines connect the dots for each covariate. Solid dots indicate SBs that are statistically significantly different from zero, and thick lines indicate the covariates for which the SB increased with weighting. For this example, we tuned GBM using the maximum SB stopping rule (es.max.ATE), as noted in the banner at the top of the plot. The plot functions in the *twang* package include the banner by default. Also by default, the plot labels the vertical axis for SB as "Absolute standard difference."

## The Multiple-Treatments Case

For the multiple-treatments example, we utilize all four treatment groups in the Schuler et al. study (BDS only, MET/CBT5, MET/CBT5 + BDS, and no treatment). We are again interested in ATE and desire weights that will balance the four treatment groups, and we aim to make each of the groups look like the overall population in our analytic sample on each of the 23 pretreatment characteristics. The left side of Figure 3.6 gives the unweighted comparison of youth in each of the four groups relative to one another. For each covariate, it plots the maximum of the pairwise SB across the six pairs of treatments. The largest pairwise SBs between the treatment groups are on race/ethnicity and variables related to the criminal justice system. In terms of raw means (not displayed), adolescents in either MET/CBT5 and MET/CBT5 + BDS groups were more likely to be white and less likely to be black (MET/CBT5: white = 51%, black = 6%; MET/CBT5 + BDS: white = 58%, black = 8%) than adolescents in either the no-treatment group or the BDS only group (BDS only: white = 36%, black = 18%; no treatment: white = 39%, black = 18%). Additionally, adolescents in either MET/CBT5 condition (with or without BDS) had lower means on the Criminal Justice System Index compared to the other groups (MET/CBT5: 0.21; MET/CBT5 + BDS: 0.33; BDS only: 0.53; no treatment = 0.35). Similarly, adolescents in the BDS only group or no-treatment group spent more days in a controlled environment in the 90 days prior to baseline (MET/CBT5 = 3; MET/CBT5 + BDS = 6; BDS only = 19; no treatment = 13). In light of these various differences, it is of interest to find propensity score weights that balance these four treatment groups.

Estimating propensity score weights with GBM for multiple treatments can be implemented in *twang* using the mnps() function (Burgette, Griffin, & McCaffrey, 2013). The mnps() function uses repeated application of the ps() function for pairs of treatments as described earlier in the chapter. In our case study, the command issued would read as follows:

```
> mnps.mult <- mnps(treat ~ bcs + cei0 + cjsi0 + cvs + e10 +
  eps7p0 + ers210 + female + ias5p0 + maxce0 + mhti30 + pos +
  prmhtx + race + recov0 + s2s20 + sdsm0 + sdsy0 + sfs8p0 +
  spsm0 + spsy0 + sri70 + tas5p0, data = data,
  estimand = "ATE", verbose = FALSE, stop.method = "es.max",
  n.trees = 10000)
```

where treat is now a factor variable that takes on four values, one for each of the treatment groups. The other specifications in the command are as described above for the ps() function, except "data" now refers to the full sample rather than just the BDS only and no-treatment groups. As in the binary treatment setting, plot(mnps.mult, plots = 1) can be utilized to assess whether n.trees is large enough to allow for proper convergence on the GBM fits.

To assess balance in our case study with more than two treatments, we focus on computing the maximize pairwise SB for each covariate. Thus, we first estimate the standard two-sample ATE SB for BDS only versus no-treatment for each variable and then repeat this for BDS only versus each of the other treatments and for all the remaining pairs of treatments.

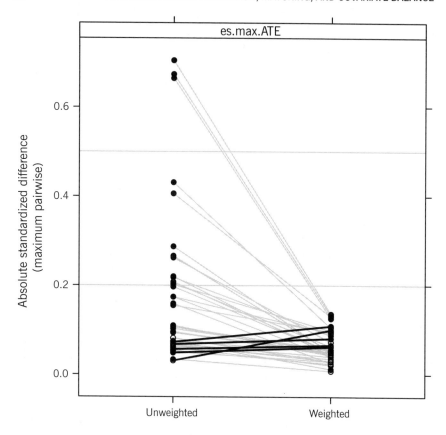

**FIGURE 3.6.** Plot generated by the plot() function in the *twang* package. Maximum pairwise SBs for the multiple treatment application, before and after weighting. Dots on the left plot values prior to weighting; dots on the right plot the absolute values after weighting; and lines connect the dots for each covariate. Solid dots indicate values that are statistically significantly different from zero, and thick lines indicate the covariates for which the values increased with weighting. For this example, we tuned GBM using the maximum SB stopping rule (es.max.ATE), as noted in the banner at the top of the plot. The plot functions in the *twang* package include the banner by default. Also by default, the plot labels the vertical axis for SB as "Absolute standard difference."

Figure 3.6 shows the maximum of the unweighted and weighted pairwise differences for each pretreatment characteristic. As shown, after weighting, the pretreatment characteristics of all four groups are well balanced with one another. Substantial reductions in the maximum SBs are observed for most variables (thin lines). Note also that SBs that were substantially above the 0.2 threshold are solidly under it after weighting. A few variables show an increase in SB after weighting (thick lines), but the increases are modest. Closed circles in the multiple-treatment setting indicate that at least one of the pairwise differences was statistically significant; many more of these occur before than afterward. Figure 3.6 was produced using the command plot(mnps.mult, plots = 3).

## OTHER CONSIDERATIONS AND CONCLUSION

Current work is being done to optimize the performance of the mnps() function and to provide a better understanding of what the best balance criteria should be in the multiple-treatment setting. Additionally, work has already been done that utilizes GBM to estimate the inverse probability of treatment weights (IPTW) when estimating marginal structural models (Griffin et al., 2014) and the causal effects of time-varying treatments. Future work will aim to expand the *twang* package with routines that implement IPTW for marginal structural models.

To summarize, PS modeling using GBM proceeds by fitting a nonparametric model of the treatment assignment and tuning the model complexity so as to optimize a chosen measure of balance. Propensity score analysis based on GBM has several key benefits. GBM can form strong predictive models with little input from the data analyst, automatically performing variable selection and accommodating nonlinear and interactive effects of the pretreatment variables on the treatment indicators. The complexity of GBM models can be tuned to optimize measures of weighted covariate balance. GBM also sensibly and automatically accounts for missing values in the pretreatment covariates. And GBM's estimated propensity scores tend to be flat at extreme covariate values if there are few observations in such regions, which may result in more stable weights than those that arise from logistic regression. As with all nonparametric methods, GBM can be less efficient than parametric models (such as standard logistic regression) when the simpler model adequately describes the data, though—in our experience—such situations are rare in applied problems.

## ACKNOWLEDGMENTS

The development of this chapter was funded by National Institute on Drug Abuse Grant Nos. 1R01DA015697 (Principal Investigator: McCaffrey) and 1R01DA034065-01A1 (Principal Investigators: Griffin/McCaffrey) and supported by SAMHSA's CSAT, Contract No. 270-07-0191. We thank the editors, Wei Pan and Haiyan Bai; an anonymous reviewer; and Rebecca Zwick and Haiwen Chen at ETS for very helpful comments; and the following grantees and their participants for agreeing to share their data to support this secondary analysis: Assertive Adolescent Family Treatment (study [AAFT]: CSAT/SAMHSA Contract Nos. 270-2003-00006 and 270-2007-00004C; grantees: TI-17589, TI-17604, TI-17638, TI-17673, TI-17719, TI-17724, TI-17728, TI-17744, TI-17765, TI-17775, TI-17779, TI-17830, TI-17761, TI-17763, TI-17769, TI-17786, TI-17788, TI-17812, TI-17817, TI-17825, TI-17864); Adolescent Residential Treatment (study [ART]: CSAT/SAMHSA Contract Nos. 277-00-6500 and 270-2003-00006; grantees: TI-14271, TI-14272, TI-14315, TI-14090, TI-14188, TI-14189, TI-14196, TI-14252, TI-14261, TI-14267, TI-14283, TI-14311, TI-14376); Adolescent Treatment Model (study [ATM]: CSAT/SAMHSA Contract Nos. 270-98-7047, 270-97-7011, 277-00-6500, and 270-2003-00006; grantees: TI-11424, TI-11432, TI-11892, TI-11894); Cannabis Youth Treatment (study [CYT]: CSAT/SAMHSA Contract Nos. 270-97-7011, 270-00-6500, and 270-2003-00006; grantees: TI-11317, TI-11321, TI-11323, TI-11324); Drug Court (study [DC]: CSAT/SAMHSA Contract Nos. 270-2003-00006 and 270-2007-00004C; grantees: TI-17433, TI-17475, TI-17484, TI-17517, TI-17434, TI-17446, TI-17486, TI-17523, TI-17535); Effective Adolescent Treatment (study [EAT]: CSAT/SAMHSA Contract No. 270-2003-00006; and grantees: TI-15413, TI-15415, TI-15421, TI-15433, TI-15438, TI-15446, TI-15447, TI-15458, TI-15461, TI-15466, TI-15467, TI-15469, TI-15475, TI-15478, TI-15479, TI-15481, TI-15483, TI-15485, TI-15486, TI-15489, TI-15511, TI-15514, TI-15524, TI-15527, TI-15545, TI-15562, TI-15577, TI-15584, TI-15586, TI-15670, TI-15671, TI-15672, TI-15674, TI-15677, TI-15678, TI-15682, TI-15686); Strengthening Communities–Youth (study [SCY]: CSAT/SAMHSA Contract Nos. 277-00-6500 and 270-2003-00006; grantees: TI-13305, TI-13313, TI-13322, TI-13323, TI-13344, TI-13345, TI-13354, TI-13356); Targeted Capacity Expansion (study [TCE] and grantees: TI-13190, TI-13601, TI-16386, TI-16400, TI-18406, TI-18723); and Young Offenders Reentry Program (study [YORP]: CSAT/SAMHSA Contract Nos. 270-2003-00006 and 270-2007-00004C; grantees: TI-16904, TI-16928, TI-16939, TI-16961, TI-16984, TI-16992, TI-17046, TI-17070, TI-17071, TI-19313). The opinions about these data are those of the authors and do not reflect official positions of the government or individual grantees.

## NOTES

1. To further reduce prediction error in the GBM, the GBM algorithm often includes a stochastic element in which a *different* random subsample of the data is selected at each iteration and only that subsample is used to estimate $h$ (Friedman,

2002). When estimating propensity scores, we typically do not include this stochastic element.

2. McCaffrey, Ridgeway, and Morral (2004) refer to the standardized bias as average standardized absolute mean difference. The *twang* package in R uses mean.es to refer to mean or maximum standardized bias.

3. McCaffrey et al. (2013) suggest comparing each group to the overall sample mean and using the maximum of this value as the assessment of balance. To ensure pairwise balance on SB of less than 0.20 using this statistic requires the difference with the overall sample mean to be less than 0.10. This can be conservative.

## REFERENCES

Breiman, L. (1998). Arcing classifiers (with discussion). *Annals of Statistics, 26*(3), 801–849.

Breiman, L. (2001). Random forests. *Machine Learning, 45*, 5–32.

Breiman, L., Friedman, J. H., Olshen, R. A., & Stone, C. J. (1984). *Classification and regression trees*. Belmont, CA: Wadsworth International Group.

Brookhart, M. A., Schneeweiss, S., Rothman, K. J., Glynn, R. J., Avorn, J., & Stürmer, T. (2006). Variable selection for propensity score models. *American Journal of Epidemiology, 163*, 1149–1156.

Bühlmann, P., & Yu, B. (2003). Boosting with the L2 loss: Regression and classification. *Journal of the American Statistical Association, 98*, 324–339.

Burgette, L. F., Griffin, B. A., & McCaffrey, D. F. (2013). Propensity scores for multiple treatments: A tutorial for the mnps function in the *twang* package. R package. Available at *http://cran.r-project.org/web/packages/twang/vignettes/mnps.pdf*.

Cochran, W. G. (1968). The effectiveness of adjustment by subclassification in removing bias in observational studies. *Biometrics, 24*, 295–313.

Cohen, J. (1998). *Statistical power analysis for the behavioral sciences* (2nd ed.). Hillsdale, NJ: Erlbaum.

Dehejia, R. H., & Wahba, S. (1999). Causal effects in nonexperimental studies: Reevaluating the evaluation of training programs. *Journal of the American Statistical Association, 98*, 1053–1062.

Dennis, M. L., Titus, J. C., White, M., Unsicker, J., & Hodgkins, D. (2003). Global Appraisal of Individual Needs (GAIN): Administration guide for the GAIN and related measures. Retrieved November 1, 2013, from *www.gaincc.org/gaini*.

Drake, C. (1993). Effects of misspecification of the propensity score on estimators of treatment effect. *Biometrics, 49*, 1231–1236.

Freund, Y., & Schapire, R. (1997). A decision-theoretic generalization of on-line learning and an application to boosting. *Journal of Computer and System Sciences, 55*(1), 119–139.

Friedman, J. H. (2001). Greedy function approximation: A gradient boosting machine. *Annals of Statistics, 29*, 1189–1232.

Friedman, J. H. (2002). Stochastic gradient boosting. *Computational Statistics and Data Analysis, 38*, 367–378.

Friedman, J. H., Hastie, T., & Tibshirani, R. (2000). Additive logistic regression: A statistical view of boosting. *Annals of Statistics, 28*, 337–374.

Griffin, B. A., Ramchand, R., Almirall, D., Slaughter, M. E., Burgette L. F., & McCaffrey, D. F. (2014). Addressing time-varying confounding when assessing the causal effects of cumulative treatments or adolescents with substance use problems. *Drug and Alcohol Dependence, 136*, 69–78.

Harder, V. S., Stuart, E. A., & Anthony, J. (2010). Propensity score techniques and the assessment of measured covariate balance to test causal association in psychological research. *Psychological Methods, 15*, 234–249.

Hastie, T., Tibshirani, R., & Friedman, J. (2009). *The elements of statistical learning* (2nd ed.). New York: Springer Science+Media.

Ho, D. E., Imai, K., King, G., & Stuart, E. A. (2007). Matching as nonparametric preprocessing for reducing model dependence in parametric causal inference. *Political Analysis, 15*(3), 199–236.

Imbens, G. W. (2004). Nonparametric estimation of average treatment effects under exogeneity: A review. *Review of Economics and Statistics, 86*(1), 4–29.

Lee, B. K., Lessler, J., & Stuart, E. A. (2010). Improving propensity score weighting using machine learning. *Statistics in Medicine, 29*, 337–346.

Lee, B. K., Lessler, J., & Stuart, E. A. (2011). Weight trimming and propensity score weighting. *PLoS ONE, 6*, e18174.

Madigan, D., & Ridgeway, G. (2004). Discussion of 'Least Angle Regression' by Efron, et al. *Annals of Statistics, 32*, 465–469.

McCaffrey, D. F., Griffin, B. A., Almirall, D., Slaughter, M. E., Ramchand, R., & Burgette, L. (2013). A tutorial on propensity score estimation for multiple treatments using generalized boosted models. *Statistics in Medicine, 32*(19), 3388–3414.

McCaffrey, D. F., Ridgeway, G., & Morral, A. (2004). Propensity score estimation with boosted regression for evaluating causal effects in observational studies. *Psychological Methods, 9*, 403–425.

Meyer, J. A., Rassen, J. A., Gagne, J. J., Huybrechts, K. F., Schneeweiss, S., Rothman, K. J., et al. (2011). Effects of adjusting for instrumental variables on bias and precision of effect estimates. *American Journal of Epidemiology, 174*, 1213–1222.

R Development Core Team. (2008). *R: A language and environment for statistical computing*. Vienna, Austria: R Foundation for Statistical Computing. Available at www.R-project.org.

Ridgeway, G. (1999). The state of boosting. *Computing Science and Statistics, 31*, 172–181.

Ridgeway, G., McCaffrey, D., Morral, A., Burgette, L., & Griffin, B. A. (2012). Toolkit for weighting and analysis of nonequivalent groups: A tutorial for the *twang* package. R package. *http://cran.r-project.org/web/packages/twang/vignettes/twang.pdf.*

Rosenbaum, P. R., & Rubin, D. B. (1983). The central role of the propensity score in observational studies for causal effects. *Biometrika, 70*(1), 41–55.

Rosenbaum, P. R., & Rubin, D. B. (1985). Constructing a control group using multivariate matched sampling methods that incorporate the propensity score. *American Statistician, 39*(1), 33–38.

Schonlau, M. (2005). Boosted regression (boosting): An introductory tutorial and a Stata plugin. *Stata Journal, 5,* 330–354.

Schuler, M., Griffin, B. A., Ramchand, R., Almirall, D., & McCaffrey, D. (2014). Effectiveness of adolescent substance abuse treatments: Is biological drug testing sufficient? *Journal of Studies of Alcohol and Drugs, 75*(2), 358–370.

Wooldridge, J. (2002). *Econometric analysis of cross section and panel data.* Cambridge, MA: MIT Press.

# CHAPTER 4

# Methodological Considerations in Implementing Propensity Score Matching

**Haiyan Bai**

Selection bias on covariates can significantly influence the accuracy of estimation of treatment effects when randomized clinical trials are not feasible (Cook & Campbell, 1979; Rosenbaum & Rubin, 1985; Shadish, Cook, & Campbell, 2002). Propensity score matching is a method used to reduce selection bias by simultaneously balancing the distributions of multiple covariates between the treatment and control groups in observational data (Luellen, Shadish, & Clark, 2005; Rosenbaum & Rubin, 1983). This technique attempts to achieve balance similar to that found in randomized trials (Gu & Rosenbaum, 1993; Stürmer et al., 2006). Therefore, propensity score matching has become a popular approach among the adjustment techniques in observational studies for causal inference (Caliendo & Kopeinig, 2008; Glynn, Schneeweiss, & Stürmer, 2006; Imai & van Dyk, 2004; Rubin, 1997). Considering the popularity of propensity score analysis in research, some existing issues should be addressed to increase the likelihood that propensity score analysis is used correctly and efficiently when making causal inferences (Bai, 2011b).

Existing literature has discussed the differences in bias reductions, comparing various propensity score matching methods; however, research findings vary. These inconsistent findings could be explained by variations in sample conditions, such as matching with replacement or without replacement, sufficient or insufficient common support, and large versus small sample sizes (or sample size ratio of treated to nontreated units [e.g., subjects]). To date, there is little literature addressing the above issues. To investigate the answers to these questions, this chapter presents 60 experimental trials on random samples from a large national dataset to investigate matching results from three commonly used propensity score matching methods. Matching with replacement versus without replacement is studied under 12 sampling conditions with different percentages of common support region, sample sizes, and sample size ratios. The chapter provides researchers with empirical evidence for the influences of sample conditions on various propensity score matching schemes and useful information for the applications of propensity score matching.

## EXISTING ISSUES AND RELATED LITERATURE

### Matching with or without Replacement

Previous research has vigorously studied the effectiveness of bias reductions from various propensity score matching methods. However, some issues are still open to discussion (Bai, 2013). One of these basic issues is whether propensity score matching should be done with or without replacement. Matching with replacement allows use of each unit in the treatment or control group as a match on propensity scores more than once, while matching without replacement allows each unit to be used as a matched unit only once.

Rosenbaum and Rubin (1985) pointed out that matching with or without replacement resulted in very different matching groups and therefore influenced the accuracy of treatment effect estimation. Other researchers (e.g., Abadie & Imbens, 2006; Dehejia & Wahba, 2002) found that matching with replacement allowed for a greater reduction of bias because it produced better matches than matching without replacement. Dehejia and Wahba (2002) stated that matching with replacement minimizes the propensity score distance between the matched nontreated units and the treated units, while matching without replacement may force a treated unit to match a nontreated unit with quite a different propensity score; therefore, matching without replacement can be very problematic when treated and nontreated units are very different. However, matching with replacement could reduce the numbers of distinct units in the control group to be counted for the counterfactual mean, and therefore to increase the variance of estimator (Smith & Todd, 2005). Further, matching with replacement can result in the lack of independence between matched sets that contain the same treated or nontreated units (Austin, 2008). In addition, the results of matching with or without replacement could also be influenced by the types of propensity score matching methods and data conditions such as common support of distributions of propensity scores for the treatment and control groups (Caliendo & Kopeinig, 2008). With the above concerns, we find few studies that conducted systematic investigation on the differences of propensity score matching results between matching with and without replacement using various propensity score matching methods under different sample conditions, such as common support, sample sizes, and sample ratio between treatment and control groups.

## Common Support

Dehejia and Wahba (2002) maintain that matching with or without replacement depends on the degree of common support for the distributions of propensity scores between the treatment and control groups, while most of the matching algorithms yield similar results when there is substantial overlap in the distributions of the propensity scores of the two groups. The common support is defined as the overlapped ranges of propensity score distributions of the treatment group and control group. A violation of the common support condition is a major source of estimation bias (Caliendo & Kopeinig, 2008; Heckman, Ichimura, & Todd, 1997). Most of the major methodological studies on propensity score matching (e.g., Caliendo & Kopeinig, 2008; Rosenbaum & Rubin, 1985; Rubin, 1977) also emphasized the necessity of sufficient common support for the distributions of the propensity scores between the treatment and control groups when using propensity score matching methods. Unfortunately, there is no standard criterion in the current literature on how much overlap of propensity scores between the groups is sufficient for propensity score matching. Rubin (2001) suggests that the means of the group propensity scores should be less than 0.5 standard deviations (*SD*) apart. While it is a measure on the propensity scores calculated from all units in samples, the common support should only account for propensity scores that overlap between treatment and control groups. Caliendo and Kopeinig (2008) introduced two methods for finding the common support region, namely, a minima and maxima comparison approach and a method of trimming to determine the common support; nevertheless, they did not specify how much common support is sufficient for propensity score matching, neither.

## Sample Size Ratio

Other research on propensity score methods (e.g., Rubin, 1979) suggests that it is easier to find sufficient matches between the units in the treatment and control groups when the sample size of the control group is considerably larger (e.g., three times as large) than the sample size of the treatment group. However, with their empirical results, Dehejia and Wahba (2002) concluded that a small sample size of a control group still performed well with some propensity score methods such as caliper matching with replacement. Again, it is not hard to see that the sample size issue is also related to different sample conditions, such as the common support and total sample sizes. Existing studies (e.g., Dehejia & Wahba, 2002) have paid attention to these issues; however, few studies have been conducted to systematically examine which propensity score matching method performs well under what data conditions.

It is reasonable for previous studies to assume that matching with or without replacement method, percent of common support, and the ratio of sample sizes of treated group to control groups are associated with the amount of bias reduced when using propensity score matching. However, it is essential to provide a clear picture for researchers to better understand how common support conditions with regards to sample size ratios between the treatment and control group and total sample sizes influence the bias reduction results using different propensity matching schemes with or without replacement. Given the lack of studies and systematic investigations that empirically supports these assumptions, this chapter examines these issues with 60 experimental trials using random samples from a national dataset. It also provides researchers with a clear and practical guidance for using propensity score matching methods effectively under various sample data conditions.

## THE 60 EXPERIMENTAL TRIALS

### Method

Sixty experimental trials were used to systematically compare three commonly used propensity score matching methods, including nearest neighbor, caliper, and optimal matching with and without replacement under various sampling conditions. Multiple samples were randomly selected from a large national educational dataset with 10 covariates according to 12 sampling conditions based on two sample sizes of the treatment group

(100 or 200), two ratios of group sample sizes (two or three times as many nontreated units as treated units), and three percentages of common support of the propensity scores between the groups (50%, 60%, 75%; see Table 4.1). The 60 experimental trials consist of: 12 (2 treatment size × 2 sample ratio × 3 common support) × 2 (nearest + caliper) × 2 (with replacement + without replacement) + 12 (2 treatment size × 2 sample ratio × 3 common support) × 1 (optimal without replacement). Samples were randomly selected using SAS 9.2, and *MatchIt* (Ho, Imai, King, & Stuart, 2007) was used to implement the matching procedures and compute adjusted outcomes.

### Data Source and Selection of Covariates

Units were randomly sampled from the Educational Longitudinal Survey of 2002 (ELS:2002). ELS:2002 was collected on 15,362 10th-grade students randomly selected from 752 schools across the United States. After conducting a missing data analysis that followed recommendations from Allison (2001) and Little and Rubin (1987), the final sample size available for this current study was $N = 6{,}152$. The data were classified into two groups by high and low parents' expectations on their child's academic attainment, with 1 indicating high expectation (i.e., beyond a college degree) and 0 indicating low expectation (i.e., up to a college degree).

TABLE 4.1. Random Samples from the ELS:2002 Data

| Samples | Sample size | Sample ratio (treat/control) | Common support |
|---|---|---|---|
| 1 |  |  | 50% |
| 2 | 300 | 100/200 | 60% |
| 3 |  |  | 75% |
| 4 |  |  | 50% |
| 5 | 400 | 100/300 | 60% |
| 6 |  |  | 75% |
| 7 |  |  | 50% |
| 8 | 600 | 200/400 | 60% |
| 9 |  |  | 75% |
| 10 |  |  | 50% |
| 11 | 800 | 200/600 | 60% |
| 12 |  |  | 75% |

According to an extensive literature review of 125 articles, parents' expectation was found to be one of the most important family factors that affected student academic outcomes (Christenson, Rounds, & Gorney, 1992), including mathematics achievement. Therefore, to serve the purpose of this investigation, parents' expectation was used as a "treatment" for increasing students' mathematics achievement. The literature also revealed that students' achievement in mathematics was related to their personal beliefs (Schommer-Aitkins, Duell, & Hutter, 2005), their peers' beliefs (Hanushek, Kain, Markman, & Rivkin, 2003), their reading abilities (Hill, Rowan, & Ball, 2005), and environmental variables (Koth, Bradshaw, & Leaf, 2008). In addition, students' mathematical performance was also related to sociodemographical variables, such as socioeconomic status and school composition (Entwisle & Alexander, 1992) as well. Therefore, 10 related covariates in the ELS:2002 dataset were selected to be modeled to systematically investigate the bias reduction effects under different sample conditions with various matching schemes. See Bai (2011a, Appendix) for variable selection and coding.

### Random Sampling Procedure

To compare the results of various matching schemes under different sampling conditions, the percentage of common support region of propensity scores between the groups was specified as 50%, 60%, and 75%, the sample size ratio of treatment and control groups as 1/2 and 1/3; and the total sample sizes as 300, 400, 600, and 800. The common support was defined as the units with the overlapped ranges of propensity scores of the treatment group and control group. The specific sample sizes and ratios were selected as fixed factors because they were likely to achieve sufficient statistical power for medium and large effect sizes for a two-group test at alpha = 0.01 (Cohen, 1992). The sample pool was 6,152 units in the ELS:2002 data with original treatment group of 2,251 units and the control group of 3,901 units.

### Checking Balance

Propensity score matching aims to create balanced groups similar to group assignment from a randomized control trial, or in other words, to create the same distributions of the covariates within the treatment and control groups after matching, which is called "balance." There are several ways to assess the balance of covariates after propensity score matching. These methods include assessing differences in means of the covariates between the treatment and control groups, standard bias reduction, and percentage bias reduction. Sometimes, researchers also use inferential tests, such as a *t*-test for continuous dependent variables and a chi-square test for categorical dependent variables, to examine the balance. However, some researchers do not recommend using statistical significance tests for checking the balance of the covariates because the significance tests can be misleading in terms of the similarity of the covariate distributions (Imai, King, & Stuart, 2008). Therefore, in this investigation, mean differences, standard bias reduction, and percentage bias reduction were used to check the balance of covariates before and after propensity score matching.

The initial difference in means between the treatment and control groups is called the selection bias ($B$) and can be expressed in the following formula from Rosenbaum and Rubin (1983, Formula 3.1, p. 49):

$$B = E(x|z = 1) - E(x|z = 0) \tag{4.1}$$

where $E(x|z = 1)$ is the expected value of each covariate or the expected value of the propensity scores (calculated from the selected covariates) for the treatment group, while $E(x|z = 0)$ is that for the control group. Rosenbaum and Rubin (1983, Formula 3.2, p. 49) also introduced the after-matching selection bias as: $B_m = E(x|z = 1) - E_m(x|z = 0)$. In this chapter, the formula was adapted as

$$B_m = E_m(x|z = 1) - E_m(x|z = 0) \tag{4.2}$$

where the subscript $m$ indicates the distribution of matched samples; $E_m(x|z = 1)$ indicates that the distribution of expected values of a covariate in the treatment group with regard to some matching schemes, such as caliper matching that may exclude some units in the treatment group resulting in the differences between $E(x|z = 1)$ and $E_m(x|z = 1)$; and $E_m(x|z = 0)$ indicates the expected value of a covariate in the control group.

To cross validate the bias reduction results, the standardized bias ($SB$; Rosenbaum & Rubin, 1985) was also used, which was defined as follows:

$$SB = \frac{B_1 - B_0}{\sqrt{\dfrac{V_1(X_1) + V_0(X_0)}{2}}} \times 100\% \tag{4.3}$$

where $V_1(X_1)$ and $V_0(X_0)$ are the variances of the covariates for the treated units and the nontreated units, respectively. After implementing propensity score matching, if the $SB$ is less than 5% of the absolute value, the matching method is considered effective in balancing the distributions of the covariate (Caliendo & Kopeinig, 2008).

Following Rosenbaum and Rubin (1983), the effectiveness of matching was also evaluated using the percent of bias reduction (*PBR*) on the covariate, for which a *PBR* larger than 80% suggests that the matching procedure is effective in reducing bias (Cochran & Rubin, 1973). *PBR* is defined as follows:

$$PBR = \frac{|B| - |B_m|}{|B|} \times 100\% \qquad (4.4)$$

where *B* is the initial mean difference and $B_m$ is the mean difference after matching.

## Matching Schemes

**Nearest Neighbor Matching.** Nearest neighbor matching matches each unit *i* in the treatment group with a unit *j* in the control group at the closest absolute distance, $d(i, j) = |l(X_i) - l(X_j)|$, where $l(X)$ is the logit of propensity score. After selecting a unit from the control group with a propensity score closest to that of each treated unit, the unit in the control group is removed from the matching pool of the control group in matching without replacement or kept in the control group for the next round of matching in matching with replacement.

**Caliper Matching.** Caliper matching matches each unit *i* in the control group with a unit *j* in the control group within a prespecified band, *b*. Based on Cochran and Rubin (1973, Table 2.3.2, p. 421), Rosenbaum and Rubin (1985) recommended $b = 0.25 \times SD[e(x)]$ for at least 90% bias reduction after caliper matching, where $e(x)$ is the propensity score. Therefore, in the experimental trials for the current investigation, 0.25 *SD* of $e(x)$ was selected to be used as the bandwidth for caliper matching. Although caliper matching easily permits matching with and without replacement, it usually discards units from both treated and control groups when there is no matched pair to be found within the specified bandwidth. This tends to result in fewer, but closer, matched pairs than in other forms of matching.

**Optimal Matching.** According to Ho et al. (2007), "optimal matching finds the matched samples with the smallest average absolute distance across all the matched pairs" (p. 11). It is worth noting that optimal matching usually selects the same set of units from the control group for the general matched samples with the set of controls selected through nearest neighbor matching without replacement, but optimal matching can minimize the average distance between matched pairs (Gu & Rosenbaum, 1993; Ho et al., 2007) while nearest neighbor matching does not. With regard to the algorithm for selecting the matching pairs, matching with replacement is not applicable to optimal matching.

There are several other matching-related methods, such as subclassification, full matching, and kernel matching, but they do not strictly form two matched samples for easily evaluating covariate balance; rather, they are usually used to combine "matching" and outcome analysis in one process. Therefore, those matching-related methods are not considered in this chapter. See Chapter 1 for an overview of all the matching and matching-related methods. *MatchIt* (Ho et al., 2007), the most efficient software for executing matching schemes in conjunction with R, was selected to conduct the experimental trials.

## Results

To compare the balance results under 12 sample conditions with nearest and caliper matching with and without replacement, and optimal matching without replacement, 60 experimental trials were conducted. Tables 4.2, 4.3, and 4.4 summarize the propensity score matching results from the 60 trials in terms of the initial or unadjusted mean differences ($B$), mean differences after matching ($B_m$), standardized mean differences ($SB$ = initial bias, and $SB_m$ = bias after matching), and percentage of bias reduction after matching ($PBR$).

Comparing the results presented in the three tables (Tables 4.2, 4.3, and 4.4), we can see that matching with replacement produced much better bias reduction results in terms of mean differences and percentage bias reduction regardless of sample sizes, percentages of common support, and sample ratios. The matching methods with replacement produced more than 90% percentage bias reduction. However, with regard to the criteria of standardized bias, the study results are inconsistent. Specifically for nearest neighbor matching, matching *with* replacement produced smaller estimates of standardized bias than matching without replacement across different sample conditions. However, for caliper matching, matching *without* replacement resulted in smaller standardized bias estimates than matching with replacement. Unfortunately, we cannot directly compare matching with and without replacement for optimal matching because matching with replacement is not applicable to optimal matching.

For matching without replacement, only caliper matching produced higher than 90% percentage bias reduction under all sample conditions

## Methodological Considerations

**TABLE 4.2. Nearest Neighbor Matching**

| | Raw data | | | Without replacement | | | | With replacement | | | |
|---|---|---|---|---|---|---|---|---|---|---|---|
| N | Common support | B | SB (%) | Treat/control | $B_m$ | $SB_m$ (%) | PBR (%) | Treat/control | $B_m$ | $SB_m$ (%) | PBR (%) |
| 300 | 50% | 0.62 | 2.56 | 100/200 | 0.49 | 1.93 | 20.39 | 100/27 | <0.01 | 1.19 | 99.73 |
| | 60% | 0.54 | 2.22 | 100/200 | 0.39 | 1.58 | 28.17 | 100/37 | 0.03 | 1.03 | 94.74 |
| | 75% | 0.43 | 1.78 | 100/200 | 0.27 | 1.15 | 36.50 | 100/45 | 0.01 | 0.69 | 98.13 |
| 400 | 50% | 0.57 | 2.44 | 100/300 | 0.38 | 1.42 | 33.00 | 100/32 | 0.03 | 1.01 | 94.71 |
| | 60% | 0.58 | 2.64 | 100/300 | 0.40 | 1.81 | 31.64 | 100/33 | <0.01 | 1.20 | 99.87 |
| | 75% | 0.38 | 1.67 | 100/300 | 0.17 | 0.66 | 55.53 | 100/48 | 0.04 | 0.76 | 90.27 |
| 600 | 50% | 0.56 | 2.32 | 200/400 | 0.41 | 1.61 | 26.01 | 200/67 | 0.01 | 1.04 | 98.30 |
| | 60% | 0.48 | 1.95 | 200/400 | 0.31 | 1.27 | 34.02 | 200/73 | 0.01 | 0.88 | 98.05 |
| | 75% | 0.33 | 1.43 | 200/400 | 0.16 | 0.73 | 50.41 | 200/95 | <0.01 | 0.68 | 99.32 |
| 800 | 50% | 0.56 | 2.45 | 200/600 | 0.36 | 1.42 | 35.51 | 200/67 | <0.01 | 1.20 | 99.48 |
| | 60% | 0.43 | 1.85 | 200/600 | 0.22 | 0.81 | 49.33 | 200/98 | 0.02 | 0.86 | 96.20 |
| | 75% | 0.32 | 1.47 | 200/600 | 0.14 | 0.55 | 57.14 | 200/99 | 0.01 | 0.65 | 97.40 |

**TABLE 4.3. Caliper Matching with Bandwidth of 0.25 *SD***

| | Raw data | | | Without replacement | | | | With replacement | | | |
|---|---|---|---|---|---|---|---|---|---|---|---|
| N | Common support | B | SB (%) | Treat/control | $B_m$ | $SB_m$ (%) | PBR (%) | Treat/control | $B_m$ | $SB_m$ (%) | PBR (%) |
| 300 | 50% | 0.62 | 2.56 | 35/35 | 0.01 | 0.05 | 97.98 | 81/28 | <0.01 | 1.05 | 99.26 |
| | 60% | 0.54 | 2.22 | 39/39 | 0.01 | 0.03 | 98.67 | 65/35 | <0.01 | 0.51 | 99.30 |
| | 75% | 0.43 | 1.78 | 54/54 | 0.01 | 0.04 | 97.87 | 87/45 | <0.01 | 0.56 | 99.72 |
| 400 | 50% | 0.57 | 2.44 | 37/37 | 0.01 | 0.07 | 99.01 | 54/34 | <0.01 | 0.43 | 99.74 |
| | 60% | 0.58 | 2.64 | 38/38 | 0.01 | 0.53 | 98.74 | 91/30 | <0.01 | 1.15 | 99.71 |
| | 75% | 0.38 | 1.67 | 60/60 | <0.01 | −0.08 | 99.26 | 69/50 | <0.01 | 0.20 | 99.40 |
| 600 | 50% | 0.56 | 2.32 | 85/85 | 0.01 | 0.01 | 98.48 | 161/64 | <0.01 | 0.78 | 99.29 |
| | 60% | 0.48 | 1.95 | 101/101 | 0.01 | 0.03 | 98.77 | 163/78 | <0.01 | 0.72 | 99.74 |
| | 75% | 0.33 | 1.43 | 128/128 | <0.01 | 0.01 | 98.73 | 180/101 | <0.01 | 0.55 | 99.59 |
| 800 | 50% | 0.56 | 2.45 | 83/83 | <0.01 | 0.06 | 99.11 | 159/70 | <0.01 | 0.91 | 99.92 |
| | 60% | 0.43 | 1.85 | 109/109 | <0.01 | 0.05 | 99.34 | 153/94 | <0.01 | 0.56 | 99.62 |
| | 75% | 0.32 | 1.47 | 132/132 | <0.01 | 0.02 | 98.84 | 156/108 | <0.01 | 0.33 | 99.88 |

*Note.* See Table 4.1 for sample ratios of treated and nontreated group in the sample pool.

**TABLE 4.4. Optimal Matching**

|  | Raw data | | | Without replacement | | | |
|---|---|---|---|---|---|---|---|
|  | Common support | $B$ | $SB$ (%) | Treat/control | $B_m$ | $SB_m$ (%) | PBR (%) |
| 300 | 50% | 0.62 | 2.56 | 100/200 | 0.49 | 1.93 | 20.39 |
|  | 60% | 0.54 | 2.22 | 100/200 | 0.22 | 1.58 | 28.17 |
|  | 75% | 0.43 | 1.78 | 100/200 | 0.27 | 1.15 | 36.50 |
| 400 | 50% | 0.57 | 2.44 | 100/300 | 0.38 | 1.42 | 33.00 |
|  | 60% | 0.58 | 2.64 | 100/300 | 0.40 | 1.81 | 31.64 |
|  | 75% | 0.38 | 1.67 | 100/300 | 0.17 | 0.66 | 55.51 |
| 600 | 50% | 0.56 | 2.32 | 200/400 | 0.41 | 1.61 | 26.01 |
|  | 60% | 0.48 | 1.95 | 200/400 | 0.31 | 1.27 | 34.02 |
|  | 75% | 0.33 | 1.43 | 200/400 | 0.16 | 0.73 | 50.41 |
| 800 | 50% | 0.56 | 2.45 | 200/600 | 0.36 | 1.41 | 35.51 |
|  | 60% | 0.43 | 1.85 | 200/600 | 0.22 | 0.81 | 49.33 |
|  | 75% | 0.32 | 1.47 | 200/600 | 0.14 | 0.55 | 57.14 |

and significant standardized bias reduction. However, the numbers of matched pairs were significantly reduced by as much as 35% of the units originally in the treated group when matching without replacement and by as much as 66% when matching with replacement. It is also evident that with replacement, caliper matching does not reduce more selection bias than without replacement; nevertheless it did retain more units from the treated group.

Furthermore, under the same data condition, a higher percentage of overlap between the treatment and control groups in most units resulted in more bias reduction as measured by both the standardized bias and percentage bias reduction. The *SB* and *PBR* were significantly improved for a majority of the trials when 75% of the propensity scores overlapped than with only 50% and 60% overlap. Especially for caliper matching which produced the best matching results for matching without replacement, 75% overlap allowed more units in the treatment and control groups to be included in the final matched data than the number of units matched when there was less overlap. As we know, the majority of the overlap of the propensity scores for the treatment and control groups indicates that the majority of the treated and nontreated units have similar distributions of covariates, namely, background characteristics. Therefore, the two groups are more likely from the same population when the overlap of the propensity scores of the treatment and control groups is sufficiently large, such as proximately over 75%.

Sample sizes influenced the matching results for most matching schemes. Nearest neighbor with and without replacement, caliper matching with replacement, and optimal matching were more responsive to the sample size changes. The matching results from these matching methods consistently showed that larger total sample sizes produced better matching results in terms of both $SB_m$ and $PBR$. However, caliper matching without replacement was not sensitive to sample sizes. While comparing to the effect of a total sample size, a larger sample size of the control group had more impact on the matching results. The results revealed that larger sample sizes of control group produced better matching results. The results also showed that under the sample conditions defined in this study there was little difference between the matching results from optimal matching and nearest neighbor matching without replacement. However, the pairs found to be matching were different from the two matching methods.

## DISCUSSION AND CONCLUSION

This chapter compared the results of propensity score matching with 60 trials for commonly used nearest neighbor matching, caliper matching with or without replacement, and optimal matching using 12 random samples. These samples are from a large empirical dataset representing hypothesized two treatment and control groups, three different percentages of common support with four different sample sizes of 300, 400, 600, and 800, and treated versus control sample size ratio of 1/2 and 1/3.

The results revealed that matching with replacement produced consistently higher bias reduction than matching without replacement. The results echoed Dehejia and Wahba's (2002) study. However, matching with replacement could create sample independent issues due to repeatedly selecting the same units for the final matched samples. The violation of the basic statistical assumption of independent observations in the final matched sample causes a serious concern. If matching with replacement is used, weighted scores should also be applied in the outcome analysis. In addition, researchers are also responsible to check the representativeness of the selected units from the control group because matching with replacement may limit the units to be selected from the control group when the sample pool is relatively small or common support is insufficient.

The results were also partially consistent with the findings from the prior study (Dehejia & Wahba, 2002). That is, if the common support is sufficient, which was suggested as approximately 75% overlapping from the results of the current investigation (see Tables 4.2, 4.3, and 4.4), the results from both matching with and without replacement were better than the results from 50% and 60% in terms of the standardized bias reduction and percentage bias reduction. Also, 75% overlapping is substantial regarding the final number of matched pairs and the population representativeness of the final selected sample. For matching with replacement, with 50% and 60% overlapping there were limited units to be selected from the control group to match the treatment group units for nearest neighbor and caliper matching (see Tables 4.2 and 4.3). For caliper matching without replacement, 50% and 60% overlapping only allows 35% to 55% of the treated units to be selected. With a large portion of the units being excluded in the final sample, the sample representativeness could be challenged.

From this investigation, the results showed that the control group sample size was more influential for the matching results than the total sample size. The larger the control group sample is, the better matching results are, which echoes the claims in the existing literature (e.g., Dehejia & Wahba, 2002; Rubin, 1997). In addition, for the control group, the percentage propensity score overlapping with the treatment group is more influential than the size of the control group pool. Larger percentage of overlapping with the treated group produced better matching results. In other words, a large pool of the control group did not guarantee a better matching result. If there are insufficient units in the control group to match the treated units, a large control group pool does not contribute to a well-matched unit selection.

Another result from this chapter echoed the claims of Ho et al. (2007) that optimal matching can be beneficial when there are limited suitable units in the control group for the treatment group. It also endorsed the argument of Gu and Rosenbaum (1993) that optimal matching generally selects the same set of units as nearest neighbor matching without replacement, while the units in some matched pairs are different.

In sum, matching with replacement is in general better than matching without replacement. The percentage of the treatment and control group overlapping and the sample size of the control group also evidently influence the matching results from all three matching methods. The larger overlapping percentage is, the better the bias reductions are in terms of $SB_m$ and PBR. The larger the sample size of the control group is, the better the matching results are.

## REFERENCES

Abadie, A., & Imbens, G. W. (2006). Large sample properties of matching estimators for average treatment effects. *Econometrica, 74*(1), 235–267.
Allison, P. D. (2001). *Missing data.* Thousand Oaks, CA: Sage.
Austin, P. C. (2008). A critical appraisal of propensity-score matching in the medical literature between 1996 and 2003. *Statistics in Medicine, 27*(12), 2037–2049.
Bai, H. (2013). A bootstrap procedure of propensity score estimation. *Journal of Experimental Education, 81*(2), 157–177.
Bai, H. (2011a). A comparison of propensity score matching methods for reducing selection bias. *International Journal of Research and Method in Education, 34*(1), 81–107.
Bai, H. (2011b). Using propensity score analysis for making causal claims in research articles. *Educational Psychology Review, 23*, 273–278.
Caliendo, M., & Kopeinig, S. (2008). Some practical guidance for the implementation of propensity score matching. *Journal of Economic Surveys, 22*, 31–72.
Christenson, S. L., Rounds, T., & Gorney, D. (1992). Family factors and student achievement: An avenue to increase students' success. *School Psychology Quarterly, 7*(3), 178–206.
Cochran, W. G., & Rubin, D. B. (1973). Controlling bias in observational studies: A review. *Sankhyā: The Indian Journal of Statistics*, Series A, 417–446.
Cohen, J. (1992). A power primer. *Psychological Bulletin, 112*(1), 155–159.
Cook, T. D., & Campbell, D. T. (1979). *Quasi-experimentation: Design and analysis issues for field settings.* Chicago: Rand McNally.
Dehejia, R. H., & Wahba, S. (2002). Propensity score-matching methods for nonexperimental causal studies. *Review of Economics and Statistics, 84*, 151–161.
Entwisle, D. R., & Alexander, K. L. (1992). Summer setback: Race, poverty, school composition, and mathematics achievement in the first two years of school. *American Sociological Review, 57*, 72–84.
Glynn, R. J., Schneeweiss, S., & Stürmer, T. (2006). Indications for propensity scores and review of their use in pharmacoepidemiology. *Basic Clinical Pharmacology Toxicology, 98*, 253–259.
Gu, X. S., & Rosenbaum, P. R. (1993). Comparison of multivariate matching methods: Structures, distances, and algorithms. *Journal of Computational and Graphical Statistics, 2*, 405–420.
Hanushek, E. A., Kain, J. F., Markman, J. M., & Rivkin, S. G. (2003). Does peer ability affect student achievement? *Journal of Applied Econometrics, 18*, 527–544.
Heckman, J. J., Ichimura, H., & Todd, P. E. (1997). Matching as an econometric evaluation estimator: Evidence from evaluating a job training program. *Review of Economic Studies, 64*, 605–654.
Hill, H., Rowan, R. B., & Ball, D. L. (2005). Effects of teachers' mathematical knowledge for teaching on student achievement. *American Educational Research Journal, 42*, 371–406.

Ho, D. E., Imai, K., King, G., & Stuart, E. A. (2007). Matching as nonparametric preprocessing for reducing model dependence in parametric causal inference. *Political Analysis, 15*(3), 199–236.

Imai, K., King, G., & Stuart, E. (2008). Misunderstandings between experimentalists and observationalists about causal inference. *Journal of the Royal Statistical Society, Series A, 171*(2), 481–502.

Imai, K., & van Dyk, D. A. (2004). Causal inference with general treatment regimes: Generalizing the propensity score. *Journal of the American Statistical Association, 99*(467), 854–866.

Koth, C., Bradshaw, C., & Leaf, P. (2008). A multilevel study of predictors of student perceptions of school climate: The effect of classroom-level factors. *Journal of Educational Psychology, 100*, 96–104.

Little, R. J. A., & Rubin, D. B. (1987). *Statistical analysis with missing data*. New York: Wiley.

Luellen, J. K., Shadish, W. R., & Clark, M. H. (2005). Propensity scores: An introduction and experimental test. *Evaluation Review, 29*, 530–558.

Rosenbaum, P. R., & Rubin, D. B. (1983). The central role of the propensity score in observational studies for causal effects. *Biometrika, 70*, 41–55.

Rosenbaum, P. R., & Rubin, D. B. (1985). Constructing a control group using multivariate matched sampling methods that incorporate the propensity score. *American Statistician, 39*, 33–38.

Rubin, D. B. (1977). Assignment to treatment group on the basis of a covariate. *Journal of Educational and Behavioral Statistics, 2*(1), 1–26.

Rubin, D. B. (1979). Using multivariate matched sampling and regression adjustment to control bias in observational studies. *Journal of the American Statistical Association, 74*(366a), 318–328.

Rubin, D. B. (1997). Estimating causal effects from large data sets using propensity scores. *Annals of Internal Medicine, 127*, 757–763.

Rubin, D. B. (2001). Using propensity scores to help design observational studies: Application to the tobacco litigation. *Health Services and Outcomes Research Methodology, 2*(3–4), 169–188.

Schommer-Aitkins, M., Duell, O. K., & Hutter, R. (2005). Epistemological beliefs, mathematical problem-solving beliefs, and academic performance of middle school students. *Elementary School Journal, 105*, 289–304.

Shadish, W. R., Cook, T. D., & Campbell, D. T. (2002). *Experimental and quasi-experimental designs for general causal inference*. Boston: Houghton Mifflin.

Smith, A. J., & Todd, P. E. (2005). Does matching overcome LaLonde's critique of nonexperimental estimators? *Journal of Econometrics, 125*(1), 305–353.

Stürmer, T., Joshi, M., Glynn, R. J., Avorn, J., Rothman, K. J., & Schneeweiss, S. (2006). A review of the application of propensity score methods yielded increasing use, advantages in specific settings, but not substantially different estimates compared with conventional multivariable methods. *Journal of Clinical Epidemiology, 59*(5), 437–461.

## CHAPTER 5

# Evaluating Covariate Balance

### Cassandra W. Pattanayak

In randomized experiments, the randomization of treatment creates treatment groups that are similar on background characteristics, in expectation. However, when treatment is not randomized, observational study design methods such as matching and subclassification can be used to create a study design that approximates the ideal, parallel, and hypothetical randomized experiment.

Methods such as matching or subclassifying on estimated propensity scores have theoretical properties that increase the chance that the resulting matches or subclasses will be balanced, in that the treatment (or "active treatment") and control (or "control treatment") groups are similar on background characteristics. For example, propensity score methods are equal percent bias reducing (Rosenbaum & Rubin, 1983). But, in practice, a particular observational study design method may be optimal for one dataset and inappropriate for another. This is true even for methods that computationally optimize the matches or subclasses based on predefined criteria for covariate balance (Iacus, King, & Porro, 2011; Zubizarreta, 2012) because the researchers' choice of predefined criteria affect which data are discarded or maintained and therefore the generalizability of the results.

Though theory is helpful for guiding the approach to observational study design, in the context of any particular dataset the goal is simply to compare active and control units (e.g., subjects or households) that are as similar to each other as possible. Potential study designs should be assessed not on the theoretical properties of the algorithms that generated them but on the similarity of the background covariates in the resulting active treatment group and control treatment group. We would not move ahead with an extremely unlucky randomized experiment where, by chance, all the men were assigned to active treatment and all the women were assigned to control treatment, even though theory shows that randomization is expected to produce balanced treatment groups on average (Rubin, 2008a). Similarly, if an unsystematic approach to selecting matches for an observational study happened to produce matches with excellent balance on the background covariates, these matches would be preferable to a less balanced design generated by a theoretically motivated algorithm.

Selecting a final design for an observational study involves iterating between (1) creating a set of potential matches or subclasses and (2) evaluating the resulting balance on key background variables. If a balance check shows that the matched or subclassified active and control groups are not similar enough on an important background variable, the matching or subclassification algorithm should be adjusted to improve balance on this variable.

This chapter focuses on how to evaluate the success of an observational study design by comparing the active treatment and control treatment groups on key background covariates. First, two examples are outlined for reference throughout the chapter, and the framework for observational study design is described. Then, best practices for evaluating balance are presented, followed by discussions on the related issues of missing data, generalizability, and the occasional need to use matching or subclassification to create covariate balance in randomized experiments.

## OBSERVATIONAL STUDY DESIGN

### Overview of Examples

This chapter refers to two empirical examples. The first is a Phase IV pharmaceutical study comparing the efficacy and side effects of a recently developed anticoagulant to the previous standard of care treatment during orthopedic surgery (Turpie et al., 2014). Subclasses of similar patients were created based on estimated propensity scores and other criteria.

The second example, used to produce the balance diagnostics shown in this chapter, is a version of the well-known and widely available job training dataset discussed by LaLonde (1986) and Dehejia and Wahba (1999). The dataset consists of 185 people who took part in the National Supported Work Demonstration and 2,490 people from a control treatment group constructed from the Population Survey of Income Dynamics.

In this chapter, one possible set of propensity score matches and one possible set of subclasses for this dataset are explored to demonstrate covariate balance diagnostics. These matches and subclasses for the LaLonde data were created to illustrate various balance diagnostics and are not intended as optimal final study designs for this dataset.

## The Rubin Causal Framework

This chapter focuses on studies with two levels of treatment, "active" and "control." The "units" are the physical entities to which treatment is applied at a particular time, such as patients in a medical study. For each unit, there are two "potential outcomes": the outcome that would be observed if the unit was assigned to active treatment, and the outcome that would be observed if the unit was assigned to control treatment. The "causal effect" is defined as a comparison between the two potential outcomes (Holland, 1986; Rubin, 1974). Of course, no more than one potential outcome can be observed for each unit (Rubin, 1978). The goal of causal inference is to impute the missing potential outcome for each unit in order to estimate the causal effect.

Most importantly for this chapter, a dataset may contain background information for each unit. These background variables are "covariates." In an observational study, researchers seek to identify pairs ("matches") or small groups ("subclasses") of units who are sufficiently similar on key covariates that their missing potential outcomes can be imputed based on the observed outcomes of units receiving the opposite treatment within the same match or subclass. Further discussion of the assumptions underlying the Rubin Causal Framework can be found in Rubin (2008c).

## Separation of Covariates and Outcomes

The first step in observational study design is to identify the time when the treatment decision was made, relative to the other variables (Rubin, 2001). Any variable that could have been affected by whether a unit received active treatment or control treatment is an outcome: this variable could take on two different potential values. Any variable that was determined before the treatment decision and therefore could not have been affected by manipulation of treatment is a covariate. The distinction between outcomes and covariates is crucial because mistakenly conditioning on an outcome as if it were a covariate can mask treatment effects (Rubin, 2000). Ideally, the covariates will be balanced between the active treatment and control treatment groups.

Observational study design and covariate balance checking should take place without access to study outcomes (Rubin, 2007, 2008b). In a randomized experiment, decisions about stratification and randomization mechanisms necessarily take place before treatment is assigned and outcomes are collected, and so it is not possible for a researcher to choose a design that favors a particular result. To ensure similar objectivity in an observational study, outcomes should be removed from the dataset before matches or subclasses are created, to avoid both real and suspected researcher bias.

## Identification and Prioritization of Covariates

A list of key covariates should be created, based on knowledge of the applied scientific context. The goal is to identify covariates that are likely correlated with both the treatment assignment and the potential outcomes, in order to create "unconfoundedness" (also called "strong ignorability"). "Unconfoundedness" is defined as independence between potential outcomes and treatment assignment, conditional on the observed covariates (Rosenbaum & Rubin, 1983). It implies that excluded or unobserved covariates do not bias treatment effect estimates.

The observed outcomes from the current study should be hidden during the design phase, to ensure that the study cannot be designed to favor any particular treatment. Also, at least half of the potential outcomes are unobserved anyway because units are assigned to the opposite treatment. Therefore, the contextual knowledge of the applied collaborator is crucial for identifying covariates importantly related to the treatment assignment and the potential outcomes. This task is similar to the task of selecting covariates for stratification in a randomized experiment. Frequently, the relationships between covariates, treatment, and potential outcomes are debatable. A simulation study by Brookhart et al. (2006) suggested that covariates related to outcomes and not treatments should be included, but that including covariates that are related to treatments and not outcomes may increase the variance of the final treatment effect estimate without improving bias. Without knowledge of the relationship between a covariate and the outcomes, though, it may be more prudent to include a covariate that is very likely related to the treatment and may or may not be important for the outcomes.

Then, the list of key covariates can be compared to the available data. If crucial covariates are not available, it may not be possible to draw causal inferences with the current dataset. Transformations of continuous covariates available in the dataset, such as squares and logs, can also be created and appended to the dataset as additional covariates. It is useful to create these transformations as separate covariates, rather than only including the corresponding terms in a propensity score model, so that it is straightforward to check balance on the transformed covariates. Including and checking balance on transformed covariates can help ensure that continuous covariates not only have similar means in the active treatment and control treatment groups but also have the same distributions in each treatment group. For example, Figure 5.1 summarizes the balance not only on the covariate "age" for the LaLonde data, but also on "Log Age" and "Age Squared," and Figure 5.2 shows the distribution of age in the matched active treatment and control groups, after including these transformations in the propensity score model.

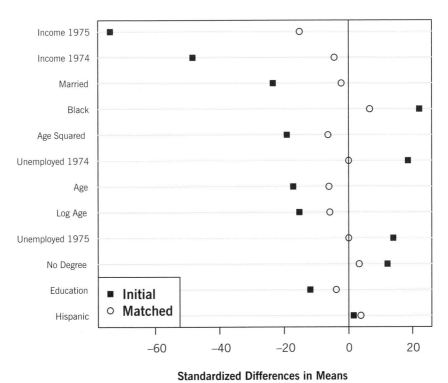

**FIGURE 5.1.** A Love Plot (Ahmed et al., 2006) summarizing the covariate balance achieved by matching for the LaLonde data.

If treatment had been randomized, we would expect the multivariate distribution of covariates to be similar between the active treatment and control treatment groups. However, propensity score methods focus on linear combinations of individual covariates rather than bivariate or multivariate covariate distributions. To address multivariate distributions, additional covariates can be created by taking the product of pairs of original covariates. For example, if "age" and "married" are both covariates, a covariate representing the interaction between age and married, age × married, might be appended to the covariate dataset. These two-way interaction covariates can then be included in the observational study design (e.g., included in a propensity score estimation model), and covariate balance can be checked by handling interaction variables as if they were any other covariates. Although this approach will not account for every aspect of a bivariate or multivariate distribution, interactions between the most

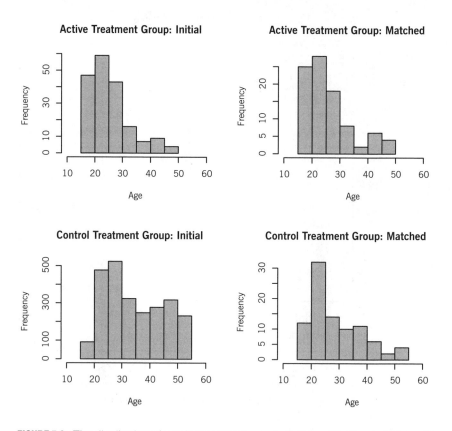

**FIGURE 5.2.** The distribution of age by treatment groups before and after matching with the LaLonde data.

# Evaluating Covariate Balance

important pairs of covariates can be addressed in this way. Figure 5.3 summarizes covariate balance on 41 two-way interaction covariates appended to the LaLonde dataset.

The most important predictors of treatment or outcomes may be functions of the covariates that originally appear in the data. For example, a dataset may include weight and height, but physicians might have taken into account body mass index when choosing a treatment. In the pharmaceutical study example, two of the most important covariates were "frailty" and "metabolic disorder," both calculated as functions of other covariates that appeared in the original dataset. Such functions of the original covariates should be calculated prior to the design of the observational study and appended to the covariate dataset for straightforward balance checking. As an example, Figure 5.1 and Table 5.1 include indicators for unemployment in 1974 and 1975, which are set equal to 1 when there is zero income in 1974 or zero income in 1975, respectively.

The key covariates should then be prioritized in the order of their expected relevance for the study at hand. One strategy, used in the

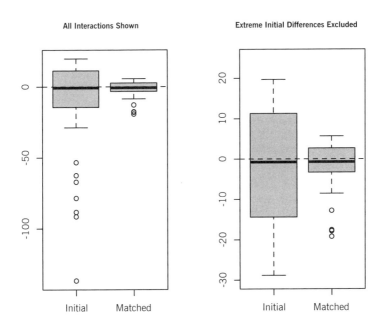

**FIGURE 5.3.** A summary of covariate balance on 41 two-way interaction covariates appended to the LaLonde data.

**TABLE 5.1. A Summary of the Covariate Balance Achieved by Matching for the LaLonde Data**

| Covariate | Mean before matching | | | Mean after matching | | |
|---|---|---|---|---|---|---|
| | Active treatment ($n = 185$) | Control treatment ($n = 2490$) | Difference in means | Active treatment ($n = 91$) | Control treatment ($n = 91$) | Difference in means |
| Married | 0.19 | 0.87 | −0.68 | 0.35 | 0.42 | −0.07 |
| No degree | 0.71 | 0.31 | 0.40 | 0.67 | 0.56 | 0.11 |
| Black | 0.84 | 0.25 | 0.59 | 0.77 | 0.59 | 0.18 |
| Hispanic | 0.06 | 0.03 | 0.03 | 0.09 | 0.02 | 0.07 |
| Education | 10.35 | 12.12 | −1.77 | 10.30 | 10.88 | −0.58 |
| Age | 25.82 | 34.85 | −9.03 | 26.07 | 29.31 | −3.24 |
| 1974 income ($) | 2096 | 19429 | −17333 | 4260 | 5865 | −1605 |
| 1975 income ($) | 1532 | 19063 | −17531 | 2826 | 6418 | −3592 |
| Unemployed 1974 | 0.71 | 0.09 | 0.62 | 0.41 | 0.41 | 0 |
| Unemployed 1975 | 0.60 | 0.10 | 0.50 | 0.31 | 0.31 | 0 |
| Estimated propensity score | 0.62 | 0.03 | 0.59 | 0.46 | 0.33 | 0.12 |

pharmaceutical study, is to divide the covariates into priority groups. Which covariates must be perfectly balanced in order for causal conclusions to be believable? Which covariates would ideally be balanced but could be sacrificed in order to achieve balance on higher priority covariates? These questions can only be answered through conversations with subject matter experts.

Covariates appended to the dataset to represent transformations of continuous covariates, two-way or higher order interactions, and functions of original covariates should be ranked by priority along with the original covariates. For example, there may be many more two-way interactions than can reasonably be included, but it may be known that treatment decisions were based on a combination of two particular covariates, and the interaction between these two covariates can be prioritized.

## Designing an Observational Study with Propensity Scores

Propensity score estimation, the focus of this book, is one of the most effective approaches to designing an observational study. The propensity score is the probability that a particular unit would have been assigned to active treatment as opposed to control treatment, conditional on that unit's covariate values. In observational studies, propensity scores can be estimated by examining the proportion of units with certain covariate values that are assigned to active treatment versus control treatment. One common approach is to run a logistic regression of the treatment assignment on the covariates, and the fitted values from this model are the estimated propensity scores. The propensity score is the "coarsest balancing score," meaning that the set of propensity scores divides the units into the smallest possible number of groups such that the active treatment and control treatment units within each group are comparable on covariates (Rosenbaum & Rubin, 1983). Propensity scores are estimated based on the prioritized covariates, including transformations, interactions, and functions of original covariates, as discussed above. After fitting a propensity score model, each unit has an estimated propensity score, just as each unit has a value for each other covariate. The estimated propensity score is a function of all the covariates used for the estimation and can be considered the most important covariate, in that it captures the extent to which each covariate differs in the active treatment and control treatment groups. Three commonly used observational study design methods are described as follows:

The first method is one-to-one or one-to-many matching on the estimated propensity score. Matching is a useful approach to creating active treatment and control groups, particularly when the original dataset contains a pool of potential controls that is much larger than the set of active treatment units, and when the goal is to generalize to a population similar to the active units (Rosenbaum & Rubin, 1985). Various forms of matching are available (as reviewed in Stuart, 2010), including methods that combine estimated propensity scores with other criteria (Diamond & Sekhon, 2013; Rosenbaum & Rubin, 1985) and optimization methods that do not rely on the estimated propensity score (Zubizarreta, 2012). See Chapter 1 for an overview of propensity score matching methods. Checking covariate balance is particularly straightforward for one-to-one matches because the sample sizes are the same in the matched active treatment and control treatment groups, and weights do not need to be taken into account.

Second, units can also be divided into subclasses based on the estimated propensity score and/or individual covariates that contain any number of active units and any number of control units. This approach, a generalization of matching, is often most appropriate when the initial active treatment and control treatment groups overlap on the ranges of the covariates or have common support (see Chapter 4 for a discussion on this topic). Subclassification assigns a weight to each unit so that summaries of the active treatment and control treatment groups refer to populations with the same covariate distributions. Various forms of subclassification have been proposed (Hansen, 2004; Rosenbaum & Rubin, 1984; Stuart, 2010), including approaches that do not rely on estimated propensity scores (Iacus et al., 2011). Subclass weights must be taken into account in covariate balance checks as well as outcome analysis.

A third and also often recommended class of methods involves weighting on the estimated propensity score (Czajka, Hirabayashi, Little, & Rubin, 1992; Hirano, Imbens, & Ridder, 2003; Imbens, 2000; Robins, Hernan, & Brumback, 2000). This method can be seen as a generalization of subclassification, where each unit is weighted accordingly to its own estimated propensity score, rather than using a subclass weight that, in essence, averages the unit's individual estimated propensity score with other, similar units' estimated propensity scores. One disadvantage of propensity score weighting is the high variance of the resulting estimators (Stuart, 2010). Units with very high or very low estimated propensity scores can be relatively influential once weighted, when actually these most extreme units are the units least likely to have counterparts in the opposite treatment group and therefore are least likely to contain useful information about causal effects.

This chapter focuses on matched and subclassified designs. However, most of the balance diagnostics discussed in this chapter also could be applied to a weighted design, where the weights are taken into account in the calculation of each balance measure.

Regardless of the method used to generate the observational study design, proposed designs should be evaluated based on the covariate balance achieved. The researcher should alternate between creating an observational study design—adjusting a propensity score estimation model, changing the matching or subclassification algorithm, incorporating additional interactions—and assessing covariate balance.

## EVALUATING COVARIATE BALANCE

Once an observational study has been designed with propensity scores, the resulting covariate balance should be compared to the initial covariate balance and to the covariate balance achieved by other proposed designs. Appropriate balance-checking strategies may differ for various types of covariates. In addition, balance-on first priority covariates can be summarized separately from balance on second-priority covariates, and so on, to inform the final choice of design. If treatment had been randomized, we would expect the active treatment and control treatment groups to be similar on every possible summary of the covariates. The goal of an observational study design is to parallel a hypothetical randomized experiment. Therefore, a broad range of balance diagnostics should be checked.

The estimated propensity score itself should be included among the continuous covariates and on the list of high-priority covariates. Even if the proposed observational study design is the result of matching or subclassifying on the estimated propensity score, various designs will lead to active treatment and control treatment groups that are balanced to a greater or lesser extent on the estimated propensity score itself.

Although observational study design would ideally lead to covariates as balanced as expected in a randomized experiment, $p$-values for hypothesis tests comparing a covariate's values in the active treatment and control treatment groups should not be used for balance checking (Imai, King, & Stuart, 2008; Stuart, 2010). The primary reason is that $p$-values are functions of sample sizes as well as the difference between treatment group means. Because sample sizes change along with treatment group means when matches or subclasses are created, it is not meaningful to compare $p$-values before and after matching or subclassification. The following discussion focuses on checking balance graphically, without hypothesis tests.

The rest of this section describes methods for assessing balance for various types of covariates. First, exact matching criteria are discussed, for which no balance diagnostic is needed. Then, the section focuses on binary covariates, followed by continuous covariates.

## Exact Matching Criteria

In many contexts, certain covariates should be matched exactly rather than incorporated into propensity score models. For each active unit, the set of potential matched controls can be limited to units with the same value on a certain covariate. Within this limited set of potential matched controls, a single match may be selected based on estimated propensity scores, to create balance on all other covariates. Similarly, units may be divided into groups based on one high-priority covariate, and subclasses may be created by further dividing units within each group. There are four common reasons that exact matching may be used. More than one of these reasons may apply.

First, a covariate might be so important that acceptable matches should have exactly the same value on that covariate. In the pharmaceutical study, patients underwent either hip surgery or knee surgery, which differ importantly, and so separate subclasses were created for hip and knee surgery patients whenever possible. Figure 5.1 and Table 5.1 reflect exact matching on the unemployment indicators in the LaLonde data.

Second, categorical covariates with many categories may be difficult or impossible to incorporate into a propensity score model. The most common example is an indicator for geography, such as country, state, site, and medical center. The researcher may believe that units and treatment decision making differ importantly between data collection sites. The simplest way to take into account such a covariate is to match units only to others within the same geographic area (however that is defined) or create subcategories that contain only units from the same geographic area. In the pharmaceutical study, subcategories were created within country and within medical site, though the site criterion was sometimes relaxed in order to prioritize other covariates. Indicators for geographic location are difficult to include in graphics or tables summarizing covariate balance, because of the large number of categories.

Third, it is often desirable to draw causal inferences for subgroups of the population. This can be accomplished by exact matching on the subgroup indicators, effectively producing separate observational study designs within each subgroup. For example, in the pharmaceutical study, the exact matching on country would allow subgroup analyses for particular regions of interest.

Last, a covariate may stand out in checks of covariate balance after matching or subclassification algorithms are applied, even after including interactions between this covariate and other covariates in the propensity score model. Although the difficulty of creating balance on this covariate may be due to the particular observed values in the dataset rather than an overarching scientific pattern, exact matching can force balance on such a covariate.

Exact matching or subclassification guarantees balance on covariates handled in this way. Still, the tables and figures included in this chapter include exactly matched covariates whenever possible, to demonstrate the balance achieved.

## Binary Covariates

It is common to examine the differences in active treatment and control treatment means. In the case of binary covariates, the mean of each binary covariate can be calculated among the matched active treatment units and among the matched control treatment units. In a study where the estimand for the outcome analysis is an odds ratio for a binary covariate rather than a difference in means, it is appropriate to calculate odds ratios from the active treatment and control treatment means. Table 5.1 includes the means for binary covariates by treatment group, before and after matching, for the LaLonde data.

# Evaluating Covariate Balance

In a subclassified design, the binary covariate means in the active treatment and control treatment can be calculated separately within each subclass. Figure 5.4 illustrates this idea with the covariate "age" based on a set of possible subclasses for the LaLonde data. Alternatively, the difference between the mean of a covariate in the active treatment group and the mean of the covariate in the control treatment group can be calculated within each subclass, and these within-subclass differences can be averaged across subclasses. To generalize to the initial study population, subclass weights are calculated as the proportion of units in that subclass overall (combining active and control units). To generalize to the initial active treatment group, subclass weights are calculated as the proportion of active treatment units in each subclass. However, any set of subclass weights can be used, as long as the same weights are used in the active treatment group and the control treatment group, and the same weights are used for the balance checking and the outcome analysis.

Covariate means can be presented both numerically (as in Table 5.1) so that readers understand the extent of the balance and the overall characteristics of the study population, and graphically (as in Figure 5.1) to

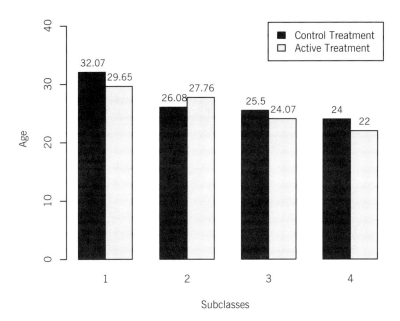

**FIGURE 5.4.** Means of the covariate "age" by treatment groups based on a set of possible subclasses for the LaLonde data.

communicate the balance as concisely as possible. Categorical covariates can be presented as a set of binary covariates indicating the factor levels, as demonstrated by the "Black" and "Hispanic" covariates in this chapter's balance diagnostics. Figure 5.1 is a Love Plot (as in Ahmed et al., 2006) summarizing the covariate balance achieved by matching for the LaLonde data. For each covariate, labeled along the y-axis, the square represents the difference between active treatment and control treatment means before matching, and the circle represents the difference between active and control means after matching. The general success of the matching method is demonstrated by the fact that the circles are closer to the vertical line at 0 than the squares are. The unemployment indicators have post-matching differences in means of zero because of exact matching. Balance did not improve on every covariate; for example, the absolute difference in means increased for the covariate "Hispanic." Final matches should be the result of comparing several proposed sets of matches and assessing balance according to covariate priority.

Figure 5.5 demonstrates another way to graphically describe a similar set of absolute differences in means. Because the covariate labels have

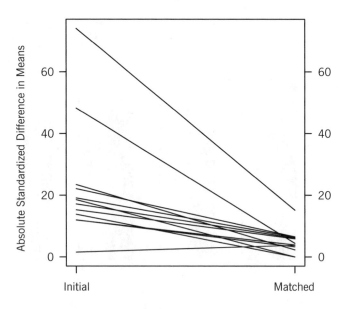

**FIGURE 5.5.** Absolute differences in means between treatment groups before and after matching for the LaLonde data.

been removed, more covariates can be included. The *MatchIt* package in R includes an interactive version of this plot that allows the user to identify the covariates (Ho, Imai, King, & Stuart, 2011).

Figure 5.3 includes the standardized differences in means for 41 pairwise products of the original covariates, before and after matching. When there are more covariates than can reasonably be summarized by a Love Plot or a graphic like Figure 5.5, box plots can show the distribution of many covariates' standardized differences in means before matching or subclassification to the distribution of these covariates' standardized differences in means after matching or subclassification. In Figure 5.3, the initial box plot shows the distribution of the 41 standardized differences in means for these interactions, before matching, and the postmatching box plot shows the distribution of the 41 standardized differences in means after matching. Graphics parallel to Figures 5.1, 5.2, 5.3, and 5.5 can also be created to compare multiple proposed observational study designs, rather than to compare the initial covariate balance to the balance achieved by one particular design. For example, by including more than two symbol types, Love Plots can communicate the balance achieved by several different designs.

In Figures 5.1, 5.3, and 5.5, the differences in means are standardized. Differences in means can be displayed with or without standardization. Standardization puts all covariate differences on the same scale. However, this choice is not always the right one. Binary covariates can always be plotted together without standardization because their means lie between zero and one, and low-frequency binary covariates can have high variances and unstable standardized means.

It is important to note that standardized differences used for covariate balance should *not* be traditional $t$-statistics. The purpose of a graphic like a Love Plot is to compare the difference in means on a particular covariate before and after matching. The purpose of standardizing is merely to compare the difference in means achieved by matching for multiple covariates simultaneously, on the same scale. However, a $t$-statistic is a function of this difference in means, along with the sample variance in each group and the sample size in each group. Comparing $t$-statistics for a particular covariate before and after matching can be misleading because any improvement in the covariate means is confounded by changes in the sample size. This is the same principle underlying the previous discussion about avoiding $p$-values when assessing covariate balance.

Instead, to standardize covariate mean differences for the purpose of balance checking, the difference in means should be divided by a denominator that is the same before and after matching for each covariate. For example, the difference in means before *and* the difference in means after matching can both be divided by the denominator for the $t$-statistic from the initial dataset, or, for matching, the differences in means before and after matching can both be divided by the standard deviation of the covariate in the initial active treatment group (Stuart, 2010). The standardized balance diagnostics shown in this chapter for the LaLonde data divide the differences in means for each covariate by the standard deviation in the initial active treatment group.

The literature provides some guidance as to the covariate balance that should be considered acceptable. In particular, a standardized difference in means less than 0.25 for each covariate has been offered as a goal, where differences in means are standardized by the initial standard deviation in the active treatment group (Rubin, 2001; Stuart, 2010). This suggestion is based on the covariate balance that would be needed in order for regression adjustment to be appropriate. However, there will always be trade-offs between the balance achieved on one covariate and the balance achieved on another, as well as trade-offs between covariate balance and generalizability. The success of a proposed study design should be evaluated in collaboration with subject matter experts based on the balance achieved on the highest priority covariates, followed by the second priority covariates, and so on.

## Continuous Covariates

Unlike binary covariates, the distribution of a continuous covariate is not completely summarized by its mean. Figure 5.2 is a graphical comparison of the full distribution of age before and after matching with the LaLonde data. The left column shows that, before matching, the active and control groups did not have the same distribution on this covariate. The right column explores whether the matched active and control treatment groups have more similar distributions on age. Figure 5.6 uses the same format to demonstrate the balance achieved on the estimated propensity score.

For a subclassified design, the full distribution of continuous covariates can be visualized for the active treatment group and the control treatment group within each subclass. Figure 5.7 shows the distribution of age by treatment groups and subclass, for a possible subclassified design for the LaLonde data. Ideally, the distributions for each treatment group within each subclass should be very similar to each other. If there are many continuous covariates and/or many subclasses, the balance achieved on continuous covariates can be assessed by examining summary statistics. The means of continuous distributions can be compared in the active

## Evaluating Covariate Balance

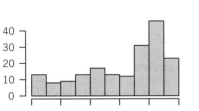
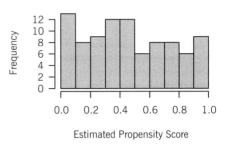
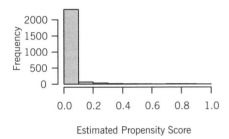
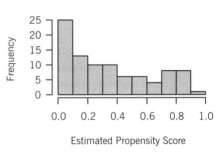

**FIGURE 5.6.** The distribution of estimated propensity scores by treatment groups before and after matching with the LaLonde data.

treatment group and the control treatment group, just as with binary covariates. With continuous covariates, it is typically necessary to standardize the covariates before showing their balance on the same graphic, to put them on the same scale. However, it is crucial to standardize these differences in means using the same denominator for each covariate before and after matching, as discussed above. Within-subclass standardized differences in means can be averaged over subclasses, based on subclass weights, just as with binary covariates, so that each covariate has one standardized difference in means before subclassification and one standardized difference in means after subclassification. Graphics parallel to Figures 5.1, 5.3, and 5.5 can then be created.

Continuous distributions can also be summarized by variance, by quantiles, or by range. Any of these statistics can be calculated for each covariate before and after matching, or compared among several proposed study designs. Rubin (2001) suggests that the ratios of the variances of each covariate within the active treatment and control treatment groups should

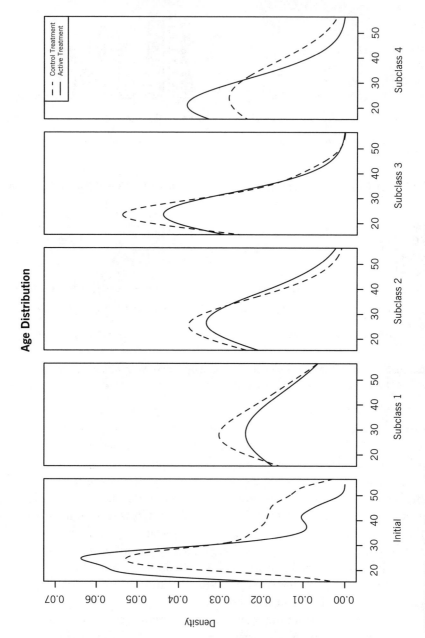

**FIGURE 5.7.** The distribution of age by treatment groups based on a set of possible subclasses for the LaLonde data.

be close to 1. There is no conventional cutoff for this ratio of variances—study designs must be chosen based on the overall balance achieved and covariate priority, but Rubin advises that the ratio of variances should not be as low as 1/2 or as high as 2. Special attention should be paid to the range of a continuous covariate. The active treatment and control treatment groups should have overlapping support on each covariate. The definition of sufficient overlap depends on the context, as illustrated by an additional example related to in vitro fertilization and birth outcomes (Pattanayak, 2011), where the active treatment group included patients who had one embryo transferred, and the control group included patients who had two embryos transferred. For an initial set of proposed matches, the youngest patient in the active treatment group was aged 18, and the youngest patient in the control group was aged 20. Physician collaborators confirmed that the fertility of 18- and 20-year-olds is similar, and so the minima of the age distributions were sufficiently similar. However, the oldest patient in the active treatment group was 44, and the oldest patient in the control group was 42. Even though this is also a 2-year difference, the fertility of a 44-year-old is importantly different from the fertility of a 42-year-old, and the maximum age in the active treatment and control treatment groups was required to be closer for the final set of proposed matches.

## ADDITIONAL CONSIDERATIONS

### Missing Data

Most datasets include missing data. Missing outcome data can be handled as in any study, for example, with multiple imputation (Rubin, 1987). Missing covariate data are more challenging. Ideally, an observational study design could produce active treatment and control treatment groups that are balanced on every aspect of the multivariate covariate distribution, including the pattern of missingness. Approaches for dealing with missing covariate data are briefly summarized below and discussed in more detail in Chapters 12, 13, and 14.

One possibility is to multiply impute missing covariate values, as in Langenskiold and Rubin (2008). If $M$ imputed covariate datasets are created, then matching or subclassification should be carried out $M$ separate times. Each of these $M$ designs requires iterating between checking covariate balance and adjusting the matches or subclasses. Each of the final $M$ designs is combined with the outcomes, and $M$ sets of results are produced, which can then be combined using the usual multiple imputation combining rules (Rubin, 1987). The disadvantages of this approach are the additional effort required to match or subclassify $M$ times and the possible lack of clarity resulting from $M$ separate study designs.

Alternatively, D'Agostino and Rubin (2000) proposed a generalized propensity score that summarizes not only the observed covariates but also the patterns of missingness on those covariates. Matches or subclasses created based on this generalized propensity score would be expected to balance active treatment and control treatment groups on both covariate values and the patterns of missingness. This approach warrants further attention and development.

A simplified but practical approach involves single imputation for covariates with negligibly missing data and missingness indicators for covariates with important levels of missingness. If, say, patient age is missing for one or two patients in a large medical study, and the researcher believes that these values cannot importantly impact the matched or subclassified design, the values can be singly imputed by drawing from the empirical distribution or by any other approach.

For each covariate that is missing for an important proportion of units, an indicator for missingness can be created and added to the dataset. Each missingness indicator can then be handled like any other covariate: its importance can be ranked relative to other covariates, interactions can be created between the missingness indicator and other covariates to reflect multivariate missingness patterns, and the missingness indicator can be used for matching or subclassification via propensity score estimation or any other method. Once a design has been proposed, the researcher can check that the rates of missingness are similar in the resulting active treatment and control treatment groups. See Chapter 12 of this volume for more discussion of this topic.

## Generalizability versus Causality

In order to achieve covariate balance, it is typical for some units to be discarded, or for subclass weights to lead to results that generalize to a population different from the population represented by the initial dataset. There is always a trade-off between the strength of causal inference and generalizability to the broadest population possible: if covariates are required to be more similar between active treatment and control treatment units, fewer available units will satisfy the balance criteria.

Fortunately, generalizability to a population with known characteristics can be checked explicitly. Often the goal is to generalize to a population similar to the initial overall population or to the initial active treatment group (as discussed in Imai, King, & Stuart, 2008). The covariate values in this initial population can be compared to the covariate values in the final observational study design, and any discrepancies can be reported and discussed.

## Randomized Experiments

This chapter focuses on observational study design because when treatment is randomized, the randomization itself is expected to create covariate balance between active treatment and control treatment groups. However, for any particular randomized experiment, only one dataset is observed. Even though randomization leads to balance on average, some datasets will be the result of relatively unlucky randomizations. The success of the randomization in creating similar active treatment and control treatment groups should be checked explicitly. In fact, any of the balance-checking practices described in this chapter thus far could be applied to a randomized experiment.

Strategies for addressing lack of covariate balance in a randomized experiment include limiting the possible random allocations by choosing a stratified or paired design; planning a rerandomization scheme that discards less desirable randomizations (Morgan & Rubin, 2012); or creating a subclassified design after data collection, as if the study were actually observational (Miratrix, Sekhon, & Yu, 2013; Pattanayak, 2011). It is also sometimes useful to regress observed outcomes on the treatment indicator and the unbalanced covariates, although the resulting estimator will be biased for finite samples, and the usual expressions for the variance of regression coefficients will not reflect the actual variance of the treatment effect estimate (Freedman, 2008a, 2008b).

## CONCLUSION

There are many ways to design an observational study with propensity scores for causal inference. A wide literature exists on the theoretical advantages and disadvantages of various methods and is crucial for creating possible observational study designs. In the context of any particular applied project, however, the goal is to generate one study design that has covariate values in the active treatment and control groups that will give the study's audience confidence in causal conclusions. Some design strategies may work better than others for a particular dataset. Diagnostics for covariate balance allow us to choose a final study design based on its success in creating similar treatment groups.

## REFERENCES

Ahmed, A., Husain, A., Love, T. E., Gambassi, G., Dell'Italia, L. J., Francis, G. S., et al. (2006). Heart failure, chronic diuretic use, and increase in mortality and hospitalization: An observational study using propensity score methods. *European Heart Journal, 27*, 1431–1439.

Brookhart, M. A., Schneeweiss, S., Rothman, K. J., Glynn, R. J., Avorn, J., & Sturmer, T. (2006). Variable selection for propensity score models. *American Journal of Epidemiology, 163*(12), 1149–1156.

Czajka, J. C., Hirabayashi, S. M., Little, R. J. A., & Rubin, D. B. (1992). Projecting from advance data using propensity score modeling. *Journal of Business and Economics Statistics, 10*, 117–131.

D'Agostino, R. B. Jr., & Rubin, D. B. (2000). Estimating and using propensity scores with partially missing data. *Journal of the American Statistical Association, 95*(451), 749–759.

Dehejia, R. H., & Wahba, S. (1999). Causal effects in non-experimental studies: Re-evaluating the evaluation of training programs. *Journal of the American Statistical Association, 94*(448), 1053–1062.

Diamond, A., & Sekhon, J. S. (2013). Genetic matching for estimating causal effects: A general multivariate matching method for achieving balance in observational studies. *Review of Economics and Statistics, 95*(3), 932–945.

Freedman, D. A. (2008a). On regression adjustments to experimental data. *Advances in Applied Mathematics, 40*, 180–193.

Freedman, D. A. (2008b). On regression adjustments to experimental data with several treatments. *Annals of Applied Statistics, 2*(1), 176–196.

Hansen, B. B. (2004). Full matching in an observational study of coaching for the SAT. *Journal of the American Statistical Association, 99*(467), 609–618.

Hirano, K., Imbens, G. W., & Ridder, G. (2003). Efficient estimation of average treatment effects using the estimated propensity score. *Econometrica, 71*(4), 1161–1189.

Ho, D. E., Imai, K., King, G., & Stuart, E. A. (2011). MatchIt: Nonparametric preprocessing for parametric causal inference. *Journal of Statistical Software, 42*(8), 1–28.

Holland, P. W. (1986). Statistics and causal inference. *Journal of the American Statistical Association, 81*(396), 945–960.

Iacus, S. M., King, G., & Porro, G. (2011). Multivariate matching methods that are monotonic imbalance bounding. *Journal of the American Statistical Association, 106*(493), 345–361.

Imai, K., King, G., & Stuart, E. A. (2008). Misunderstandings between experimentalists and observationalists about causal inference. *Journal of the Royal Statistical Society, Series A, 171*(2), 481–502.

Imbens, G. W. (2000). The role of the propensity score in estimating dose-response functions. *Biometrika, 87*(3), 706–710.

LaLonde, R. J. (1986). Evaluating the econometric evaluations of training programs. *American Economic Review, 76,* 604–620.
Langenskiold, S., & Rubin, D. B. (2008). Outcome-free design of observational studies: Peer influence on smoking. *Annales d'Economie et de Statistique, 91/92,* 107–125.
Miratrix, L. W., Sekhon, J. S., & Yu, B. (2013). Adjusting treatment effect estimates by post-stratification in randomized experiments. *Journal of the Royal Statistical Society, Series B, 75*(2), 369–396.
Morgan, K. L., & Rubin, D. B. (2012). Rerandomization to improve covariate balance in experiments. *Annals of Statistics, 40*(2), 1263–1282.
Pattanayak, C. W. (2011). *The critical role of covariate balance in causal inference with randomized experiments and observational studies.* Doctoral dissertation, Harvard University, Cambridge, MA.
Robins, J. M., Hernan, M. A., & Brumback, B. (2000). Marginal structural models and causal inference in epidemiology. *Epidemiology, 11*(5), 550–560.
Rosenbaum, P. R., & Rubin, D. B. (1983). The central role of the propensity score in observational studies for causal effects. *Biometrika, 70*(1), 41–55.
Rosenbaum, P. R., & Rubin, D. B. (1984). Reducing bias in observational studies using subclassification on the propensity score. *Journal of the American Statistical Association, 79*(387), 516–524.
Rosenbaum, P. R., & Rubin, D. B. (1985). Constructing a control group using multivariate matched sampling methods that incorporate the propensity score. *American Statistician, 39*(1), 33–38.
Rubin, D. B. (1974). Estimating causal effects of treatments in randomized and nonrandomized studies. *Journal of Educational Psychology, 66*(5), 688–701.
Rubin, D. B. (1978). Bayesian inference for causal effects: The role of randomization. *Annals of Statistics, 6*(1), 34–58.
Rubin, D. B. (1987). *Multiple imputation for nonresponse in surveys.* New York: Wiley.
Rubin, D. B. (2000). Statistical issues in the estimation of the causal effects of smoking due to the conduct of the tobacco industry. In J. Gaswirth (Ed.), *Statistical science in the courtroom* (pp. 321–351). New York: Springer-Verlag.
Rubin, D. B. (2001). Using propensity scores to help design observational studies: Application to the tobacco litigation. *Health Services and Outcomes Research Methodology, 2,* 169–188.
Rubin, D. B. (2007). The design versus the analysis of observational studies for causal effects: Parallels with the design of randomized trials. *Statistics in Medicine, 26*(1), 20–36.
Rubin, D. B. (2008a). Comment: The design and analysis of gold standard randomized experiments. *Journal of the American Statistical Association, 103*(484), 1350–1353.
Rubin, D. B. (2008b). For objective causal inference, design trumps analysis. *Annals of Applied Statistics, 2*(3), 808–840.

Rubin, D. B. (2008c). Statistical inference for causal effects, with emphasis on applications for epidemiology and medical statistics. In C. R. Rao, J. P. Miller, & D. C. Rao (Eds.), *Handbook of statistics 27: Epidemiology and medical statistics* (pp. 28–63). Amsterdam, The Netherlands: Elsevier.

Stuart, E. A. (2010). Matching methods for causal inference: A review and a look forward. *Statistical Science, 25*(1), 1–21.

Turpie, A. G., Haas, S., Kreutz, R., Mantovani, L. G., Pattanayak, C. W., Holberg, G., et al. (2014). A non-interventional comparison of rivaroxaban with standard of care for thromboprophylaxis after major orthopaedic surgery in 17,701 patients with propensity score adjustment. *Thrombosis and Haemostasis, 111*(1), 94–102.

Zubizarreta, J. R. (2012). Using mixed integer programming for matching in an observational study of kidney failure after surgery. *Journal of the American Statistical Association, 107*(500), 1360–1371.

# PART III

# Weighting Schemes and Other Strategies for Outcome Analysis after Matching

# CHAPTER 6

# Propensity Score Adjustment Methods

## M. H. Clark

Researchers use propensity scores to balance nonrandomized groups on background characteristics or covariates through a variety of statistical adjustments. The four most commonly used propensity score methods (or propensity score adjustment methods) are matching, subclassification, weighting, and covariate adjustment (Austin, 2010; Stuart, 2010). These adjustment methods should provide unbiased treatment effects if all of the covariates that contribute to selection bias are included in the propensity score model. Despite their increased popularity, it is not clear under which conditions each adjustment method is most appropriate. This chapter describes and compares the four propensity score adjustment methods in their ability to balance covariates and reduce selection bias in treatment effects for both continuous and categorical outcome variables.

## PROPENSITY SCORE ADJUSTMENT METHODS

### Matching

Matching pairs or groups similar units (e.g., subjects) from experimental and control groups based on the proximity of their propensity scores. Propensity scores from each group can be matched using a variety of algorithms, including exact, optimal, greedy, Mahalanobis matching, and groupings, which include paired (one-to-one) or ratio (one-to-many) matching (Bai, 2013; Caliendo & Kopeinig, 2008; Stuart, 2010). Adjustments can be made using a paired samples $t$-test, if matching a treatment unit to a single control unit (Austin, 2008); a generalized estimating equation (GEE), in which the matches are random effects (Austin & Mamdani, 2006; Clark & Cundiff, 2011); or a McNemar's test, if the dependent variable is dichotomous (Falconer, Clark, & Parris, 2011), among others (Hill, 2008). However, some matching strategies result in dropping units when restricting the distance of matches between propensity scores (caliper matching) or limiting the number of matches for each unit. Although caliper matching forces more comparable groups, if the propensity score distributions between the treatment and control groups do not overlap well, many of the units from the sample will be dropped because they do not have suitable matches.

## Subclassification

Subclassification, which is also referred to as stratification or blocking, divides the samples into strata based on propensity scores so that each stratum includes participants from the treatment and control groups. Although strata can be defined using a variety of criteria (Luellen, Shadish, & Clark, 2005), Cochran (1968) proposed that five strata of equal sample sizes could account for 90% of the bias from the observed covariates. Like matching there are several ways to compute adjusted effects using subclassification. The simplest method may be to use a treatment-by-strata factorial analysis of variance (ANOVA) to account for the stratified propensity scores. However, many researchers compute a between-subjects analysis for each stratum and average effect sizes across strata (Austin & Mamdani, 2006; Shadish, Clark, & Steiner, 2008). If the dependent variable is dichotomous, some of these analyses, such as ANOVAs or $t$-tests, are not appropriate and Chi-square or multiway frequency analyses should be employed instead.

While similar to matching, subclassification may allow for more common support between the treatment and control groups, which would result in fewer dropped units. Unfortunately, because units are grouped by propensity scores, converting the continuous propensity scores to a categorical matching variable will likely reduce the precision of the matched units. Furthermore, if there is little overlap between the propensity score distributions of the treatment and control groups, the strata across the groups will have unequal sample sizes, which may result in reduced statistical power.

## Weighting

Although there are several propensity score weighting estimators (Kang & Schafer, 2007; McCaffrey, Ridgeway, & Morral, 2004; Schafer & Kang, 2008), in general, weighting multiplies observations by a derivative of the propensity score to balance the treatment and control groups. The most common propensity score weighting procedures use the inverse probability of treatment weighted (IPTW) estimator to find either (1) the average treatment effect (ATE) by weighting all of the participants or (2) the average treatment effect for the treated (ATT) by weighting only those who were treated (Kurth et al., 2006; Stone & Tang, 2013). To find the ATE, the IPTW estimator weights observations for the treated group by the inverse of the propensity score and weights the untreated observations by the inverse of one minus the propensity score. To find the ATT, observations from the treatment group are weighted by one, and observations in the control group are weighted by the propensity score and the inverse of one minus the propensity score (e.g., Stone & Tang, 2013).

Although some studies have found that propensity score weighting can be effective in reducing bias (Austin, 2010; Harder, Stuart, & Anthony, 2010; Stone & Tang, 2013), Rubin (2001) suggests that it may not be an appropriate procedure when many propensity scores are very close to one or zero. Likewise, others have demonstrated that propensity scores must accurately model selection bias for propensity score weighting to be effective (Freedman & Berk, 2008; Kang & Schafer, 2007). Otherwise, weighting may actually increase selection bias.

## Covariate Adjustment

Covariate adjustment uses propensity scores as a covariate in an analysis of variance (ANCOVA) or a multiple regression rather than (or in addition to) including covariates as individual predictors (Rosenbaum & Rubin, 1983; Shah, Laupacis, Hux, & Austin, 2005). Therefore, covariate adjustment removes bias by accounting for the correlation between the propensity scores and the outcome variable. Like weighting, some studies have found that covariate adjustment is an effective method for removing bias (Austin & Mamdani, 2006; Kang & Schafer, 2007). However, others do not recommend this method when variances among covariates are heterogeneous (D'Agostino, 1998; Rubin, 2001) or when covariates or propensity scores are not linearly related to the outcome (Rosenbaum, 2001). Others have found that covariate adjustments may not sufficiently reduce bias even when variances are homogeneous and nonlinear terms have been included in adjustment models (Shadish et al., 2008).

## PREVIOUS STUDIES COMPARING PROPENSITY SCORE ADJUSTMENT METHODS

Within the past 30 years, propensity score use has increased exponentially (Bai, 2011). In many studies, propensity scores reduce bias and balance covariates as well as or better than traditional covariate adjustments (Shah et al., 2005; Stürmer et al., 2006). Propensity score matching is often the adjustment method of choice in behavioral science, and covariate adjustment on propensity scores is frequently used in medical research. However, there are conditions in which other adjustment methods are at least as or more effective in reducing bias (Austin, 2010; Harder, Stuart, & Anthony, 2010; Schafer & Kang, 2008; Shadish et al., 2008).

Austin and Mamdani (2006) compared the four propensity score adjustment methods described above to traditional covariate adjustments (i.e., ANCOVA or multiple regression with controlling for covariates) with respect to their ability to reduce bias in treatment effects for statins on the risk of mortality. Matching ($OR$ = .85) and covariate adjustment using propensity scores ($OR$ = .81–.84) resulted in treatment effects most similar to those found from randomized clinical trials ($OR$ = .84), whereas subclassification ($OR$ = .77), weighting ($OR$ = .77), and traditional covariate adjustment ($OR$ = .75) tended to overestimate treatment effects. Although matching and subclassification were both effective in balancing the individual covariates, matching was better. Unfortunately, the matching procedure dropped 22.47% of the treated units and 60.96% of the control units, which may have limited the external validity of the results from the matched sample.

Kurth et al. (2006) compared traditional covariate adjustment to propensity score matching, covariate adjustment, and two types of weighting (ATE and ATT) on mortality risk of stroke victims when treated with a tissue plasminogen activator. They found that all adjustment methods except the ATE weighting decreased the estimated treatment effects. However, they were only able to find effects similar to those obtained from randomized clinical trials when adjustments were made using propensity score matching or ATT weighting. Just as the particular type of weighting procedure can make a difference, the type of matching procedure may also vary. When estimating marginal odds ratios, Austin (2007) found that under most conditions, matching using a GEE model or a 2 × 2 contingency table was more effective than matching using a conditional logistic regression, subclassification, or covariate adjustment using propensity scores. However, when the true odds ratio was one, covariate adjustment and the conditional logistic regression matching procedures were just as effective in reducing bias as the other two matching procedures.

Several studies found that combining adjustment procedures reduced bias better than a single method (Kang & Schafer, 2007; Schafer & Kang, 2008; Shadish et al., 2008). Researchers often do not know either the true selection model (all the reasons why people select a particular treatment condition) or all of the cofactors that contribute to a treatment effect. Therefore, Kang and Schafer (2007) examined doubly robust models in which propensity scores and traditional covariate adjustments were used concurrently to reduce bias due to measurement attrition. They found that as long as either the propensity score model or the traditional covariate adjustment model was correctly specified, they could obtain an unbiased treatment effect. However, when both models were misspecified or only one misspecified model was used, treatment effects remained biased. When the models were correctly specified and statistical adjustments were made with only the propensity scores, weighting provided better estimates than subclassification. Using doubly robust models, in which at least one model was correctly specified, weighting and regression procedures performed better than subclassification. Although there was little difference in adjustments made with weighting and regressions when the sample size was small and both covariate and propensity score models were correct, the regression model using residual bias correction was superior when sample sizes were large and propensity scores were correctly modeled.

Shadish et al. (2008) compared traditional covariate adjustments; propensity score subclassification, weighting, and covariate adjustments; and models that combined propensity score adjustments with individual covariates on treatment effects from two interventions. For the mathematics training intervention, subclassification was more effective in reducing bias than weighting or covariate adjustment using propensity scores. However, the traditional covariate adjustment reduced more bias than any of the propensity score adjustments alone. The most bias (96%) was removed when individual covariates and stratified propensity scores were included in an adjustment model. For the vocabulary intervention, weighting reduced the most bias, followed by traditional covariate adjustment. However, including individual covariates as an adjunct to propensity score adjustments did not always reduce more bias than the propensity score adjustments alone in the vocabulary samples. Similarly, Schafer and Kang (2008) found little improvement when using dual-model strategies with propensity score adjustments. In general, they found that subclassification on propensity scores and traditional covariate adjustments were the most effective adjustment methods, while matching and weighting by the inverse of the propensity score reduced the least amount of bias and were less consistent in their estimations over several trials. Using doubly robust models was still effective in reducing bias, but these models did not have much of an advantage over adjustments using propensity scores or covariates alone. However, this may be because the propensity scores were properly modeled to begin with. Although propensity scores model different relationships with covariates than traditional covariate adjustment, this helps to explain why some researchers have found little differences between traditional covariate adjustments and propensity score adjustments.

Other studies have found that covariate selection can moderate the relationship between adjustment method and bias reduction. Austin, Grootendorst, and Anderson (2007) compared four different propensity scores models using propensity score matching and subclassification. The first model (PS1) computed propensity scores from all available covariates that were related to treatment assignment, and PS2 computed propensity scores from covariates that were related to the outcome. Models 3 and 4 computed propensity scores from covariates that were related to both treatment assignment and outcome (PS3) or all available covariates (PS4), respectively. In general, matching provided better covariate balance than subclassification, and it substantially reduced selection bias regardless of the model used to compute the propensity scores. However, the propensity score model moderated the effectiveness of propensity score subclassification. Subclassification on propensity scores was more effective in balancing covariates when using models computed from only those covariates that correlated with the outcome (PS3 or PS2) than when using models that included covariates other than those relating to outcome (PS1 or PS4).

Steiner, Cook, Shadish, and Clark (2010) examined 19 different propensity scores models using four adjustment methods: traditional covariate adjustment, propensity score matching, subclassification, and covariate adjustment. In general, models with more covariates were better able to reduce bias. Although it wasn't necessary to include all available covariates in the propensity score models, the best models were those that included covariates that measured how well participants liked the topic of the intervention (mathematics training) and a proxy-pretest of the outcome measure (math skills). When these covariates were included, all adjustment methods were able to reduce at least 90% of the bias. However, both traditional covariate adjustment and covariate adjustments using propensity scores sometimes overcorrected bias when these covariates were included.

Finally, it is worth considering the statistical procedures used to compute the propensity scores. Luellen et al. (2005) found that logistic regression estimated better propensity scores than classification trees or bagging when subclassifying on propensity scores. Likewise, Stone and Tang (2013) found that propensity score matching was better at reducing bias when propensity scores were computed using logisitic regression rather than boosted modeling or Bayesian logisitic regression. However, boosted modeling estimates propensity scores that are often better suited for weighting (Lee, Lessler, & Stuart, 2010; Stone & Tang, 2013). In a study that compared three propensity score estimation methods (logistic regression, logistic regression using a saturated model, generalized boosted modeling [GBM]) with five propensity score adjustments (one-to-one matching, full matching, subclassification, weighting by the odds, IPTW), Harder et al. (2010) found that how propensity scores were computed moderated how well statistical adjustments reduced selection bias. In general, one-to-one matching and IPTW produced the lowest median estimates of bias; however, these estimates were not consistent across all measured covariates. While the median differences between the propensity score estimation methods varied by very little for these two propensity score adjustment methods, logistic regression and GBM were a little more consistent in balancing covariates. However, only two specific conditions sufficiently balanced all of the covariates: (1) weighting by the odds when propensity scores were estimated using GBM and (2) subclassification using propensity scores computed from a logistic regression that included higher-order covariates.

## A FURTHER COMPARISON OF PROPENSITY SCORE ADJUSTMENT METHODS FOR BOTH CONTINUOUS AND CATEGORICAL OUTCOMES

The literature has shown that many of the results and conclusions about propensity score adjustment methods varied between the studies reviewed above. Because propensity scores are modeled based on the specific data for each study, it is difficult to make generalizations about the conditions under which each method is most effective. By continuing to test each method under various conditions and data sets, we may more clearly predict optimal conditions for each adjustment procedure. The current chapter examines which type of propensity score adjustment method is most effective in (1) reducing bias in both continuous and categorical outcomes and (2) balancing covariates with strong levels of bias. Existing data from a program evaluation of an orientation seminar for first-year college students are used to illustrate how bias could be reduced using caliper matching, ATE weighting, subclassification, and covariate adjustment using propensity scores. While this chapter uses many of the same adjustment methods as described in the literature above, it applies those adjustments to educational outcomes with varying scales of measurement using a sample known to be highly affected by selection bias. However, it is not expected that educational data, in general, will provide different results from those found using psychological (e.g., Harder et al., 2010) or medical data (e.g., Hirano & Imbens, 2001).

## Hypotheses

Based on previous findings, it is expected that all four propensity score adjustment methods will improve covariate balance and change the treatment effects for the two dependent variables. However, the adjustment methods will differ in their ability to reduce selection bias. Given that many studies have consistently found that matching reduces bias better than most of the other adjustment methods (Austin, 2007; Austin & Mamdani, 2006; Kurth et al., 2006), matching on the propensity scores is expected to be one of the better methods for balancing the covariates. Although the results for weighting on the propensity score are not as consistent as those from matching, several studies have shown that weighting is often one of the better methods under certain circumstances (Austin, 2010; Freedman & Berk, 2008; Shadish et al., 2008 ; Stone & Tang, 2013). Although some researchers have found that using ATT weighting may be preferable to ATE weighting, especially when propensity scores are estimated with logistic regression (Kurth et al., 2006; Lee et al., 2010; Stone & Tang, 2013), the particular weighting procedure used for this comparison study normalizes the weights, which may provide better adjustments than many weighting procedures (Hirano & Imbens, 2001). Therefore, it is expected that weighting will balance covariates better than propensity score subclassification or covariate adjustment. Although previous propensity score researchers have examined adjustment methods on both continuous and dichotomous outcomes, it is not clear that there will be any differences in the results from students' academic performance and second-year retention due to their scales of measurement.

## Methods

### Data Source

The original data consisted of a sample of 435 first-year undergraduate college students who were recruited to take part in a study to examine how first-year seminar courses and cognitive and noncognitive factors related to academic performance and retention. Data were collected on demographic characteristics, Big Five personality traits, academic motivation, loneliness, depression, locus of control, institutional commitment, participation in first-year seminars and learning communities, first-year grade point average (GPA), and second-year retention. Clark and Cundiff (2011) provide a more detailed description of these participants and the instruments used to collect the data. The institutional review board at the university where the original human subjects' data were collected reviewed and approved the data collection procedures.

The independent variable used in this comparison study was whether or not students voluntarily elected to enroll in a first-year seminar course, and the dependent variables were first-year GPA and second-year retention. GPA was the cumulative grade point average for each student's first two semesters in college, measured on an interval scale that ranged from 0 to 4. Second-year retention was measured by whether or not students enrolled for courses in the fall semester following their first year of college. Only participants who had complete data on all the variables used as covariates in this study were retained. Therefore, data from only 379 participants were used for this study, of which, 92 students were in the treatment group and 287 were in the control group.

### Computing Propensity Scores and Estimating Selection Bias

Of the 25 available covariates, 10 were selected for the propensity score model based on their relationships to program participation and either first-year GPA or second-year retention. Covariates were considered to be related to the outcomes or program participation if these relationships were statistically significant at $p < .25$. Covariate imbalance was also measured for each covariate using a standardized measure of bias ($SB$; see Equation 6.1), similar to that used by Austin (2008) and Rosenbaum and Rubin (1985):

$$SB = (M_T - M_C)100 / \sqrt{\left[s_T^2(n_T - 1) + s_C^2(n_C - 1)\right] / (n_T + n_C - 2)} \qquad (6.1)$$

where $M_T$ is the mean of the treatment group, $M_C$ is the mean of the control group, $s_T^2$ is the variance of the treatment group, $s_C^2$ is the variance of the control group, and $n_T$ and $n_C$ are the sample sizes of the treatment and control groups, respectively. Odds ratios that were computed for the categorical covariates, such as Caucasian and African American, were converted to standardized estimates of bias using a formula similar to Hasselblad and Hedges's (1995):

$$SB = \left[100\ln(OR)\sqrt{3}\right]/\pi \qquad (6.2)$$

Table 6.1 includes the covariates that met the inclusion criterion, statistics supporting the relationships between the covariates and the outcome variables, means and standard deviations for each treatment condition, and an estimate of the selection bias. In this study, a covariate was considered biased if its *SB* exceeded 5 (Bai, 2013; Harder et al., 2010).

A logistic regression was used to estimate the predicted probabilities that participants would select into the first-year seminar from the covariates that were related to either GPA or second-year retention. To improve linear modeling, the resulting probabilities from the regression were rescaled using a logit transformation (logit($e_i$) = log[$e_i/(1 - e_i)$]; Rubin, 2001, p. 172), and all statistical adjustments were made using these linear propensity scores.

## Statistical Adjustments with Propensity Scores

*Matching.* A caliper matching procedure was used to match each student in the treatment group to three students in the control group. Using a greedy matching algorithm, the closest matches were selected first, and progressively farther matches were selected for the remaining treated units (Guo & Fraser, 2010). Each treated unit could be matched to as many as three control units as long as each match was within a specified distance (Stuart, 2010). The distance between matches was no more than $0.4s_p$ to reduce 95% of the bias when the variances between the treatment groups of the propensity score were homogeneous (Cochran & Rubin, 1973). Once units were matched, a mixed-effects linear regression in SPSS v.20 was used to assess the difference between groups on GPA and covariates measured on a continuous scale. A mixed-effects logistic regression in SAS 9.2 was used to assess the difference between groups on second-year retention and covariates measured on a dichotomous scale.

TABLE 6.1. Measures of Selection Bias and Covariate Imbalance

|  |  |  |  | Treatment | | Comparison | | |
| --- | --- | --- | --- | --- | --- | --- | --- | --- |
| Variable | Univ101[a] | GPA[b] | Retention[a] | M | SD | M | SD | SB |
| High school GPA | -.349*** | .499*** | .133*** | 2.935 | 0.573 | 3.503 | 0.681 | -86.512 |
| ACT | -.377*** | .298*** | .053 | 19.815 | 2.828 | 23.176 | 3.75 | -94.691 |
| Extraversion | .106** | -.041 | .034 | 2.604 | 0.78 | 2.424 | 0.711 | 24.717 |
| Agreeableness | .092* | .198*** | .076* | 3.003 | 0.509 | 2.891 | 0.527 | 21.427 |
| Neuroticism | -.059* | .012 | -.092* | 1.821 | 0.699 | 1.922 | 0.751 | -13.671 |
| IM to accomplish | .081* | .139*** | .086* | 3.378 | 1.28 | 3.126 | 1.346 | 18.942 |
| IM to experience | .093* | .043 | .097* | 2.405 | 1.238 | 2.123 | 1.304 | 21.888 |
| Loneliness | -.104** | -.019 | -.117** | 0.897 | 0.551 | 1.033 | 0.561 | -24.346 |
| Caucasian | -.090* | .212*** | -.022 | 0.652 | 0.479 | 0.746 | 0.436 | -24.644 |
| African American | .134*** | -.226*** | .051 | 0.283 | 0.453 | 0.16 | 0.367 | 39.971 |

[a]Point Biserial correlations are reported for all covariates except Caucasian and African American; Phi coefficients are reported for these covariates.
[b]Pearson correlations are reported for all covariates except Caucasian and African American; Point Biserial correlations are reported for these covariates.
*$p < .25$; **$p < .05$; ***$p < .01$.

Subclassification. Propensity scores were divided into five strata, in which each stratum contained 20% of the units. The strata and interaction between strata and treatment conditions were included in the statistical models to partial out the variance for the propensity score strata. A two-factor ANOVA was used to compute the adjusted treatment effect for GPA and continuous covariates, and a logistic regression was used to compute the adjusted effect for retention and dichotomous covariates.

Weighting. Despite the mixed results on the effectiveness of ATE weighting, an IPTW estimator (Austin, 2010; Harder et al., 2010; Kurth et al., 2006) was used. This particular estimator normalizes the weights "so that they add up to one in each treatment group" (Hirano & Imbens, 2001, p. 264), which may provide better adjustments than those that divide the sum of the weighted observations by the group sample size. Equation 6.3 was used to obtain the weighted mean difference between the treatment and control groups, which was used as the numerator in an independent measures $t$-test for each of the dependent variables and covariates.

$$\hat{\tau} = \frac{\sum_{i=1}^{N} r_i z_i / e(\mathbf{x}_i)}{\sum_{i=1}^{N} z_i / e(\mathbf{x}_i)} - \frac{\sum_{i=1}^{N} r_i (1 - z_i) / (1 - e(\mathbf{x}_i))}{\sum_{i=1}^{N} (1 - z_i) / (1 - e(\mathbf{x}_i))} \quad (6.3)$$

where $r_i$ is the dependent variable, $z_i$ is the treatment condition, and $e(\mathbf{x}_i)$ is the propensity score.

Covariate Adjustment. Propensity scores were used as a single covariate in either (1) a between-subjects ANCOVA to compare the difference between the treatment and control groups on GPA and each continuous covariate, or (2) in a logistic regression to assess the adjusted difference in retention and for each dichotomous covariate.

## Results

### Propensity Scores and Covariate Balance

The propensity scores themselves were tested for balance across treatment conditions using an independent samples Kolmogorov–Smirnov test (Gilbert, Grobman, & Landon, 2012). Perhaps because the covariates included in the propensity score equation were strong predictors of selection, the propensity score distributions were not equal between the treatment and control groups, $Z = 4.743$, $p < .001$. Figure 6.1 illustrates the distributions

## Propensity Score Adjustment Methods

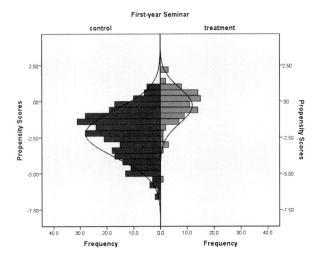

**FIGURE 6.1.** Propensity score distributions for control and treatment groups.

for each group. Although the lack of propensity score balance will not result in optimal statistical adjustments, the resulting propensity scores can still be effective in reducing selection bias from the treatment effects and improve individual covariate imbalance.

The standardized bias estimates were computed on the individual covariates for each statistical adjustment method to evaluate how the adjustments improved covariate balance. Using the statistical procedures described in the Methods section, each covariate was tested for differences between the treatment and control groups before and after each statistical adjustment. Although not tested for statistically significant differences, the SB estimates in Table 6.2 indicate that all of the covariates were less biased after the propensity score adjustments. While these estimates suggest that weighting reduced the most bias, the point estimates and standard errors in Table 6.3 suggest that the variability of the weighted observations may be responsible for the smaller SBs. While covariate adjustment using propensity scores had smaller standard errors than the other methods and still had very small SBs, it was also the most likely adjustment method to overcorrect the biases. Subclassification on propensity scores appeared to be the least effective method in balancing the covariates. Although the standard errors for the stratified estimates were slightly smaller than those for matching, the adjusted sample size for the matched groups was much smaller, thereby inflating the standard errors.

**TABLE 6.2. Standardized Bias Estimates for Covariates after Each Statistical Adjustment**

| Covariate | No adjustments | Matched | Subclassification | Weighted | Covariate adjusted[a] |
|---|---|---|---|---|---|
| High school GPA | −86.512 | 7.115 | 32.236 | 0.000 | 6.882 |
| ACT | −94.691 | **0.000** | 0.619 | 0.000 | −2.963 |
| Extraversion | 24.717 | 5.883 | −5.477 | 0.000 | −2.700 |
| Agreeableness | 21.427 | 8.881 | 0.950 | 0.000 | −2.921 |
| Neuroticism | −13.671 | −5.147 | −11.619 | −0.000 | −8.255 |
| IM to accomplish | 18.942 | −8.900 | 12.950 | 0.001 | −4.978 |
| IM to experience | 21.888 | **0.234** | 10.747 | −0.001 | −2.249 |
| Loneliness | −24.346 | −6.223 | −12.479 | 0.001 | −10.246 |
| Caucasian | −24.644 | 9.461 | 19.848 | 0.012 | **0.165** |
| African American | 39.971 | −8.876 | −20.123 | −0.001 | −6.726 |

*Note.* Standardized bias estimates in **bold** are those that meet the requirements for covariate balance ($SB < 5$).
[a]Covariate adjusted used either an ANCOVA to account for propensity scores for continuous covariates or a logistic regression to account for propensity scores for dichotomous covariates.

**TABLE 6.3. Mean Differences, Regression Estimates, and Standard Errors for Covariates after Each Statistical Adjustment**

| Covariate | No adjustments | | Matched | | Subclassified | | Weighted | | Covariate adjusted | |
|---|---|---|---|---|---|---|---|---|---|---|
| | MΔ/B | SE | MΔ/B | SE | MΔ/B | SE | MΔ | SE | MΔ/B | SE |
| High school GPA | −0.568 | 0.079 | 0.056 | 0.136 | 0.234 | 0.087 | −0.205 | 13.625 | 0.041 | 0.071 |
| ACT | −3.361 | 0.425 | 0 | 0.454 | 0.020 | 0.387 | 3.304 | 103.524 | −0.074 | 0.299 |
| Extraversion | 0.180 | 0.087 | 0.059 | 0.173 | −0.056 | 0.123 | 0.397 | 17.314 | −0.023 | 0.102 |
| Agreeableness | 0.112 | 0.063 | 0.067 | 0.130 | 0.007 | 0.088 | 0.371 | 15.550 | −0.018 | 0.074 |
| Neuroticism | −0.101 | 0.089 | −0.056 | 0.188 | −0.122 | 0.126 | −0.616 | 5.310 | −0.072 | 0.104 |
| Internal motivation to accomplish | 0.252 | 0.159 | −0.17 | 0.330 | 0.245 | 0.227 | 1.199 | 22.684 | −0.078 | 0.188 |
| Internal motivation to experience | 0.282 | 0.154 | 0.004 | 0.295 | 0.196 | 0.219 | −3.012 | 7.461 | −0.034 | 0.181 |
| Loneliness | −0.136 | 0.067 | −0.046 | 0.128 | −0.097 | 0.093 | 0.282 | 3.455 | −0.067 | 0.078 |
| Caucasian | −.447 | 0.257 | 0.172 | 0.379 | 0.360 | 0.481 | 0.450 | 3.754 | 0.003 | 0.313 |
| African American | 0.725 | 0.282 | −0.161 | 0.428 | −0.365 | 0.498 | −0.445 | 1.843 | −0.122 | 0.338 |

*Note.* MΔ is the mean difference between the treated and untreated estimates, B is the logistic regression estimate, and SE is the standard error of the mean differences or regression estimates. MΔ is reported for the continuous covariates, and B is the effect estimate for Caucasian and African American except when weighting by the inverse of the propensity score.

## Changes in Outcomes

First-Year GPA. Without adjusting for selection bias, those who participated in the first-year seminar had significantly lower first-year GPAs than those who did not, $t(377) = -2.995$, $p = .003$. After a three-to-one greedy caliper matching procedure, a mixed model ANOVA indicated that there was no difference in GPA averages between those who had taken the first-year seminar course and those who had not, $F(1,147.254) = 0.056$, $p = .814$. Although only 45 (49%) of the treatment units were matched to 132 control units (202 units were dropped because they did not have suitable matches), similar results were found using other statistical adjustment methods. Neither subclassification, $F(1, 369) = 0.292$, $p = .589$; weighting, $t(1490) = 0.354$, $p = .724$; nor accounting for propensity scores in an ANCOVA, $F(1, 375) = 0.212$, $p = .646$; indicated that the program had an effect on first-year GPA. Like the results from the covariate balancing, weighting had the largest mean differences and standard errors (shown in Table 6.4) and covariate adjustment had the smallest. However, all standardized mean differences were close to zero ($d = 0.019 - 0.065$).

Second-Year Retention. Without any propensity score adjustments, there was no significant difference in the proportion of students who returned to the university for a second year when comparing those who participated

TABLE 6.4. Mean Differences, Regression Estimates, Standard Errors, and Effect Sizes for Treatment Effects after Each Statistical Adjustment

| Statistical adjustment | First-year GPA | | | Second-year retention | | |
|---|---|---|---|---|---|---|
| | MΔ | SE | d | B/MΔ | SE | d |
| No adjustments | −0.304 | 0.102 | −0.359 | 0.315 | 0.302 | 0.174 |
| Matched | 0.036 | 0.161 | 0.040 | 1.039 | 0.478 | 0.573 |
| Subclassified | 0.104 | 0.192 | 0.065 | −0.260 | 0.607 | −0.143 |
| Weighted | 1.295 | 3.662 | 0.019 | 0.023 | 1.178 | 0.001 |
| Covariate adjusted | 0.009 | 0.015 | 0.071 | 0.601 | 0.353 | 0.331 |

Note. MΔ is the mean difference between the treated and untreated estimates; negative values indicate that the untreated group had higher scores than those who received the intervention. SE is the standard error of the mean differences between the treated and control estimates, d is the standardized mean difference between the treated and untreated estimates, and B is the logistic regression estimate. B is used as the effect estimate for all adjustment methods when computing second-year retention except weighting, which uses MΔ. Although this study focuses on effect sizes rather than hypothesis tests, t-tests can be estimated by $t = MΔ/SE$ and Wald $\chi^2 = (B/SE)^2$.

in the first-year seminar and those who didn't, Wald $\chi^2(1)$ = 1.088, $p$ = .298, $OR$ = 1.370. However, after matching on propensity scores, those who had taken the first-year experience course were 2.826 times as likely as the control group to return for a second year, $t(131)$ = 2.170, $p$ = .031. This effect was not as strong using the other propensity score adjustments. There were still no significant differences in the retention rate between treatment and control groups after subclassification, Wald $\chi^2(1)$ = 0.184, $p$ = .668, $OR$ = 0.771; weighting, $t(1490)$ = 0.020, $p$ = .984, $OR$ = 1.002; or accounting for propensity scores in a logistic regression, Wald $\chi^2(1)$ = 2.900, $p$ = .088, $OR$ = 1.823. Despite the lack of statistical significance for most of these effects, the standardized mean differences (shown in Table 6.4) varied considerably, depending on the propensity score adjustment methods used. While matching and covariate adjustment on propensity scores estimated moderate effect sizes that favored the intervention, subclassification indicated that those in the treatment group would be less likely to return to college the following year. As usual, weighting estimated a standardized mean difference of nearly zero; but in this case, it may not have been strictly due to its high standard error, as the mean difference between the treatment and control groups was also close to zero.

## Discussion

### Outcome Effects

Before adjusting for selection bias, those who participated in the first-year seminar had lower GPAs than those who did not participate, making it appear that the seminar hurt (rather than helped) students' academic performance. After propensity score adjustments, there were no differences in GPA between those who participated in the seminar and those who didn't regardless of the adjustment method used. Not only were there no *significant effects* for the seminar on GPA, but all of the effect sizes were very close to zero. Unlike the consistency found with GPA, the change in retention rates varied depending on the type of propensity score adjustment method that was used. Without any adjustments, there was a small (but not statistically significant) effect for the seminar on second-year retention. While the effect sizes and the regression estimates increased after propensity score matching and covariate adjustment, the treatment effects decreased after weighting and subclassification. Although we do not know the unbiased effect size for *this* sample, Strumpf and Hunt (1993) found a large effect on second-year retention ($OR$ = 2.264, $d$ = 0.450) for a college orientation seminar when they randomly assigned students to conditions.

Assuming that the results of their study can be generalized to the population used here, then matching and covariate adjustment using propensity scores provided the best estimates for retention.

## Covariate Balance

Based on the measures of standardized bias for each covariate prior to making the propensity score adjustments, it was clear that these observed characteristics were not balanced across treatment groups. The average standardized bias[1] was 37.08% for these covariates; and all of them exceeded the acceptable 5% of selection bias. Although all of the adjustment methods improved the balance on each of the covariates, only weighting on propensity scores appeared to have sufficiently balanced all of the covariates so that no covariate had more than 5% bias remaining. However, it is very likely that this small amount of bias may be due to the relatively large standard errors associated with propensity score weighting. Covariate adjustment using propensity scores balanced six of the ten covariates, and the remaining four covariates had less than 10% bias remaining. Although only two covariates were sufficiently balanced after matching on the propensity score, the remaining eight covariates had less than 10% bias remaining, and the average standardized bias was 5.67% for all covariates. Subclassification on the propensity score was the least effective in balancing the covariates. Like matching, it only sufficiently balanced two covariates, but only one of the remaining eight covariates had less than 10% bias remaining. Most still had between 10 and 20% bias, and the average remaining bias was 12.70%.

## Other Considerations

**Propensity Score Balance.** One of the first concerns with these data is that the propensity scores that were computed from the 10 covariates were not evenly distributed across treatment groups. Before making any statistical adjustments, propensity score distributions with and without the logit transformations were examined. Although the unadjusted propensity scores (those that had not been transformed) had better overlap between the treatment and control groups than the logit transformed propensity scores, the unadjusted propensity scores were skewed. The propensity scores were not well balanced in either scale, but using the propensity scores as unadjusted predicted probabilities may have produced different results for matching and weighting.

Furthermore, because the propensity scores were not balanced, the conditions under which propensity score adjustment were made were not ideal. Some researchers purport that to balance covariates with propensity score adjustments, the propensity scores themselves should be balanced (Austin & Mamdani, 2006; Rubin, 2001). However, other studies have found that propensity score adjustments can still effectively reduce bias even when the propensity scores are not balanced between groups (Clark & Hoffman, 2014). Although Clark and Hoffman found that matching and covariate adjustment were least effected by propensity score imbalance, Rubin warns that covariate adjustment is likely to result in unreliable treatment effects if the propensity scores are not balanced. Caliendo and Kopeinig (2008) suggest that propensity score imbalance in matching may not affect the internal validity of the adjusted results, but the lack of common support reduces the external validity. However, the internal validity of propensity score imbalance may be affected for other adjustment methods. While it is not clear how this influenced the weighting procedure, propensity score imbalance was a particular concern in this comparison study for subclassification. There were very few participants in the first three strata for the treatment group, which meant that only a few (between one and nine) treatment units were estimating the effects for the three of the five strata.

**Estimate of Treatment Effects.** Although the primary benchmark for determining bias reduction in this comparison study was by how well propensity score adjustments balanced the observed covariates, the ultimate goal in using these adjustments is to estimate an unbiased treatment effect. While using real-world data provides realistic effects and covariates, the design used to collect the data for this comparison study did not include a sample that would allow an estimation of the unbiased treatment effects. Typically, researchers know the true effects in biased studies by using computer simulations to generate their data (Austin et al., 2007; Kang & Schafer, 2007; Lee et al., 2010). Other researchers have used doubly randomized preference trials in which participants are randomly assigned to either a randomized or comparable quasi-experiment so that they can obtain both biased and unbiased treatment effects (Clark & Hoffman, 2014; Luellen et al., 2005; Pohl, Steiner, Eisermann, Soellner, & Cook, 2009). Without these estimates, the adjusted outcomes were compared to those from a separate randomized study that used a similar intervention (Strumpf & Hunt, 1993). Although the randomized study did provide an unbiased estimate for second-year retention, it did not include one for first-year GPA. Furthermore, it is not clear that the samples were comparable, since Strumpf and Hunt restricted their sample to students who were in good academic standing and this study did not. Therefore, it is very likely that the true effect from this sample is smaller than the one from their sample.

**Covariate Selection.** One of the primary assumptions when computing propensity scores is that all non-ignorable covariates are included in the propensity score model. Although all of the available linear covariates related to selection and at least one of the outcomes were included, there may be several unobserved variables that contributed to the selection bias that were not included. Not only was this study limited to the 25 covariates that were available, but nonlinear or interactive terms in the propensity score models were not included. While this more restricted modeling is not unusual (Thoemmes & Kim, 2011), some researchers have found that including higher-order terms improves propensity score estimates (Harder et al., 2010; Schafer & Kang, 2008). Therefore, it is possible that the variables that were included did not sufficiently account for the selection bias that affected these outcomes.

Another potential problem is that the same propensity scores, which are data specific, were used to adjust effects for two different dependent variables. Although GPA and second-year retention were related, not all of the covariates that predicted GPA also predicted retention. It had been assumed that covariates that were not related to one of the outcomes would not affect the propensity score adjustments any more than including these types of covariates in a traditional adjustment approach. However, Austin et al. (2007) found that propensity score subclassification was better at reducing bias when the propensity scores were computed with *only* those covariates that related to the outcomes. Therefore, including covariates in the propensity score model that were not related to both outcomes may also be responsible for the unusual results found when using propensity score subclassification for second-year retention.

**Adjustment Computations.** As discussed in the literature review, there is more than one way to compute each of the adjustment methods used here. Those presented here were the ones expected to provide the best results; however, it is quite possible that a different subclassification method or weighting algorithm would have provided different results. Bai (2013) and Austin (2009) found that some matching methods are better at reducing bias than others; however, both agreed that caliper matching was one of the better methods. There are fewer variations in how covariate adjustments can be computed; however, there are several ways they could be modeled. In this example, there was not a significant quadratic relationship between the propensity scores and GPA, but this could have been included in the model to improve the fit (Shadish et al., 2008). Similarly, using doubly robust adjustments to model both selection and outcome could have provided better estimates (Kang & Schafer, 2007; Schafer & Kang, 2008).

In this study, subclassification and weighting had the most unusual results, particularly when estimating effects for second-year retention. Weighting is one of the more sensitive adjustment methods and could have been influenced by both the particular weighting equation and method of estimating the propensity scores. For GPA, a normalized ATT estimator (McCaffrey et al., 2004) provided a similar treatment effect ($d = 0.022$) to the one obtained from the ATE procedure ($d = 0.019$). Using a more common ATT estimator (e.g., Stone & Tang, 2013) resulted in a negative, but still very small, effect size ($d = -0.024$). Effect sizes from second-year retention were also similar when comparing the ATE estimator ($d = .001$) to the normalized ($d = -0.011$) and more common ATT estimators ($d = 0.005$). However, none of these came close to the randomized effect found by Strumpf and Hunt (1993).

The subclassification procedure used in this study accounted for the interaction between the strata and the treatment condition in a factorial ANOVA, rather than through the more common propensity score subclassification procedure, which computes the between-subjects effects for each stratum and averages the effects across strata. Although the method used here appears to have underestimated the true treatment effect, perhaps due to a lack of common support in the first three strata, the more common approach would have overestimated the treatment effect. Computing treatment effects for each stratum resulted in the following effect sizes for second-year retention: $d = 10.775, 11.062, 0.472, 0.527$, and $-0.143$. Because the effects from the first two strata are very different from the effects of the last three strata, it is unlikely that the true treatment effect would be reflected by the mean effect size, 4.539. However, the effect found for the middle strata is very similar to the randomized effect found by Strumpf and Hunt (1993).

## CONCLUSION AND RESEARCH IMPLICATIONS

At first glance, it appears that weighting may have been the most effective method in reducing bias, since it considerably changed both of the outcome variables and completely balanced all of the observed covariates.

However, it is worth pointing out that weighting obtained the same results regardless of the comparison (i.e., it nullified every variable). Since units with extremely large or small propensity scores result in especially large weights, weighting often inflates standard errors and standard deviations, which may explain the reduced effect sizes and $t$ values. Although normalizing the propensity score distributions is meant to control this, even a few logit propensity scores close to one can impact the variance of the weighted observations. Had units with propensity scores close to one been removed from the sample, the estimates may have been more reasonable. However, Harder et al. (2010) advise against this, as these units are often good predictors of the outcome. In this sample, many of these units were those in the control group who had characteristics very similar to those in the treatment group. Therefore, it may not be prudent to conclude that weighting was the best adjustment method for these data. Subclassification was also an unreliable adjustment method for this particular sample. Not only was it ineffective in balancing the covariates, but it very likely *increased* the bias for second-year retention.

Although the true treatment effects for this sample were unknown, matching and covariate adjustment using propensity scores provided similar estimated effects for both outcomes. While they reduced approximately the same average amount of bias across all 10 covariates, most of the individual covariates were balanced better after the covariate adjustment procedure than matching. Furthermore, matching on propensity scores dropped 53.3% of the sample, whereas covariate adjustment retained all of the units in the sample. Therefore, covariate adjustment using propensity scores appears to be the most reliable procedure for this particular sample.

It is clear from this comparison study and many others that propensity score adjustments improve covariate balance in quasi-experiments; however, the most effective method depends on the specific data parameters. While it was encouraging to find similar results from each adjustment method when assessing GPA, the results were less consistent for retention. Therefore, the measurement scale of the outcome variable and specific adjustment equations (i.e., ATE vs. ATE weighting) should be considered when selecting a propensity score adjustment method. It is also very likely that other factors that were not specifically tested in this comparison study, such as hidden bias (i.e., including other covariates), propensity score modeling (i.e., including higher-order terms), propensity score scaling (i.e., not using a logit transformation), sample size or group sample size ratio, contributed to these estimates as well.

As with many other studies, matching was a consistently good estimator for both continuous and dichotomous outcomes; but it may not provide generalizable results when a large percent of units is dropped (Austin, 2007; Austin & Mamdani, 2006; Austin et al., 2007). While propensity score covariate adjustment may not always provide valid results (Rosenbaum, 2001; Rubin, 2001), it can be a good estimator—even when the propensity scores are not well balanced. While weighting or subclassification with these specific data are not recommended, many researchers consider these to be very good adjustments under different circumstances (Lee et al., 2010; Shadish et al., 2008; Schafer & Kang, 2008; Stone & Tang, 2013). Had propensity scores been estimated using generalized boosted modeling rather than logistic regression, much more favorable outcomes for weighting or subclassification may have been found.

## ACKNOWLEDGMENTS

The data used in this chapter were previously reported in Clark and Cundiff (2011). I would like to thank Matthew Herman, Vinetha Belur, Steven Middleton, Deborah Racey, Alen Avdic, and Blake Hutsell for their assistance in collecting the data.

## NOTE

1. This average was obtained by taking the average of the absolute value of the *SB* estimates (Bai, 2013).

## REFERENCES

Austin, P. C. (2007). The performance of different propensity score methods for estimating marginal odds ratios. *Statistics in Medicine, 26,* 3078–3094.

Austin, P. C. (2008). A critical appraisal of propensity-score matching in the medical literature between 1996 and 2003. *Statistics in Medicine, 27,* 2037–2049.

Austin, P. C. (2009). Some methods of propensity score matching had superior performance to others: Results of an empirical investigation and Monte Carlo simulation. *Biometrical Journal, 51,* 171–184.

Austin, P. C. (2010). The performance of different propensity score methods for estimating differences in proportions (risk differences or absolute risk reductions) in observational studies. *Statistics in Medicine, 29,* 2137–2148.

Austin, P. C., Grootendorst, P., & Anderson, G. M. (2007). A comparison of the ability of different propensity score models to balance measured variables between treated and untreated subjects: A Monte Carlo study. *Statistics in Medicine, 26,* 734–753.

Austin, P. C., & Mamdani, M. M. (2006). A comparison of propensity score methods: A case study estimating the effectiveness of post-AMI statin use. *Statistics in Medicine, 25,* 2084–2106.

Bai, H. (2011). Using propensity score analysis for making causal claims in research articles. *Educational Psychology Review, 23,* 273–278.

Bai, H. (2013). A bootstrap procedure of propensity score estimation. *Journal of Experimental Education, 81,* 157–177.

Caliendo, M., & Kopeinig, S. (2008). Some practical guidance for the implementation of propensity score matching. *Journal of Economic Surveys, 22*(1), 31–72.

Clark, M. H., & Cundiff, N. L. (2011). Assessing the effectiveness of a college freshman seminar using propensity score adjustments. *Research in Higher Education, 52,* 616–639.

Clark, M. H., & Hoffman, N. G. (2014). *An examination of the relationship between propensity score balance and bias reduction in quasi-experiments.* Manuscript submitted for publication.

Cochran, W. G. (1968). The effectiveness of adjustment by subclassification in removing bias in observational studies. *Biometrics, 24,* 295–313. Retrieved from www.jstor.org/stable/2528036.

Cochran, W. G., & Rubin, D. B. (1973). Controlling bias in observational studies: A review. *Sankhya, Series A, 35,* 417–446.

D'Agostino, R. B. (1998). Tutorial in biostatistics: Propensity score methods for bias reduction in the comparison of a treatment to a non-randomized control group. *Statistics in Medicine, 17,* 2265–2281.

Falconer, M. K., Clark, M. H., & Parris, D. (2011). Validity in an evaluation of Healthy Families Florida: A program to prevent child abuse and neglect. *Children and Youth Services Review, 33,* 66–77.

Freedman, D. A., & Berk, R. A. (2008). Weighting regressions by propensity scores. *Evaluation Review, 32,* 392–409.

Gilbert, S. A., Grobman, W. A., & Landon, M. B. (2012). Elective repeat cesarean delivery compared with spontaneous trial of labor after a prior cesarean delivery: A propensity score analysis. *American Journal of Obstetrics and Gynecology, 206,* 311.e1–311.e9.

Guo, S. Y., & Fraser, M. W. (2010). *Propensity score analysis: Statistical methods and applications.* Thousand Oaks, CA: Sage.

Harder, V. S., Stuart, E. A., & Anthony, J. C. (2010). Propensity score techniques and the assessment of measured covariate balance to test causal associations in psychological research. *Psychological Methods, 15,* 234–249.

Hasselblad, V., & Hedges, L. V. (1995). Meta-analysis of screening and diagnostic tests. *Psychological Bulletin, 117,* 167–178.

Hill, J. (2008). Discussion of research using propensity-score matching: Comments on "A critical appraisal of propensity-score matching in the medical literature between 1996 and 2003." *Statistics in Medicine, 27,* 2055–2061.

Hirano, K., & Imbens, G. W. (2001). Estimation of causal effects using propensity score weighting: An application to data on right heart catheterization. *Health Services and Outcomes Research Methodology, 2,* 259–278.

Kang, J. D. Y., & Schafer, J. L. (2007). Demystifying double robustness: A comparison of alternative strategies for estimating a population mean from incomplete data. *Statistical Science, 22,* 523–539.

Kurth, T., Walker, A. M., Glynn, R. J., Chan, K. A., Gaziano, J. M., Berger, K., et al. (2006). Results of multivariable logistic regression, propensity matching, propensity adjustment, and propensity-based weighting under conditions of nonuniform effect. *American Journal of Epidemiology, 163,* 262–270.

Lee, B. K., Lessler, J., & Stuart, E. A. (2010). Improving propensity score weighting using machine learning. *Statistics in Medicine, 29,* 337–346.

Luellen, J. K., Shadish, W. R., & Clark, M. H. (2005). Propensity scores: An introduction and experimental test. *Evaluation Review, 29,* 530–558.

McCaffrey, D. F., Ridgeway, G., & Morral, A. R. (2004). Propensity score estimation with boosted regression for evaluating causal effects in observational studies. *Psychological Methods, 9*(4), 403–425.

Pohl, S., Steiner, P. M., Eisermann, J., Soellner, R., & Cook, T. D. (2009). Unbiased causal inference from an observational study: Results of a within-study comparison. *Educational Evaluation and Policy Analysis, 31,* 463–479.

Rosenbaum, P. R. (2001). Observational studies. In N. J. Smelser & P. B. Baltes (Eds.), *International encyclopedia of social and behavioral sciences* (pp. 10,808–10,815). Oxford, UK: Elsevier Science.

Rosenbaum, P. R., & Rubin, D. B. (1983). The central role of the propensity score in observational studies for causal effects. *Biometrika, 70,* 41–55.

Rosenbaum, P. R., & Rubin, D. B. (1985). Constructing a control group using multivariate matched sampling methods that incorporate the propensity score. *American Statistician, 39,* 33–38.

Rubin, D. B. (2001). Using propensity scores to help design observational studies: Application to the tobacco litigation. *Health Services and Outcomes Research Methodology, 2,* 169–188.

Schafer, J. L., & Kang, J. (2008). Average causal effects from nonrandomized studies: A practical guide and simulated example. *Psychological Methods, 13,* 279–313.

Shadish, W. R., & Clark, M. H. (2002). An introduction to propensity scores. *Metodologia de las Ciencias del Comportamiento Journal, 4*(2), 291–298.

Shadish, W. R., Clark, M. H., & Steiner, P. M. (2008). Can nonrandomized experiments yield accurate answers? A randomized experiment comparing random to nonrandom assignment. *Journal of the American Statistical Association, 103,* 1334–1344.

Shah, B. R., Laupacis, A., Hux, J. E., & Austin, P. C. (2005). Propensity score methods gave similar results to traditional regression modeling in observational studies: A systematic review. *Journal of Clinical Epidemiology, 58,* 550–559.

Steiner, P. M., Cook, T. D., Shadish, W. R., & Clark, M. H. (2010). The differential role of covariate selection and data analytic methods in controlling for selection bias in observational studies: Results of a within-study comparison. *Psychological Methods, 15,* 250–267.

Stone, C. A., & Tang, Y. (2013). Comparing propensity score methods in balancing covariates and recovering impact in small sample educational program evaluations. *Practical Assessment, Research and Evaluation, 18*(13), 1–12. Available at *http://pareonline.net/getvn.asp?v=18&n=13*.

Strumpf, G., & Hunt, P. (1993). The effects of an orientation course on the retention and academic standing of entering freshmen, controlling for volunteer effect. *Journal of the Freshman Year Experience, 5,* 7–14.

Stuart, E. A. (2010). Matching methods for causal inference: A review and a look forward. *Statistical Science: A Review Journal of the Institute of Mathematical Statistics, 25,* 1–21.

Stürmer, T., Joshi, M., Glynn, R. J., Avorn, J., Rothman, K. J., & Schneeweiss, S. (2006). A review of the application of propensity score methods yielded increasing use, advantages in specific settings, but not substantially different estimates compared with conventional multivariable methods. *Journal of Clinical Epidemiology, 59,* 437–447.

Thoemmes, F. J., & Kim, E. S. (2011). A systematic review of propensity score methods in the social sciences. *Multivariate Behavioral Research, 46,* 90–118.

# CHAPTER 7

# Propensity Score Analysis with Matching Weights

**Liang Li**
**Tom H. Greene**
**Brian C. Sauer**

In this chapter, we introduce the method of matching weights (MWs), a propensity score weighting method proposed by Li and Greene (2013), as an analogue to pair matching, a widely used propensity score matching method. They are analogous because they have similar estimands and covariate distributions. Therefore, the MW method is applicable where pair matching is used. The MW combines the positive attributes of both weighting and pair matching methods. Similar to traditional weighting methods, the MW supports straightforward computation of the sampling error of the estimated propensity scores, simple asymptotic analysis, and double robust estimation. Like pair matching, the computation of the MW estimator avoids the numerical instability that plagues some other weighting methods. We also provide theoretical justification and empirical results to show that the MW estimator is more efficient than the pair matching estimator, and has more accurate variance estimation and notably better covariate balance. In addition, we introduce the mirror histogram as a useful graphical tool to visualize the overlap of propensity score distributions for both pair matching and MW methods, and a test of model misspecification to formally diagnose whether adequate covariate balance is achieved in the propensity score model development. This chapter provides a nontechnical expository presentation of the work presented by Li and Greene (2013), as well as practical guidance for the implementation of the MW methodology through the use of three examples representing three contrasting propensity score distribution scenarios.

## NOTATION AND DEFINITION

We first introduce some notation and definitions. Let $\{r_i, z_i, X_i, i = 1, 2, \ldots, n\}$ denote a random sample of $n$ units (e.g., subjects), where $r_i$ is the outcome, $z_i$ is an indicator of the treatment ($z_i = 1$) or control ($z_i = 0$) group, and $X_i$ is a vector of covariates to be adjusted for in the propensity score analysis. The individual causal effect is ($\Delta_i = r_{1i} - r_{0i}$), where $r_{1i}$ and $r_{0i}$ are potential outcomes for unit $i$ under the treatment and control, respectively. Our goal is to estimate the average treatment effect $E(\Delta_i)$, where the expectation is taken over a population of research interest. The methodology in this chapter relies on two typical assumptions for propensity score analysis: the stable unit treatment value assumption and the strong ignorability assumption (i.e., no unmeasured confounding). For more details on these assumptions and the potential outcome framework, please refer to Chapter 1. Under these assumptions, Rosenbaum and Rubin (1983) proved that the treatment and the covariates are conditionally independent given the propensity score, which is defined as $e_i = \Pr(z_i = 1 | X_i)$. The propensity score is a function of the covariates. It is often calculated for each unit from a logistic regression model of $X$ on $z$.

It is important to understand that different propensity score methods may have different estimands. In other words, they estimate different characteristics of the population from which the data are sampled. Commonly used estimands include the population average treatment effect (PATE), $\tau_{PATE} = E(\Delta_i) = \lim_{n \to \infty} n^{-1} \sum_{i=1}^{n} \Delta_i$, and the population average treatment effect for the treated (PATT), $\tau_{PATT} = E(\Delta_i | z_i = 1) = \lim_{n \to \infty} \sum_{i=1}^{n} \Delta_i z_i / \sum_{i=1}^{n} z_i$. The former estimand pertains to the mean difference in the outcome between the two hypothetical scenarios where all units in the study population are assigned to the treatment or the control; the latter is the mean difference defined on the subpopulation of treated units.

## PAIR MATCHING

The MW method was proposed by Li and Greene (2013) as a weighting analogue to pair matching, a propensity score matching method that currently is widely used in medicine and other research areas. A recent survey shows that 83% of the surveyed medical publications that used propensity score matching methods chose pair matching (Austin, 2008, 2009b). For a discussion of the propensity score matching methods in general, please refer to Chapters 4 and 5 in this book. Pair matching is more specifically defined as one-to-one matching on the propensity score without replacement. In pair matching, treatment and control units with similar propensity scores, according to certain criteria, are selected to form a matched pair (one-to-one matching); once a unit is selected into a pair, that unit can no longer be selected into other pairs (without replacement); the selection process goes on until no more matched pairs can be identified within the criteria. Quite often a small positive constant, called the caliper, is used as part of the criteria. A treated unit and a control can be matched only when the difference in their propensity scores is smaller than the caliper. Sometimes a nearest neighbor matching is used in place of a caliper matching, where each treated unit is matched to an available control with the nearest propensity score.

## The Estimand of Pair Matching

Pair matching is often used to estimate the PATT (Imbens & Wooldridge, 2009). However, a sometimes overlooked fact is that this is feasible only when (1) the propensity score distribution of the controls overlaps sufficiently with that of the treated units and (2) within the neighborhood of every propensity score stratum, there are at least as many controls as treated units so that every treated unit can be matched. The mirror histogram, proposed by Li and Greene (2013), is a useful tool to illustrate this point (Figure 7.1). Above the horizontal line is the propensity score histogram of the control group ($z = 0$) and below, the treatment group ($z = 1$). Nested inside them are the histograms of the pair matched units in the control (light green, above) and treatment (dark green, below) groups. The vertical axis must be on the frequency instead of probability scale so that the histograms of the matched data strictly reside inside the histograms of the original dataset, because only a subset of the units are selected into a matched dataset (matching without replacement). The mirror histogram shows how many treated and control units are matched within each propensity score stratum. Heuristically speaking, on any propensity score stratum between 0.5 and 1, there are by definition more treated units than the controls. Consequently, in a dataset that includes units with propensity scores between 0.5 and 1, not all treated units may be matched, in which case the estimand may deviate from the PATT. In principle, as long

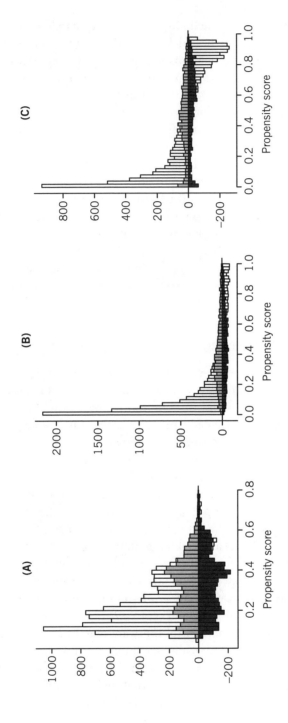

**FIGURE 7.1.** Mirror histograms to illustrate the pair matching for the three examples. The PS model includes all the covariates without additional interaction or nonlinear terms. The caliper equals to 0.2 times the standard deviation of the PSs of all the units on the logit scale.

as there are at least as many untreated units as there are treated units in the data, we could match all the treated units with propensity scores between 0.5 and 1 by using a very large caliper or a nearest neighbor algorithm. However, doing so would cause these treated units to be matched to controls with systematically smaller propensity scores, resulting in inaccurate control of confounding. When a small caliper is used, matching all the treated units requires that almost all the propensity scores be less than 0.5, but this is not the case in many applications. Hence, the estimand of pair matching often deviates from the PATT in practice.

Deviation in estimands from the PATT (or PATE) may often be acceptable or even desirable, for at least two reasons. First, there is little motivation for focusing on the PATT or PATE (Imbens & Wooldrige, 2009). For example, suppose the goal of the research is to study whether there is any protective or detrimental effect of intraoperative blood transfusion on cardiac surgery patients, adjusting for differences in preoperative patient characteristics. The PATT (or PATE) contrasts the average potential outcomes under the scenarios in which the blood is either provided to or withheld from all the currently transfused subjects (or all the cardiac surgery patients in the population from which the sample is drawn). While it is convenient to study these contrasts mathematically, they are not useful in guiding the practice. It is unlikely that blood transfusion could be given or withheld from all the patients as treatment policy alternatives. Exceptions are always made, particularly for those units with propensity scores close to 0 or 1. These are likely the unmatched units in a pair matching analysis. Leaving such units unmatched may be more clinically relevant because the analysis would then focus on subjects with greater equipoise (Li, Zaslavsky, & Landrum, 2007), that is, subjects whose characteristics are associated with reasonably high probabilities both of receiving and of not receiving the treatment. In this sense, these units with propensity scores in the middle range bear more similarity with the target population of randomized clinical trials, as physicians are likely to have greater comfort randomizing units with propensity scores close to 0.5 than randomizing units with propensity scores close to 0 or 1.

Second, the objective of a propensity score analysis is usually to gain generalizable knowledge on whether the treatment has an effect. The exact quantification of the unweighted average treatment effect is often of secondary importance because the average treatment effect often varies, with subpopulations characterized by measured as well as unmeasured patient factors. When many factors are involved, it is impossible to characterize the full spectrum of treatment effect heterogeneity. The effect of blood transfusion might depend on patient-level factors. Different investigators carrying out propensity score analysis using data from different hospitals may arrive at different average treatment effect estimators because both the patient mixes and the treatment assignment pattern (propensity score model) vary from hospital to hospital. However, as long as the blood transfusion truly has a sizeable protective or detrimental effect, these analyses should generally be consistent and all contribute to our generalizable knowledge about blood transfusion. There is no special standing for the patient mix of a particular hospital and hence the corresponding PATT or PATE, though it is important to present adequate descriptive statistics on both the original and matched samples, as will be shown later in Table 7.1.

## Some Methodological Issues with Pair Matching

Despite its widespread application, there remain important unresolved methodological problems with pair matching, highlighted in a discussion paper in *Statistics in Medicine* (see Austin, 2008 and discussions therein). One issue concerns variance estimation. An unresolved debate persists over whether a paired or unpaired analysis of the outcome is more appropriate for statistical inference. The actual situation may be even more complicated because the estimated propensity scores calculated from a fitted logistic regression model are correlated and different matching algorithms using these estimated propensity scores introduce additional correlations between and within matched pairs. The sampling distribution of the matching estimator is very complicated and not yet well understood (Abadie & Imbens, 2006, 2008, 2009). It has been observed from empirical research that not accounting for the sampling error of the estimated propensity scores often results in conservative statistical inference (Stuart, 2010). Another issue is related to the covariate balance check. The typical propensity score analysis requires reformulating the propensity score model until adequate covariate balance is achieved, but the definition of "adequate covariate balance" is unclear. As a rule of thumb, it has been suggested that the standardized difference of every covariate should be within 10% (Austin, 2009a). It is plausible, however, that the optimal threshold should decrease with increasing sample size as greater precision becomes feasible. Since the sample distributions of the covariates between the matched groups can almost never be identical, it is generally unclear to the data analyst whether the observed imbalance is due to random error, inadequate formulation of the propensity score model, or suboptimal implementation of the matching procedure. In the latter two cases, modification to the propensity score model or the matching algorithm is warranted; otherwise, any further modification is futile. Therefore, the

**TABLE 7.1. Descriptive Statistics of the Unadjusted, Pair-Matched, and MW-Weighted Data in Example C**

| Variable | Unadjusted | | | Pair matching | | | MW | | |
|---|---|---|---|---|---|---|---|---|---|
| | Z = 1 (n = 3,422) | Z = 0 (n = 4,842) | SDF | Z = 1 (n = 1,310) | Z = 0 (n = 1,310) | SDF | Z = 1 | Z = 0 | SDF |
| Age | 57 (6.65) | 45.36 (16.66) | 91.8 | 55.32 (8.19) | 54.82 (8.7) | 6 | 55.13 (8.4) | 55.11 (8.32) | 0.2 |
| Body mass index | 24.08 (4.16) | 24.09 (5.33) | −0.1 | 24.8 (4.22) | 25.01 (4.55) | −4.9 | 24.88 (4.29) | 24.84 (4.62) | 0.8 |
| Log creatinine | −0.19 (0.32) | −0.2 (0.39) | 1.4 | −0.14 (0.33) | −0.13 (0.36) | −2.2 | −0.13 (0.34) | −0.13 (0.35) | 1.2 |
| FEV1 | 24.67 (15.53) | 43.27 (21.08) | −100.5 | 34.92 (20.63) | 38.71 (21.46) | −18 | 37.39 (21.3) | 37.54 (21.15) | −0.7 |
| Female | 50.7 | 44 | 13.6 | 49.2 | 48.5 | 1.4 | 48.3 | 48.6 | −0.7 |
| Diabetes | 4.6 | 18.1 | −43.4 | 8.4 | 8.5 | −0.3 | 8.8 | 8.5 | 0.8 |
| Hypertension | 23.3 | 20.6 | 6.4 | 23.6 | 25.6 | −4.6 | 23.4 | 23.8 | −1.1 |
| Double lung transplantation | 41 | 68 | −56.2 | 50.8 | 52.7 | −3.7 | 51.7 | 52.1 | −0.8 |

*Note.* For continuous variables, the mean (standard deviation) is presented; for binary variables, the percentage is presented. The results are based on the final selected PS model.

practical users of propensity score analysis need theoretically justified guidelines on covariate balance diagnosis.

For pair matching with a caliper, there is the additional issue of optimal caliper selection. The caliper has considerable influence on the matching results. While it is likely that a smaller caliper may be more beneficial when the sample size is large, a theoretically justified guideline on the optimal choice of the caliper—taking into account covariate balance, bias, statistical efficiency, and the specifics of the matching algorithm—is not yet available (Austin, 2010).

## MATCHING WEIGHT

MW method was developed in part to address the above-described methodological issues of pair matching. The MW for unit $i$ is defined as

$$W_i = \frac{\min(1-e_i, e_i)}{z_i e_i + (1-z_i)(1-e_i)} \quad (7.1)$$

The MW estimator of the treated effect is

$$\hat{\Delta}_{MW} = \frac{\sum_{i=1}^{n} W_i z_i r_i}{\sum_{i=1}^{n} W_i z_i} - \frac{\sum_{i=1}^{n} W_i (1-z_i) r_i}{\sum_{i=1}^{n} W_i (1-z_i)} \quad (7.2)$$

Here is the intuition behind MW in details. Suppose we focus on a small stratum around propensity score $e_0$ on the mirror histogram (e.g., Figure 7.1) with $m_0$ units. On average, we would expect $e_0 m_0$ treated and $(1 - e_0)m_0$ control units within this stratum. When $e_0 < 0.5$, all treated units can be matched, but only a fraction of the controls $e_0/(1 - e_0)$ can be matched. Therefore, the probability of being selected into the matched data is 1 for a treated unit and $e_0/(1 - e_0)$ for a control in that stratum. Put in another way, each control unit contributes "a fraction" of itself to the matched dataset. When $e_0 > 0.5$, the probability of being selected into the matched data is $(1 - e_0)/e_0$ for a treated unit and 1 for a control in that stratum; for example, each treated unit contributes "a fraction" of itself to the matched dataset. As we can see from Equation 7.1, the MW can be viewed as the probability of being selected into the matched data, or the "fraction" of each unit contributed to the matched dataset. Of course, the actual probability of being matched is much more complicated due to use of the caliper, the specifics of the matching algorithms, and so on. The heuristic arguments above only illustrate the motivation behind the MW from a probabilistic perspective.

## The Estimand of Matching Weight

Once the MW is defined, it can be shown that the MW and pair matching estimator have the same asymptotic limit when the propensity score is defined on an arbitrary discrete scale (Li & Greene, 2013). If we regard this limit as the estimand, then they have the same estimand. For example, if we assume the propensity scores follow a discrete distribution on the 99-value discrete scale {0.01, 0.02, ... , 0.99}, and if we pair match on the propensity score exactly, then when the sample size is large, the MW and pair matching have the same estimand. When the logistic propensity score model involves continuous covariates, the propensity score is also continuous. A theoretical result on the asymptotic limit of pair matching estimator is not yet available, but the argument above suggests that its estimand should be similar to that of the MW estimator, particularly when the sample size is large and the caliper is small.

As long as the propensity score model is correctly specified, the covariate distributions of the treated and control groups, after weighting by the MWs, are asymptotically the same, because

$$\lim_{n\to\infty} \frac{\sum_{i=1}^{n} W_i z_i g(X_i)}{\sum_{i=1}^{n} W_i z_i} = \lim_{n\to\infty} \frac{\sum_{i=1}^{n} W_i (1-z_i) g(X_i)}{\sum_{i=1}^{n} W_i (1-z_i)}$$

for any function $g(X_i)$ of the covariates. Any finite sample imbalance can be attributed to random sampling error. This represents a special case of a general difference between weighting and matching methods for propensity score adjustment. With matching, even when the true propensity score is known, the finite sample imbalance may be due to either random sampling error or suboptimal implementation of the matching algorithm. This can cause difficulty in balance diagnosis.

The estimand of MW estimator is

$$\Delta_0 = \frac{E\{\min(1-e_i, e_i)\Delta_i\}}{E\{\min(1-e_i, e_i)\}}$$

It is a weighted average of individual treatment effects, but with more weight given to the units with propensity scores close to 0.5, that is, those with more "equipoise" of receiving either treatment. From this perspective, it is similar to the "population-overlap weight" (Li, Zaslavsky, & Landrum, 2007), which is Equation 7.1 with the numerator replaced by $e_i/(1-e_i)$. When the numerator of Equation 7.1 is 1, it is the inverse probability weight (IPW; Lunceford & Davidian, 2004). When the numerator is $e_i$, Equation 7.1 becomes the weight for estimating PATT (Hirano & Imbens, 2001). When all treated units are matched, a condition nearly equivalent to all the propensity scores less than 0.5, the numerator of Equation 7.1 is $e_i$ and the MW automatically becomes the PATT weight of Hirano and Imbens (2001). In this situation, the estimands of pair matching and MW are both the PATT. When some treated units are unmatched, a condition nearly equivalent to some propensity scores greater than 0.5, the estimands of pair matching and MW are still similar to each other but are generally different from the PATT.

A widely known drawback of the IPW and the PATT weights is that when the propensity score is close to 0 or 1, the weight may be very large, causing bias and numerical instability (Kang & Schafer, 2007). For example, the PATT weight is 1 for treated units and $e_i/(1 - e_i)$ for controls. On a propensity score stratum very close to 1, a small fraction $(1 - e_i)$ of the units are controls, but their weights could be very large. The PATT weight weights the controls to create a counterfactual population as if all the treated units had been assigned to the control group. This is difficult on strata where there is poor overlap in the propensity scores between the treated and control groups. The large weights in part reflect the data sparsity due to poor overlap on propensity score strata close to 1, and in part reflect the fact that the logistic regression model is often inaccurate when the estimated probability is very large or very small, as it involves extrapolation on its linear predictors. However, the pair matching estimator is usually numerically quite stable because it retains a one-to-one matching ratio throughout the range of propensity scores by allowing a deviation of the estimand from the PATT or PATE when that task is difficult due to inadequate overlap. As an analogue to pair matching, the MW is also numerically very stable. The unstandardized MW in Equation 7.1 is confined between 0 and 1, with a substantial proportion of units receiving a weight of 1. After standardization (Equation 7.2), the MWs are never excessively large for only a small fraction of units. The numerical stability makes MW an attractive choice for problems where there is limited overlap in propensity scores between the treatment groups.

There is an interesting relationship between the unstandardized IPW and MW. The IPW is always greater than 1, indicating that each unit contributes "multiple copies" of themselves to create the counterfactual populations needed to calculate the PATE; the MW is between 0 and 1, indicating that each unit contributes "a fraction" of itself to mimic the pair matched dataset, which is a subset of the original data. From this perspective, the IPW and MW are mirror reflections of each other.

## Estimation and Statistical Inference

The MW estimator has a closed-form expression and is easy to calculate. For the purpose of estimating its variance while incorporating the sampling error of the estimated propensity score, we can view the MW estimator as a solution to the following estimating equation:

$$0 = \sum_{i=1}^{n} \phi_i(\theta) = \sum_{i=1}^{n} \begin{bmatrix} W(X_i, z_i, \beta) z_i (r_i - \mu_1) \\ W(X_i, z_i, \beta)(1 - z_i)(r_i - \mu_0) \\ S_\beta(X_i, \beta) \end{bmatrix} \quad (7.3)$$

$S_\beta(X_i, \beta)$ is the score equation of the logistic regression model for the propensity score, with $\beta$ being the regression coefficient. We express $W_i$ as $W(X_i, z_i, \beta)$ to emphasize its dependence on $\beta$. The unknown parameters in this equation include $\theta = (\mu_1, \mu_0, \beta^T)^T$. Solving this equation is equivalent to estimating $\beta$ by fitting a logistic regression in a first step and estimating $\mu_1$ and $\mu_0$ by $\hat{\mu}_1 = \sum_{i=1}^{n} W_i z_i r_i / \sum_{i=1}^{n} W_i z_i$ and $\hat{\mu}_0 = \sum_{i=1}^{n} W_i (1-z_i) r_i / \sum_{i=1}^{n} W_i (1-z_i)$, respectively, in a second step. The MW estimator is $\hat{\Delta}_{MW} = \hat{\mu}_1 - \hat{\mu}_0$. Hence, essentially no equation solving is needed for the point estimator. Equation 7.3 is needed only for estimating the variance of $\hat{\Delta}_{MW}$ using the sandwich method:

$$\widehat{var}(\hat{\theta}) = \left[\sum_{i=1}^{n} \frac{\partial \phi_i(\theta)}{\partial \theta}\right]^{-1} \left[\sum_{i=1}^{n} \phi_i(\theta) \phi_i(\theta)^T\right] \left[\sum_{i=1}^{n} \frac{\partial \phi_i(\theta)}{\partial \theta}\right]^{-T}, \theta = \hat{\theta}$$

Since $\hat{\Delta}_{MW}$ is a linear combination of $\hat{\theta}$, its variance can be easily calculated from the variance matrix above. Note that there is a discontinuity point in $W(X_i, z_i, \beta)$ with respect to the parameters, due to the $\min(1 - e_i, e_i)$ function in the numerator of the formula for the MW. Details on dealing with this technical issue when calculating the derivatives can be found in Li and Greene (2013).

The sandwich variance calculation is computationally simple but does require derivation of the score equations and their derivatives. Another approach is to use the bootstrap. One can randomly sample the data with replacement, fit the propensity score model, and calculate the MW point estimator in closed form. The process is repeated a large number of times, and the sample variance of the point estimators is taken to be an estimate of the variance of $\hat{\Delta}_{MW}$. Since the MW point estimator has a closed form expression, the programming is straightforward and no derivative calculation is required. The bootstrap is justified for the MW method because the

MW estimator is an M-estimator, but it is not applicable to pair matching (Abadie & Imbens, 2008).

Li and Greene (2013) demonstrated through simulations that the MW estimator can be considerably more efficient than the pair matching estimator. A heuristic explanation is as follows. Suppose we focus on a very small neighborhood around a propensity score $e_0$ on the mirror histogram, with $m_1$ treated units and $m_0$ controls ($m_1/m_0 \approx e_0/(1 - e_0)$). Without loss of generality, let $m_1 < m_0$. In pair matching, all $m_1$ treated units are matched, and $m_1$ of the $m_0$ controls are matched. In the MW method, all $m_1$ treated units receive weight 1, and all the $m_0$ control units receive equal weights $e_0/(1 - e_0)$. With MW, more units contribute to the averaging, reducing the variance of the estimator.

The simulations of Li and Greene (2013) also show that the variance estimator of pair matching, regardless of whether paired or unpaired analysis is used, can exhibit a severe conservative bias. This phenomenon has been observed by other researchers (Stuart, 2010) and seems to be an issue with matching methods in general. By contrast, the MW estimator has the correct variance estimator and confidence interval coverage.

### Double Robust MW Estimator

In addition to the propensity score model, we can also fit a pair of regression models to relate the outcome variable $r$ to X using the data from the treated and control units separately. Denote the conditional expectations of the outcome by $m_1(X_i, \alpha_1) = E(r_i|X_i, z_i = 1)$ for the treated units and $m_0(X_i, \alpha_0) = E(r_i|X_i, z_i = 0)$ for the controls, where $\alpha_1$ and $\alpha_0$ are the corresponding model parameters. We define the double robust MW estimator as

$$\hat{\Delta}_{MW,DR} = \frac{\sum_{i=1}^{n} W_i \{m_1(X_i, \alpha_1) - m_0(X_i, \alpha_0)\}}{\sum_{i=1}^{n} W_i} + \frac{\sum_{i=1}^{n} W_i z_i \{r_i - m_1(X_i, \alpha_1)\}}{\sum_{i=1}^{n} W_i z_i} - \frac{\sum_{i=1}^{n} W_i (1 - z_i) \{r_i - m_0(X_i, \alpha_0)\}}{\sum_{i=1}^{n} W_i (1 - z_i)}$$

The double robust MW estimator is consistent for $\Delta_0$, as long as either the propensity score model is correctly specified or the two conditional expectations from the outcome regression models are correctly specified. In most statistical methods, if the model is specified incorrectly, the estimator is biased. Even if one part of the model fails, the double robust MW estimator will obtain a consistent result as long as the other part of the model holds. Therefore, the data analyst has two chances, instead of one, to achieve consistent estimation. This is why this estimator is called the double robust estimator. The incorporation of additional outcome models requires extra work, but it also offers a benefit: when the outcome models are correctly specified, the double robust MW estimator can be more efficient than the MW estimator in Equation 7.2.

The variance of the double robust MW estimator is estimated with the sandwich method. A difference is that additional score equations corresponding to the two outcome regression models must be incorporated into the estimating equations. Again, a computationally simpler alternative is to use the bootstrap, which avoids deriving and programming the score equations and their derivatives.

Of note, double robustness has not been established theoretically for estimators based on matching methods, though Ho, Imai, King, and Stuart (2007) argued, based on empirical studies, that fitting a regression model on the outcome on the dataset matched on the propensity score, instead of the original dataset, results in double robust estimation. The simulations of Li and Greene (2013) support this concept to a limited extent. In those simulations, the procedure of Ho et al. (2007) appeared to be approximately doubly robust in the sense that a small bias remained when the outcome model was misspecified. The double robust MW estimator has the double robust properties as guaranteed by the theory, and it is more efficient than the estimator from the procedure of Ho et al. (2007).

## Balance Checking

The ability to check covariate balance between the treatment groups is an important advantage of the propensity score methods over direct regression-based estimation of the treatment effect. Lack of balance suggests that the treatment comparison may not be feasible on certain subgroups of units without extrapolation, or that there may be bias due to a misspecification of the propensity score regression model. In general, the covariate distributions, after applying the MWs, can be checked by comparing weighted covariates between the treatment groups:

$$\frac{\sum_{i=1}^{n} W_i z_i g(X_i)}{\sum_{i=1}^{n} W_i z_i} \text{ and } \frac{\sum_{i=1}^{n} W_i (1-z_i) g(X_i)}{\sum_{i=1}^{n} W_i (1-z_i)}$$

where the function $g(\cdot)$ can be any prespecified functions of the covariates. For example, we can let $g(x) = x$ or $g(x) = x^2$ to check the balance in means or second moments, and let $g(x) = 1\{x \leq x_0\}$ to check the balance in the cumulative distribution functions at $x_0$. We can define weighted means and variances of a covariate $X_i$ as $\bar{x}_{(1)} = \sum W_i z_i X_i / \sum W_i z_i$,

$\bar{x}_{(0)} = \sum W_i(1-z_i)X_i / \sum W_i(1-z_i)$, $s_{(1)}^2 = \sum W_i z_i (X_i - \bar{x}_{(1)})^2 / (\sum W_i z_i - 1)$, $s_{(0)}^2 = \sum W_i(1-z_i)(X_i - \bar{x}_{(0)})^2 / (\sum W_i(1-z_i) - 1)$, and calculate the standardized difference (SDF) of each covariate by

$$\frac{100 \times (\bar{x}_{(1)} - \bar{x}_{(0)})}{\sqrt{(s_{(1)}^2 + s_{(0)}^2)/2}}$$

The SDF quantifies the mean difference while adjusting for the variation in the data. These balance-checking formulas can be applied to pair matching by defining $W_i$ to be 0 for the unmatched units and 1 for the matched units.

As we discussed previously, the MW estimator has less variation than the pair matching estimator. This advantage is also shown in the SDFs of covariates. In typical applications of pair matching, the SDFs in a good match are in the magnitude of a few percent. It has been advocated that 10% should be used as the threshold for claiming balance (Austin, 2009a). As shown in the applications of this chapter, the SDFs from the MW method are often below 1%. Therefore, the MW method may lead to substantially better covariate balance than pair matching.

A limitation of an ad hoc threshold such as 10% is that it does not distinguish systematic differences due to bias in the estimated propensity scores or suboptimal matching from the random sampling error in the data. Formal hypothesis tests of balance have generally been considered undesirable in the propensity score literature (Imai, King, & Stuart, 2008; Austin, 2008), as balance is a property of the sample but not the underlying population. Some data analysts present two-group tests on covariates before and after matching and argue that if the *p*-values are nonsignificant after matching, then balance is achieved. This approach is problematic because the null hypothesis is unclear and the *p*-values are expected to be larger after matching because the matched dataset is a subset of the original data.

The section of the Estimand of Matching Weight in this chapter shows that, within the MW framework, as long as the propensity score model is correctly specified, any observed imbalance in the weighted covariate data is due to the sampling error. Therefore, we can recast the balance test as a test for model misspecification (Hansen & Bowers, 2008; Lee, 2013; Shaikh, Simonsen, Vytlacil, & Yildiz, 2009). In this formulation, the null hypothesis can be appropriately expressed as stipulating that the propensity score model is correctly specified. The alternative hypothesis is that the model is misspecified. In theory, any goodness-of-fit test for logistic regression can serve this purpose, when the logistic regression is used as the propensity score model. However, different goodness-of-fit test statistics are sensitive to different deviations from the null. For the purpose of balance checking, we prefer test statistics that are direct measures of imbalance, so that a large test statistic indicates both imbalance and deviation from the null. The widely used Hosmer–Lemeshow test, for example, would not be an appropriate choice in this context. The test of misspecification is much more difficult to implement with pair matching because even if the model is correctly specified, there could still be systematic imbalance due to suboptimal implementation of the matching procedure. As we stated at the beginning of the section Notation and Definition, we make the ignorability assumption throughout this chapter. Hence, the proposed test of "misspecification" of the propensity score model evaluates only the incorrect specification of the propensity score regression equation; it does not address the question of whether the ignorability assumption is violated, such as when a confounder is omitted.

Li and Greene (2013) used the following test statistic as a measure of propensity score model misspecification:

$$T = \hat{\mathbf{B}}^T \hat{\Sigma}_B^{-1} \hat{\mathbf{B}}$$

where

$$\hat{\mathbf{B}} = \frac{\sum_{i=1}^n W_i z_i g(X_i)}{\sum_{i=1}^n W_i z_i} - \frac{\sum_{i=1}^n W_i (1-z_i) g(X_i)}{\sum_{i=1}^n W_i (1-z_i)}$$

and $\hat{\Sigma}_B$ is the estimated variance covariance matrix of $\hat{\mathbf{B}}$. This statistic measures a rescaled squared distance in covariates between the treatment groups and hence is a direct measure of imbalance. Under the null hypothesis, the test statistic has an asymptotic central chi-square distribution with degrees of freedom equal to the rank of $\hat{\Sigma}_B$. A large value indicates imbalance. The test accounts for the sampling error in the estimated propensity score by incorporating the score equation of the propensity score model into calculating the variance covariance matrix $\hat{\Sigma}_B$, similar to the approach in the section Estimation and Statistical Inference.

## EXAMPLES

### Introduction to the Three Data Examples

We present three real data examples to illustrate the use of the MW method. They represent situations where there is sufficient overlap in propensity score distributions between the two comparison groups (Example

A), some nonoverlap (Example B), and serious imbalance (Example C). The mirror histograms in Figure 7.1 visualize these distributions. Since the overlap (or equivalently, imbalance) in propensity score distributions between the comparison groups has strong influence on the propensity score analysis, these three examples show the performance of the MW method in various practical situations.

### Example A

The dataset includes 13,353 patients admitted to the intensive care unit who were mechanically ventilated for more than 48 hours and treated with one of two classes of sedative agents, propofol (9,831 patients, $z = 0$) and benzodiazepine (3,522 patients, $z = 1$). The outcome is hospital length of stay. There are 21 covariates (Figure 7.2). Figure 7.1A shows that the propensity score distributions between the treated ($z = 1$) and control ($z = 0$) groups overlap well and most propensity scores are less than 0.5. As a result, almost all treated units are matched in a pair matching.

### Example B

The dataset includes 12,649 cardiac surgery patients, of whom 3,105 received red blood cell transfusion in the operating room and 9,544 did not. The goal is to compare whether intraoperative red blood cell transfusion affects the ICU length of stay. There are 24 covariates (Figure 7.3). Figure 7.1B shows that there is moderate overlap in the propensity score distributions and that many treated units with propensity scores between 0.6 and 1.0 cannot be matched in pair matching.

### Example C

The dataset includes 8,264 lung transplantation patients, of whom 3,422 had chronic obstructive pulmonary disease (COPD) or asthma ($z = 1$) and 4,842 did not ($z = 0$). The scientific objective is to study the effect of COPD/asthma on posttransplantation survival. The analysis adjusted for seven covariates (Figure 7.4). Figure 7.1C shows that the overlap is poor and that only a small proportion of treated and control units can potentially be matched in pair matching. This is the situation where the PATT and PATE are difficult to estimate due to the data sparsity in at least one comparison group at the two ends of the propensity score range. Since many units have propensity scores close to 0 and 1, the inverse probability weights may be excessively large for some units, causing unstable computation and bias when the inverse probability weighting method is applied.

## Propensity Score Model Development and Balance Checking

For each example, we always used the same propensity score model when comparing the results between pair matching and MW. For pair matching, we used a caliper of 0.2 times the standard deviation of the propensity score on its logit scale, as recommended by Austin (2010). When the outcome regression model is used for double robust estimation, we include all covariates in the model as linear terms with no additional interaction terms. Since the analysis of the outcome variable is straightforward with the MW method once the propensity score model is chosen, the following discussion focuses mainly on propensity score model formulation and balance checking.

Example A

We started the propensity score analysis by fitting a logistic regression of the treatment group indicator on all 21 covariates. No interactions or nonlinear terms were considered at this stage. The test of propensity score model misspecification produced a $p$-value of 1.2e–20, indicating notable imbalance in covariates. Note that most covariates had SDFs less than 1%, based on the MW. This test result indicates that when there is a large sample size as in this example, even 1% SDF is considered excessive; there is a need to reformulate the propensity score model to further reduce imbalance. The covariate "General Medicine" (admitted to Department of General Medicine) had the highest SDF, at 2.7%. We reformulated the propensity score model by adding interactions between "General Medicine" and all other covariates. The $p$-value of the misspecification test improved to 2.3e–7. Now the covariate "Instable HEMO" (hemodynamic instability prior to surgery) had the highest SDF, at 1.4%, and all other covariates, including "General Medicine," were below 1%. We further reformulated the propensity score model by adding interactions between hemodynamic instability ("Instable HEMO") and other covariates. The $p$-value of the misspecification test increased to .0007. All SDFs were now within 1%, and two covariates had the highest SDF at 0.8%: "Hospital type 2" and "Managed by critical care team". Different ICUs may handle the sedative agent differently, and not all ICUs operate using a well-defined multidisciplinary critical care team. We added cross-product interactions between these two covariates and others into the propensity score model. The final propensity score model had 90 covariate and interaction terms. The misspecification test $p$-value was .07. Most SDFs under MW are less than 0.5%, with only two SDFs at 0.6% and one at 0.7%. We concluded that under this propensity score model, the observed imbalance is indistinguishable from the sampling error. In contrast, the SDFs from pair matching using the same propensity score model were much larger in magnitude, ranging from 1 to 6%. From the first propensity score model to the last one, the chi-square test statistic decreased from 145.6, 71.1, 48.0, down to 31.1, indicating improvement in overall covariate balance under the MW approach.

Figure 7.2 shows the mirror histograms of pair matching and MW as well as the plot of SDFs, based on the final selected propensity score model. Note that the mirror histogram of the MWs is constructed in a similar way as that of pair matching. The only difference is that the height of the bars is not the frequency count of the treated or control units in each stratum, but the summation of the unstandardized MWs of those units. The pair matching and MW produce very similar mirror histograms. The SDFs are substantially larger with pair matching, as expected based on the arguments in the section on Balance Checking.

Adding interactions is an effective way of reformulating the propensity score model and reducing imbalance associated with covariates (Rosenbaum & Rubin, 1984). In this example, the covariates with high SDFs are all binary. Incorporating their interactions with all other covariates is equivalent to specifying different propensity score models on subgroups defined by these covariates. When the covariate is continuous, we might consider adding nonlinear terms, such as polynomial or splines. This will be illustrated in the next two examples. Example A has 13,353 observations and 3,522 treated units. The sample size is large enough to avoid convergence problems in the logistic regression. In studies with smaller sample size, adding too many interaction terms may cause quasi-complete separation of logistic regression, and hence it may be necessary to remove certain interaction terms that cause this problem. However, as with all goodness-of-fit tests or test of model misspecification, with smaller sample size comes lower statistical power, so that it is possible to reach statistical nonsignificance without adding too many terms to the propensity score model. Regardless of the sample size, we always recommend using both the test and standardized differences to guide the formulation of the propensity score model. Example B also illustrates this point.

## Example B

This dataset was studied in Li and Greene (2013). (Please refer to that paper for details in propensity score model development.) In recapitulation, we started with a propensity score model with all 24 covariates and no interactions or nonlinear terms. That model passed the misspecification test with a $p$-value of .5. Therefore, no further model reformulation

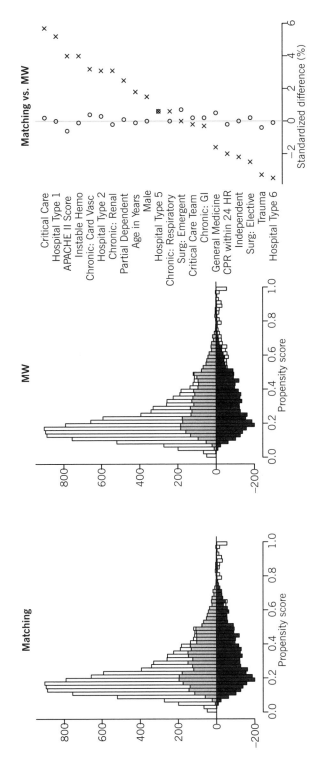

**FIGURE 7.2.** The mirror histograms of pair matching and MW and the plot of SDFs. Open circle, MW; cross, pair matching. The results are based on the final selected PS model for Example A.

was needed. However, a prognostically important covariate ("preoperative hematocrit") had the largest SDF, at 1.6%, while most other covariates' SDFs were below 0.5%. We added two spline terms of this continuous covariate and their interactions with other variables. The misspecification test for the final propensity score model had a $p$-value of .9, and the SDF of hematocrit was reduced to 0.7%. This example shows that we can use both the misspecification test and SDFs to guide the choice of propensity score models. If more than one propensity score model passes the misspecification test, we recommend choosing the one with the smaller SDFs. Figure 7.3 shows the mirror histograms and the SDF plot from the final propensity score model. The pair matching and MW produce very similar mirror histograms, and the SDFs are much smaller with MW.

### Example C

We again started from the propensity score model with all eight covariates and no interactions or nonlinear terms. The covariates were highly unbalanced after being weighted by the MWs, with a test $p$-value of 4.9e–73 and the SDFs ranging from 1% to 10%. Age and FEV1 (a continuous measure of lung function) had the highest SDFs (8.7 and 10.2%, respectively). For these two covariates, we added spline terms in the form of $\max(x - \tau, 0)$, where $x$ is the covariate and $\tau$ is an internal knot. We used three knots for each covariate, valued at the 25%, 50%, and 75% quantiles. The propensity score model passed the misspecification test with a $p$-value of .13, indicating that there was probably a strong nonlinear relationship between age, FEV1, and treatment assignment, not captured by the first propensity score model. Figure 7.4 shows the mirror histograms and the SDF plot. Again, the pair matching and MW produce very similar mirror histograms, and the SDFs are generally much smaller with MW.

### Descriptive Statistics

It is very important to describe characteristics of the matched sample in a pair matching analysis. Likewise, we can do the same thing with the MW-weighted sample. Table 7.1 compares the summary statistics of each covariate for the unadjusted data, pair matched data, and MW-weighted data from Example C. First, the summary statistics from the MW method are very similar to those from pair matching, another indication that the MW is analogous to pair matching. Second, the covariates appear to be more balanced in the MW method, as evidenced by the summary statistics as well as the SDFs. The same observation was also made in Examples A

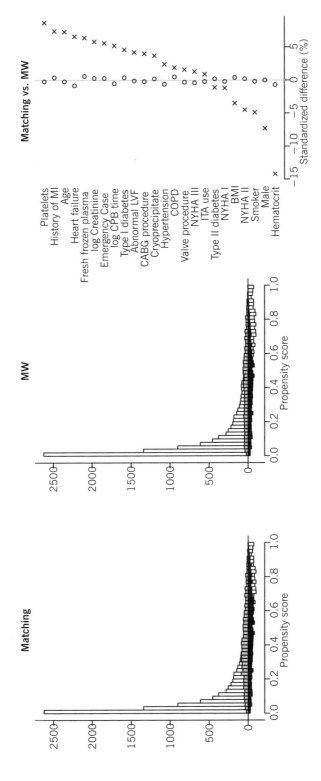

**FIGURE 7.3.** The mirror histograms of pair matching and MW and the plot of SDFs. Open circle, MW; cross, pair matching. The results are based on the final selected PS model for Example B.

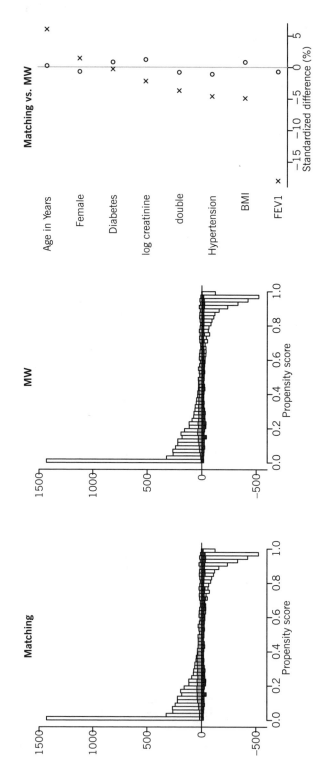

**FIGURE 7.4.** The mirror histograms of pair matching and MW and the plot of SDFs. Open circle, MW; cross, pair matching. The results are based on the final selected PS model for Example C.

and B. With more than 20 covariates, those tables are very large, and we omitted them for brevity.

## Analysis of Outcome

### Example A

The expected mean difference (sandwich standard error, $p$-value) in log hospital length of stay is estimated to be 0.0216 ($SE$ = 0.0190, $p$ = .26) for pair matching, 0.0246 ($SE$ = 0.0165, $p$ = .13) for the MW method, and 0.0240 ($SE$ = 0.0164, $p$ = .14) for the double robust MW method. In contrast, the unadjusted difference is 0.0681. The MW estimator has smaller standard errors than its pair matching counterpart and is therefore more efficient. The reduction in the standard error from 0.0190 to 0.0165 represents a relative efficiency of 1.33, indicating that the "effective sample size" obtained by the MW weight method was around 33% higher than that obtained by pair matching. The bootstrap standard errors are 0.0166 for both MW and double robust MW estimator, very close to the sandwich standard errors.

### Example B

Details on the analysis of outcome can be found in Li and Greene (2013).

### Example C

The outcome is time to death, which is subject to censoring. Figure 7.5 shows the survival probability curves of the two comparison groups, with the data being weighted by the MWs. The vertical bars are 95% confidence intervals at selected time points, calculated from the bootstrap. A Cox model was fit to the MW-weighted data to obtain the estimated hazard ratio. Contrasting that estimated hazard ratio with its bootstrap standard error, we had a Wald-type test $p$-value of 0.00012, indicating significant difference between the two groups. Of note, the hazard ratio is problematic in some respects as a causal estimand, as the hazard ratio at later follow-up times requires conditioning on survival to those times. A causal treatment effect on a survival outcome may be better expressed as a contrast of each subject's potential times to event under alternative treatment groups. The double robust method in this chapter is directly applicable to continuous and binary outcome data but is generally not applicable to time to event data due to censoring. This problem will be studied in future research.

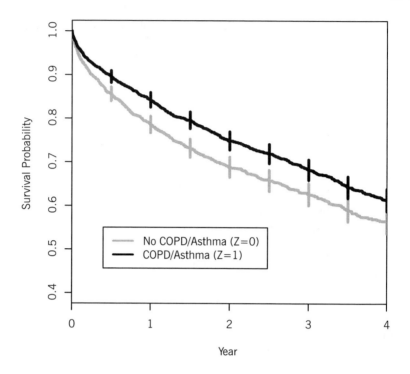

**FIGURE 7.5.** Survival probability curves of the comparison groups, weighted by the MWs (Example C). The vertical bars indicate 95% confidence intervals at selected time points.

## On the Ignorability Assumption

We have not discussed how to assess the ignorability assumption or how to select covariates into the propensity score model. For more discussion on these issues and sensitivity analysis, please refer to Chapters 13 and 14 in this book. The three examples were chosen to illustrate the use of the MW method under various overlap conditions. It is possible that some confounders were left out of these analyses, as the assumption of ignorability cannot be verified with the data. Even when this assumption is violated, the propensity score analysis can still work well as a tool to achieve balance in the observed covariates. In that case, the estimated treatment effect is not the causal effect but a measure of the adjusted association between the treatment and the outcome that may, in some conditions, approximate the treatment effect better than an unadjusted estimate.

## CONCLUSION

In this chapter, we described the MW method as an analogue to pair matching with respect to its estimand, weighted covariate distributions, and mirror histograms. Because the MW method and pair matching have similar estimands, the MW approach can also be used wherever pair matching is applicable. The original motivation of the MW method was to develop a method to avoid several of the methodological complications of pair matching (Austin, 2008) while preserving its estimand. The MW method is simple to implement and generally more efficient than the pair matching estimator. It offers accurate variance estimation, improved covariate balance, and double robust estimation. It also comes with a misspecification test for balance checking purposes.

Figure 7.6 describes the procedure to implement the MW method. Of note, we recommend checking balance through the use of both a test

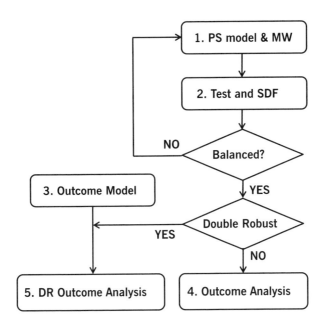

**FIGURE 7.6.** Flowchart of matching weight analysis. Step 1 is to fit the PS model and calculate the MWs in close form. Step 2 is to perform balance check through the test for PS model misspecification and standardized differences (SDF). If balance is achieved, proceed with either the two-group outcome analysis (Step 4) or double robust (DR) outcome analysis (Step 5), otherwise, return to Step 1 and reformulate the PS model. Due to the double robustness, the specification of the outcome regression model (Step 3) is not essential, though some model diagnosis in this step is helpful.

of misspecification and examination of standardized differences, as illustrated in the three examples, particularly Example B. When multiple propensity score models pass the test, the model with the smallest standardized differences in key covariates should generally be selected. We generally recommend double robust outcome analysis. The MW and double robust MW estimator can be easily calculated with standard software. While standard errors may be estimated by numerically solving appropriate estimating equations, the standard errors can be obtained without the use of specialized software by employing the bootstrap resampling. The test of propensity score model misspecification does require some programming, and we are in the process of developing an R package for it. The standardized differences are easy to calculate in closed form.

One limitation of the MW method is that, like pair matching, its estimand may deviate from the PATT or PATE, and hence may not be suitable in studies where the PATT or PATE are of scientific interest. We argued in this chapter that such deviation is sometimes desirable in studies where generalizable knowledge about the treatment effect in various heterogeneous populations is sought, particularly when there is inadequate overlap in the propensity score distributions between the original treated and control groups.

## REFERENCES

Abadie, A., & Imbens, G. W. (2006). Large sample properties of matching estimators for average treatment effects. *Econometrica, 74*(1), 235–267.

Abadie, A., & Imbens, G. W. (2008). On the failure of the bootstrap for matching estimators. *Econometrica, 76*(6), 1537–1557.

Abadie, A., & Imbens, G. W. (2009). Matching on the estimated propensity score. *NBER Working Paper Series*, w15301. Available at *http://ssrn. com/ abstract=1463894*.

Austin, P. C. (2008). A critical appraisal of propensity-score matching in the medical literature between 1996 and 2003. *Statistics in Medicine, 27*, 2037–2049.

Austin, P. C. (2009a). Balance diagnostics for comparing the distribution of baseline covariates between treatment groups in propensity-score matched samples. *Statistics in Medicine, 28*, 3083–3107.

Austin, P. C. (2009b). Some methods of propensity-score matching had superior performance to others: Results of an empirical investigation and Monte Carlo simulations. *Biometrical Journal, 51*, 171–184.

Austin, P. C. (2010). Optimal caliper widths for propensity-score matching when estimating differences in means and differences in proportions in observational studies. *Pharmaceutical Statistics, 10*, 150–161.

Hansen, B. B., & Bowers, J. (2008). Covariate balance in simple, stratified and clustered comparative studies. *Statistical Sciences, 23*, 219–236.

Hirano, K., & Imbens, G. W. (2001). Estimation of causal effects using propensity score weighting: An application to data on right heart catheterization. *Health Services and Outcomes Research Methodology, 2*, 259–278.

Ho, D. E., Imai, K., King, G., & Stuart, E. A. (2007). Matching as nonparametric preprocessing for reducing model dependence in parametric causal inference. *Political Analysis, 15*, 199–236.

Imai, K., King, G., & Stuart, E. A. (2008). Misunderstandings among experimentalists and observationalists in causal inference. *Journal of the Royal Statistical Society Series A, 171*, 481–502.

Imbens, G. W., & Wooldridge, J. M. (2009). Recent developments in the econometrics of program evaluation. *Journal of Economic Literature, 47*(1), 5–86.

Kang, J. D. Y., & Schafer, J. L. (2007). Demystifying double robustness: A comparison of alternative strategies for estimating a population mean from incomplete data (with discussions and rejoinder). *Statistical Science, 22*, 523–539.

Lee, W. S. (2013). Propensity score matching and variations on the balancing test. *Empirical Economics, 44*, 47–80.

Li, F., Zaslavsky, A. M., & Landrum, M. B. (2007). Propensity score analysis with hierarchical data. *JSM Proceedings, Section on Statistics in Epidemiology*, 2474–2481. American Statistical Association, Alexandria, VA.

Li, L., & Greene, T. (2013). A weighting analogue to pair matching in propensity score analysis. *International Journal of Biostatistics, 9*(2), 215–234.

Lunceford, J. K., & Davidian, M. (2004). Stratification and weighting via the propensity score in estimation of causal treatment effects: A comparative study. *Statistics in Medicine, 23*, 2937–2960.

Rosenbaum, P. R., & Rubin, D. B. (1983). The central role of the propensity score in observational studies for causal effects. *Biometrika, 70*, 41–55.

Rosenbaum, P. R., & Rubin, D. B. (1984). Reducing bias in observational studies using subclassification on the propensity score. *Journal of the American Statistical Association, 79*(387), 516–524.

Shaikh, A. M., Simonsen, M., Vytlacil, E. J., & Yildiz, N. (2009). A specification test for the propensity score using its distribution conditional on participation. *Journal of Econometrics, 1*, 33–46.

Stuart, E. (2010). Matching methods for causal inference: A review and a look forward. *Statistical Science, 25*, 1–21.

# CHAPTER 8

# Robust Outcome Analysis for Propensity-Matched Designs

**Scott F. Kosten**
**Joseph W. McKean**
**Bradley E. Huitema**

This chapter focuses on the design and statistical analysis of the matched-pairs observational study. We begin with a general overview of the role of the propensity score in observational studies and describe the nature of the estimands associated with these designs. Then we turn to the matched-pairs version of observational study and present evaluative evidence regarding the adequacy of many methods of outcome analysis for this design. The remainder of the chapter introduces new methods of outcome analysis and provides an example that illustrates the advantages of one method over competing approaches. The recommended analysis is a recently developed robust method that we label as the *RW* method. Input and output for new software that computes this analysis (and several competing alternatives) is provided in the Software section of this chapter.

## ROLE OF THE PROPENSITY SCORE IN OBSERVATIONAL STUDIES

The propensity score may have a role in (1) the design, (2) the outcome analysis, or (3) both the design and the outcome analysis of an observational study. The design refers to the method of selecting and assembling the comparison units (e.g., subjects), whereas the outcome analysis refers to the method of estimating the outcome effect after the study has been designed and carried out. A brief description of the role of propensity scores in design, the outcome analysis, and both is presented below. See Chapters 1 and 6 of this book for detailed discussions of this topic.

## Design

Many observational studies are designed using the propensity score as either a *blocking* variable to form blocks or subgroups that contain treated and control units with similar propensity scores, or a *matching* variable to form matched pairs of treated and control units with similar propensity scores. In these situations, the propensity score is used exclusively in the design; it has no direct role in the outcome analysis.

## Outcome Analysis

In contrast, the propensity score may play no role in the design of the study, but may be used in the outcome analysis. For example, the propensity score may be used as a covariate in an analysis of covariance (ANCOVA). Use of the propensity score in this role has been found not to be as desirable as was once believed; it is no longer recommended (Imbens & Wooldridge, 2009).

## Both Design and Outcome Analysis

The propensity score can play dual roles. That is, it may be applied in both the design and analysis stages of a single study. This occurs in situations in which an important design element includes the elimination of certain units from the comparison groups. For example, it may be desirable to eliminate units having propensity scores close to zero or one because few comparison units are available at these extremes. This use of the propensity score seeks to assemble groups that can be more meaningfully and precisely compared after dropping units than before doing so. Once the ultimate comparison groups are assembled, the propensity score may be used in the outcome analysis for weighting purposes. That is, each observation may be weighted using a function (usually based on inverse probability weights) of the propensity score.

## ESTIMANDS

The estimand is the parameter one attempts to estimate. The treatment effect estimands associated with the various applications of the propensity score mentioned above are not all the same. In most cases the estimand is the effect of the treatment on the treated population, but both the design and the analysis are relevant in identifying whether this is so.

### Effect of the Treatment on the Treated

When the design is based on blocking or matching, the outcome analysis usually provides an estimate of the *average treatment effect on the treated*. (If covariates are included in the analysis, the estimand may be described more specifically as the average treatment effect on the treated, *conditional on the covariates*; this is a distinction we will not pursue.) Because these designs usually use the propensity score to identify control units that are similar to the treated units, it makes sense to claim that the relevant estimand is associated with the treated population; that is, the treatment effect estimate generalizes to units in a population of the treated.

### Effect of the Treatment on the Total Population Sampled

Consider a design in which all available treated and control units are included in the analysis without additional structure imposed (e.g., no blocking or matching of units on the basis of the propensity score). In this case, the estimand is not the effect of the treatment on the treated. Instead, designs of this type when analyzed using common estimation procedures, such as inverse probability weighting (IPW) estimation (Hernan & Robins, 2006; Robins, Hernan, & Bromback, 2000), multiple ANCOVA, picked-points analysis (e.g., Huitema, 2011), and doubly robust estimation (Bang & Robins, 2005), provide estimates of the population average treatment effect. This refers to the treatment effect that would be obtained if the treatment were applied to all units in the total population sampled (rather than just the units in the treated population).

### Effect of the Treatment on the Control

If the treatment units are matched to the controls (perhaps because the treated sample is much larger than the control sample), the estimand is the effect of the treatment on the control population. Studies based on this design are not common.

## Multiple Estimands

Although a single estimand is usually specified for a given analysis, it is sometimes possible to modify standard analyses to provide estimates of more than one estimand. Abadie and Imbens (2006) describe such an approach for matched designs. Another approach, picked-points analysis (PPA), may be used to provide more than one type of estimate in the case of unmatched designs. The specific version of PPA that can be used in this situation has been described as generalized PPA (Huitema, 2011).

Other estimands may be conceptualized and estimated. Suppose that the design involves a method of selecting participants that restricts the values of the propensity score on which matches are based. For example, Crump, Hotz, Imbens, and Mitnik (2009) suggest discarding observations with propensity scores that are outside the bounds of an interval having limits determined by a function of the marginal distribution of the propensity score. These limits often work out to be approximately 0.10 and 0.90. In this case, the estimand is the treatment effect in a population specified to have no units with propensity scores outside the interval (0.10, 0.90).

## MATCHED-PAIRS OBSERVATIONAL DESIGN

Although the propensity score is worthwhile in all of the applications mentioned above, the approach we prefer is to use it in the design (not the analysis) of matched-pairs observational studies. These studies are designed (assembled) through the following steps:

1. Identify the sample of $n_T$ treated units.

2. Obtain treatment group measures on many covariates (**X**) that are believed to correlate with the dependent variable and/or the treatment group indicator variable.

3. Recruit many nontreated participants who are believed to be similar to the treated units; this collection is the *full control sample* of $n_{FC}$ participants.

4. Obtain covariate information (on the same covariates as are measured on the treatment group) from the full control sample.

5. Estimate the propensity score for the combined sample of treated and full control participants.

6. Match the estimated propensity score for each unit in the treatment group to the closest propensity estimate available in the

full control group; the collection of control units identified in the matching process is the *matched control sample* of $n_{MC}$ units.

7. Obtain scores on the dependent variable from all treated and matched control units.

Because the advantages of the matched-pair design generally increase as the size of the full control sample increases, the researcher should devote substantial time and effort identifying and recruiting participants for this sample. Two points should be kept in mind when recruiting participants for the full control sample: (1) it will be necessary to obtain complete covariate information on all of them and (2) it will *not* be necessary to obtain outcome information for all full control participants.

Outcome scores are required for *only* the $n_{MC}$ participants selected as matches for the treated; there are no more than $n_T$ of these. Because only covariate data are required on the full control sample, studies of this type can be relatively economical to carry out. Covariate information is usually both widely available and inexpensive to obtain, whereas outcome data are often expensive to collect. This means that it is often possible to obtain a much larger full control sample than treated sample. Although there is no clear definition of "much larger," we recommend that the size of the full control group be *at least* twice as large as that of the treatment group.

If this is impossible and the number of units in the full control group is of the same order as the number of treated units, it may be preferable to not use the matched pairs design; in this case, one of the so-called doubly robust estimation methods for the outcome analysis may be more appropriate than the method recommended here. The conditions under which one of these approaches to design and analysis is preferable to the other require further investigation. We are currently engaged in research that may shed light on this issue. Our conjecture is that doubly robust estimation may have higher power because the associated design is such that all available control units are used in estimating the treatment effect; this is usually not true in the case of propensity-matched designs.

## Propensity Score Estimation

Matching a treated unit to a control requires one to first obtain an estimate of the propensity score $e(X)$ for each unit in both the treatment and full control groups. This is accomplished by first regressing (usually using logistic regression) the treatment indicator variable (0 for control, 1 for treated) on all covariates X; this analysis is carried out on the combined sample of all treated and full control units. The coefficients from this analysis are then applied to provide the propensity score estimate for each treated and full control unit included in the logistic regression analysis using

$$\hat{p} = \hat{e}(\mathbf{X}) = \{1 + \exp[-(\hat{\beta}_0 + \hat{\beta}_1 X_1 + \hat{\beta}_2 X_2 + \cdots + \hat{\beta}_m X_m)]\}^{-1}$$

$$= \frac{e^{\hat{\beta}_0 + \hat{\beta}_1 X_1 + \hat{\beta}_2 X_2 + \cdots + \hat{\beta}_m X_m}}{1 + e^{\hat{\beta}_0 + \hat{\beta}_1 X_1 + \hat{\beta}_2 X_2 + \cdots + \hat{\beta}_m X_m}}$$

See Chapters 1 and 3 for additional coverage regarding the estimation and diagnosis of propensity models.

## Matching

Once the propensity scores (or some function of them) are estimated, they are used as the basis for matching. The matching method recommended here is known as *one-to-one matching with replacement*. This method has been shown to provide greater bias reduction than simply matching to the closest remaining full control unit (Dehejia & Wahba, 2002). It involves matching control unit $j$ to treatment unit $i$ if

$$|\hat{p}_i - \hat{p}_j| < |\hat{p}_i - \hat{p}_k|$$

where $\hat{p}$ is the propensity score estimate, $k = 1, \ldots, j-1, j+1, \ldots, n_{FC}$, and $n_{FC}$ is the number of participants in the full control sample.

Once a specific control has been selected from the full control sample as a match, it is returned to the sample; it may be selected again as the match for one (or more) additional treated unit; that is, the matching is performed with replacement. It is also possible to have two or more control participants with the same propensity score estimate; in this case the matched participant is randomly selected from the set of participants with identical propensity score estimates. Software to perform this method of matching is described in the Appendix at the end of the chapter.

## OUTCOME ANALYSIS ALTERNATIVES

Once the treatment and matched control pairs have been assembled during the design stage, an outcome analysis must be selected and applied in order to estimate the treatment effect. Although there are many reasonable parametric and nonparametric choices for this purpose, we propose a new robust method designed specifically for the matched-pairs observational design. The reasons for recommending the proposed analysis rest on the results of a large simulation study of 18 methods for the outcome analysis of this design (Kosten, 2010; Kosten, McKean, & Huitema, 2014).

## Simulation Design

A list of the 18 outcome analysis methods is provided in Table 8.1. All but the last six methods listed in the table were investigated in an earlier well-known study (Hill & Reiter, 2006) of various analyses for this design. No clear winner emerged in this study. In general, the methods included

**TABLE 8.1. 18 Outcome Analysis Methods Applied to Simulated Matched-Pairs Observational Designs**

| Method | Label |
|---|---|
| 1. Matched pairs $t$ (NCA) | M |
| 2. Weighted two-sample $t$ (NCA) | T |
| 3. Weighted least squares (NCA) | S |
| 4. Weighted least squares (CA) | s |
| 5. WLS robust sandwich variance (NCA) | R |
| 6. WLS robust sandwich variance (CA) | r |
| 7. Bootstrap—variance (NCA) | D |
| 8. Bootstrap—variance (CA) | d |
| 9. Bootstrap—percentile (NCA) | B |
| 10. Bootstrap—percentile (CA) | b |
| 11. Hodges–Lehmann aligned rank (NCA) | H |
| 12. Hodges–Lehmann aligned rank (CA) | h |
| 13. Block-adjusted least squares (NCA) | L |
| 14. Block-adjusted least squares estimation (CA) | l |
| 15. Block-adjusted Wilcoxon estimation (NCA) | W |
| 16. Block-adjusted Wilcoxon estimation (CA) | RW |
| 17. Wilcoxon estimation on Rubin differences, (CA) | x |
| 18. Least-squares estimation on Rubin differences (CA) | y |

*Note.* CA, covariate adjusted; NCA, non-covariate adjusted.

in the evaluation were not specifically developed for application to studies designed using the propensity score; they included classic, normal theory, and bootstrap methods for two-group comparisons. No additional description of those methods (i.e., Methods 1–12 in the table) is provided here. The Hill and Reiter article and the references cited earlier in this section provide full details.

Methods 13–16 were specifically proposed for the analysis of matched-pair observational studies designed using propensity scores (Kosten, 2010; Kosten et al., 2014). These four methods are based on either the *RW* design matrix (subsequently described in detail) or a reduced version of this matrix. Method 18 is a covariate-adjusted method that was proposed by Rubin (1979) for the analysis of observational matched-pair studies designed using multivariate (i.e., discriminant and Mahalanobis) matching methods. This outcome analysis is carried out by regressing (using least-squares estimation) the column of outcome differences (between treatment and control groups) on the columns of treatment minus control differences on the covariates. The adjusted treatment effect estimator is provided by the intercept. Method 17 is the same as the Rubin approach, except that robust Wilcoxon estimation is used in place of least squares.

In addition to the inclusion of Methods 13–18, our simulation study differed from that of Hill and Reiter (2006) in that (1) the method of propensity score estimation (used in identifying matched controls) was based on logistic regression rather than probit regression and (2) three types of error distribution were studied rather than just the normal. A brief description of the additional distributions and other aspects of the simulation design is presented next.

## Factors Investigated

The simulation study included three response surfaces, three error distributions (normal, contaminated normal, and Cauchy), and four different degrees and types of overlap between treatment and control covariate distributions. Hence, there were $(3 \times 3 \times 4) = 36$ conditions.

The response surfaces included (1) linear parallel surfaces that are separated by a constant distance of four units (the true treatment effect) regardless of the covariate score, (2) nonlinear parallel surfaces separated by four units regardless of covariate score, and (3) nonlinear nonparallel surfaces in which the distance (the treatment effect) is a function of the covariate value.

The three error distributions were chosen so that the degree of tail thickness included thin (normal), moderately thick (contaminated normal), and very thick (Cauchy) tails. The contaminated normal distribution had a 20% rate of contamination; the scale ratio of the contaminated part to the normal part was set at four. The inclusion of these distributions in the simulation allowed an examination of the sensitivity of the various analyses to both heavy tails and extreme outliers (associated with Cauchy distributions). An analysis that has poor inferential properties in the presence of thick-tailed distributions and/or outliers is considered nonrobust. Both of these departures from normality occur in practice; it is of considerable importance to know how well alternative methods hold up in these situations.

Because observational studies are characterized by selection bias, it is of interest to see how well analytic methods perform under different degrees of covariate imbalance. Four levels of covariate imbalance were included in the simulation study: (1) strong overlap (the treatment and control covariate means were equal), (2) moderate overlap (a portion of each group (43%) was sampled from covariate distributions with equal means, and the remaining portion was sampled from covariate distributions that differ by two standard deviations), (3) weak overlap (simulated as described above for moderate overlap, but the proportion of each group sampled from treatment and control distributions with equal covariate means was only 14%), and (4) uneven overlap (relatively few treated units were compared to controls for low covariate values, and the opposite was true for high covariate values).

Each of the 18 outcome methods was investigated under all 36 conditions described above. The number of simulations under each condition was 10,000 except for the four computationally intensive bootstrap methods; 1,000 simulations were carried out for them.

The major criteria used to evaluate the methods include (1) treatment effect bias (i.e., the size of the discrepancy between the true treatment effect and the average estimate provided by the analysis), (2) the proportion of the time that the confidence intervals capture the true treatment effect, and (3) the average length of the CIs. Additional detail on the simulation design is presented elsewhere (Kosten, 2010; Kosten et al., 2014).

## Simulation Results

All methods were essentially unbiased under the ideal condition combination of strong overlap, parallel response surfaces, and normal errors; this was true whether or not covariates were included. The size of the population mean difference (i.e., the estimand) was set at 4.00, and the empirical mean estimate obtained for each method was 4.00. The empirical confidence coefficients for nominal 95% intervals, however, ranged from approximately 0.90 for the Rubin method to 1.00 for two of the bootstrap methods; the *RW* and *l* methods were essentially exact, both having empirical confidence coefficients of 0.95.

The situation changed dramatically under most other conditions. Table 8.2, for example, presents the results for all methods under the following condition combination: linear response surface, strong overlap, and Cauchy errors. It can be seen that there are dramatic differences in the adequacy of the various methods. The mean treatment effect ranges from −8.54 to 4.21 (whereas the true effect value is 4.00), the mean CI length ranges from 1.24 to 90.56, and the mean CI coverage ranges from 0.93 to 1.00.

The results shown in this table constitute only a small portion of the data used in the overall evaluation of the methods. The overall evaluation was based on data simulated in all 36 condition combinations included in the design.

## Acceptable Contenders

Based on the criteria of freedom from bias and coverage of the CIs in all 36 conditions, the following seven methods were identified as acceptable: *r* (robust sandwich variance estimator, with covariates), *H* and *h* (the Hodges–Lehman aligned-rank methods, without and with covariates), and *L*, *l*, *W*, and *RW* (the block-adjusted methods without and with covariates). All seven methods on this list had overall empirical confidence coverage coefficients that fell in the interval (0.93, 0.97); the empirical confidence coverage coefficients for all of the other methods were excessively liberal, excessively conservative (e.g., all bootstrap methods), or liberal under some conditions and conservative under others (Method S).

The methods that survived the first cut were then evaluated with respect to empirical efficiency. This was measured as the ratio of the mean length of the CI for a specified method, over the mean length of the CI for method *l* (i.e., the block- and covariate-adjusted least-squares method).

## The Winner

The clear winner among the 18 methods was a robust approach that we label as the *RW* method. This method is defined by (1) an atypical design matrix and (2) a parameter estimation procedure that is based on what are known as Wilcoxon scores (described in McKean & Sheather, 1991). This is the method recommended here. It was easily the most robust procedure in the study. Furthermore, under normal error conditions it was only slightly less efficient than was the least-squares *l* method (just as theory predicts), which is based on the same design matrix.

RW is essentially a type of robust analysis of covariance that simultaneously incorporates blocking information, covariate information, and an approach that allows multiple-treatment units to be matched to a single control unit within any block. Advantages of this method are that (1) it provides high power, (2) it reduces bias associated with differences between treatment and matched control covariate distributions that is likely to remain after matching, and (3) it is robust to both outliers present on the outcome measure and to some more general types of non-normality (such as thick-tailed distributions). The nonrobust version of the *RW* method (the *l* method) is also recommended if normality is well approximated.

Two other approaches that performed well in the simulation (but not as well as the *RW*) are labeled as the *W* and *L* methods. They are the no-covariate analogues to the *RW* and *l* methods; both of them are block-adjusted, but they do not adjust the treatment estimate for residual bias that may be measured by the covariates. They are reasonable alternatives to *RW* and *l* when the number of covariates is very large and the number of units is very small. It may be impossible to compute *RW* and *l* in this situation because there may be no degrees of freedom for error.

## THE *RW* METHOD

A brief description of the problems associated with least-squares methods and a common effort to solve them is presented next. Then the general ideas associated with the *RW* estimation method are presented, the required design matrix is described, and an example is worked out.

### Problem with Least-Squares Estimates

The reason the *RW* method is far more robust to bias in the treatment effect estimate than are conventional parametric approaches can be understood by considering the criterion used in fitting the regression coefficients. Recall that when a conventional regression model is fitted it meets the following least-squares criterion: The residual sum of squares

$$\sum_{i=1}^{N}(Y_i - \hat{Y}_i)^2$$

is minimum. That is, the regression coefficient estimates have the property that they minimize the sum of the squared differences between the observed outcome $Y_i$ and the predicted outcome

$$\hat{Y}_i = \hat{\beta}_0 + \hat{\beta}_1 X_{1_i} + \hat{\beta}_2 X_{2_i} + \ldots + \hat{\beta}_m X_{m_i}$$

For a given dataset it is impossible to identify a set of coefficients that will produce a smaller residual sum of squares; hence, the least-squares criterion is met. In many applications, it is reasonable to estimate the coefficients using this criterion because sample data often appear to reasonably well conform to the assumptions of the regression model.

But it is not unusual to encounter outcome data that do not approximate the properties assumed by the model. For example, when an outlier is present in the outcome distribution, it often has a larger biasing influence on the regression coefficient estimates than one might expect because it is the *squared* residuals that are minimized. Consequently, coefficients based on least-squares estimation often inadequately estimate the major patterns present in the underlying population distribution. For example, in the case of an observational study, a single outlier can have a major influence on the size of both the coefficient for the treatment effect and the error variance estimate. This implies that in many applications least-squares methods can produce highly biased treatment effect estimates and poor inferential properties. This was repeatedly demonstrated in the simulation study mentioned earlier. A quick glance at the variation in the size of the average treatment effect estimates provided by different methods shown in Table 8.2 dramatically illustrates the potential effects of outliers. These characteristics lead to interest in more robust methods of estimation and inference for observational studies.

## Problems with Rank Transformation as a Solution

One simple approach for reducing the influence of outlying observations is to simply transform the outcome variable to ranks. Although this approach is popular (especially in the social sciences) because it sometimes effectively reduces the influence of outliers, it is accompanied by two major disadvantages. The parameter estimates from such an analysis often do not reasonably describe the phenomena of interest, and conventional methods of model diagnostics are rendered useless or misleading.

In most studies, there are good reasons for choosing a specific outcome metric; coefficients obtained on the chosen measure are usually

**TABLE 8.2. Simulation Results for 18 Outcome Methods under the Conditions of Linear Response Surfaces, Strong Covariate Overlap, and Cauchy Errors (True Effect = 4.00)**

| Method | Simulations | Mean Treatment effect estimate | Mean CI length | CI coverage |
|---|---|---|---|---|
| M | 10,000 | −3.3493 | 68.6362 | 0.9509 |
| T | 10,000 | −3.3493 | 80.4983 | 0.9828 |
| S | 10,000 | −3.3493 | 73.3368 | 0.9703 |
| s | 10,000 | −3.2156 | 73.3443 | 0.9679 |
| R | 10,000 | −3.3493 | 71.4843 | 0.9805 |
| r | 10,000 | −3.2156 | 70.4908 | 0.9775 |
| B | 1,000 | −8.0489 | 78.7349 | 0.9910 |
| b | 1,000 | −8.0274 | 80.5161 | 0.9920 |
| D | 1,000 | −8.5442 | 90.5564 | 0.9990 |
| d | 1,000 | −8.2768 | 90.3321 | 0.9990 |
| H | 10,000 | 4.0055 | 1.8241 | 0.9626 |
| h | 10,000 | 4.2109 | 4.8378 | 0.9609 |
| L | 10,000 | −4.5475 | 76.6634 | 0.9746 |
| l | 10,000 | −4.8745 | 77.1002 | 0.9739 |
| W | 10,000 | 4.0057 | 1.6887 | 0.9576 |
| RW | 10,000 | 4.0046 | 1.2403 | 0.9421 |
| x | 10,000 | 4.0040 | 1.1147 | 0.9328 |
| y | 10,000 | −3.6848 | 69.1166 | 0.9500 |

more relevant to the phenomenon studied and are more easily communicated than are coefficients based on rank transformations of these outcomes. Often, ranked outcomes completely obliterate the crucial descriptive properties the researcher is attempting to demonstrate. An example of this can be seen elsewhere (see Huitema, 2011, pp. 315–317).

For these reasons it is useful to seek an efficient method that will (1) allow use of the desired untransformed outcome metric, (2) provide meaningful parameter estimates that are not highly sensitive to outliers (or several other departures from normality), (3) provide improved inferential properties relative to least-squares methods (i.e., narrower CIs and more powerful tests), and (4) provide useful diagnostic methods to evaluate the adequacy of the model.

The *RW* method incorporates both an atypical design matrix and an estimation method that differs substantially from ordinary least squares. The estimation method provides the features listed in the previous paragraph. *RW* was specifically developed for matched-pairs observational studies that have been designed using a matching method that allows a control to be matched to more than one treated unit. The estimation method is briefly described next.

## Parameter Estimation

Instead of using the least-squares criterion in the estimation of the regression coefficients, the parameter estimates are optimized so that they minimize another criterion (known as the dispersion function) using the so-called R-estimation method that is based on "Wilcoxon scores." (This method has nothing to do with the well-known Wilcoxon signed rank and independent samples tests.) Details on R-estimation and Wilcoxon scores are not provided here; they can be found in Hettmansperger and McKean (2011), Kloke and McKean (2012, 2013), and McKean (2004). The essential idea is that the regression coefficients are estimated by minimizing the following dispersion function:

$$\sum_{i=1}^{N} \frac{\sqrt{12}}{N+1} \left[ R(Y_i - \hat{Y}_i) - \frac{N+1}{2} \right] (Y_i - \hat{Y}_i)$$

where $\hat{Y}_i = \hat{\beta}_1 X_{1_i} + \hat{\beta}_2 X_{2_i} + \ldots + \hat{\beta}_p X_{p_i}$, $R(Y_i - \hat{Y}_i)$ is the rank of the residual $(Y_i - \hat{Y}_i)$ among the residuals $(Y_1 - \hat{Y}_1), (Y_2 - \hat{Y}_2), \ldots, (Y_N - \hat{Y}_N)$ and $N$ = number of rows in the design matrix.

Note that there is no intercept in the equation used to obtain the $Y$ estimates. This equation is estimated first; the intercept is estimated in a second step after the residuals of the original equation are computed. The median of these residuals is the estimator for the intercept.

## Design Matrix

The required design matrix **X** contains columns for the following: the intercept *1*, the treatment indicator variable *T* (0 for matched control, 1 for treatment), the $n_{UC} - 1$ indicator variables $(I_2 \ldots I_{n_{UC}})$ that identify blocks $2 \ldots n_{UC}$, and the $C$ covariates. The set of these columns is represented as

$$[1 \; T \; I_2 \; I_3 \; \ldots \; I_{n_{UC}} \; X_1 \; X_2 \; \ldots \; X_C]$$

Each block contains one control unit and one or more treatment units to which that control has been matched. Because a single control can be the best match for more than one treated unit, the number of unique controls $n_{UC}$ (which is equal to the number of blocks) may be less than the number of treated units. That is, the number of blocks is equal to the number of treated units minus the number of instances ($n_{instances}$) in which control units are matched to more than one treated unit: $(n_T - n_{instances}) = n_{UC}$ = number of blocks. If there are no instances of a control unit being matched to more than one treated unit, the number of blocks = $n_T$. The total number of rows $N$ in the required design matrix is equal to the number of treated units $n_T$ plus the number of unique controls $n_{UC}$.

## Example

An example of the RW analysis is presented here. It is assumed that the data collection, the propensity score estimation, the matching, and the diagnostics regarding the adequacy of the propensity model have already taken place. The required X matrix is shown in Table 8.3 for a tiny study. Both the treatment group sample size ($n_T = 10$) and the number of covariates ($C = 3$) are unrealistically small for an observational study; however, this small dataset may facilitate an understanding of how the design matrix is formed.

There are 13 columns in the X matrix. The first is a column of ones. The second column (the treatment indicator) indicates that there are 10 treated units and 9 unique controls. Columns three through 10 are the eight block indicators $I_2 \ldots I_9$. Notice that the block indicator variable column entries are all zeros in rows 1 and 11. These rows identify the first treated unit and the first matched control unit, respectively. An inspection of column three (which is $I_2$) shows that the second treated unit is matched to the second control unit. Similarly, column four shows that the third treated unit (row three) is matched to the third control unit. This pattern continues for the remaining indicator variable columns; however, the last indicator column (column 10) is slightly different in that it contains three ones, whereas the other block indicator columns contain only two. Note that this column indicates that treated units 9 and 10 are both matched to control unit 9. This is the only instance in which a control is matched to more than one treated unit; hence, one is subtracted from $n_T$ to obtain the number of unique control units: $(n_T - 1) = n_{MC} = 9$. Columns 11, 12, and 13 are the covariate columns. The $N = 19$ outcome measures appear in the Y vector.

**TABLE 8.3. Example Design Matrix X and Outcome Vector Y for *RW* and *l* Analyses**

$$X = \begin{bmatrix} 1 & 1 & 0 & 0 & 0 & 0 & 0 & 0 & 0 & 0 & 11 & 7 & 144 \\ 1 & 1 & 1 & 0 & 0 & 0 & 0 & 0 & 0 & 0 & 41 & 30 & 627 \\ 1 & 1 & 0 & 1 & 0 & 0 & 0 & 0 & 0 & 0 & 9 & 6 & 129 \\ 1 & 1 & 0 & 0 & 1 & 0 & 0 & 0 & 0 & 0 & 40 & 27 & 520 \\ 1 & 1 & 0 & 0 & 0 & 1 & 0 & 0 & 0 & 0 & 2 & 2 & 33 \\ 1 & 1 & 0 & 0 & 0 & 0 & 1 & 0 & 0 & 0 & 48 & 23 & 537 \\ 1 & 1 & 0 & 0 & 0 & 0 & 0 & 1 & 0 & 0 & 5 & 4 & 51 \\ 1 & 1 & 0 & 0 & 0 & 0 & 0 & 0 & 1 & 0 & 27 & 17 & 563 \\ 1 & 1 & 0 & 0 & 0 & 0 & 0 & 0 & 0 & 1 & 22 & 12 & 317 \\ 1 & 1 & 0 & 0 & 0 & 0 & 0 & 0 & 0 & 1 & 30 & 21 & 478 \\ 1 & 0 & 0 & 0 & 0 & 0 & 0 & 0 & 0 & 0 & 32 & 8 & 455 \\ 1 & 0 & 1 & 0 & 0 & 0 & 0 & 0 & 0 & 0 & 3 & 7 & 43 \\ 1 & 0 & 0 & 1 & 0 & 0 & 0 & 0 & 0 & 0 & 4 & 4 & 12 \\ 1 & 0 & 0 & 0 & 1 & 0 & 0 & 0 & 0 & 0 & 3 & 4 & 23 \\ 1 & 0 & 0 & 0 & 0 & 1 & 0 & 0 & 0 & 0 & 29 & 17 & 375 \\ 1 & 0 & 0 & 0 & 0 & 0 & 1 & 0 & 0 & 0 & 22 & 6 & 308 \\ 1 & 0 & 0 & 0 & 0 & 0 & 0 & 1 & 0 & 0 & 35 & 12 & 479 \\ 1 & 0 & 0 & 0 & 0 & 0 & 0 & 0 & 1 & 0 & 40 & 15 & 465 \\ 1 & 0 & 0 & 0 & 0 & 0 & 0 & 0 & 0 & 1 & 34 & 20 & 480 \end{bmatrix} \quad Y = \begin{bmatrix} 37 \\ 152 \\ 34 \\ 98 \\ 20 \\ 92 \\ 25 \\ 67 \\ 62 \\ 64 \\ 69 \\ 7 \\ 6 \\ 1 \\ 58 \\ 45 \\ 69 \\ 73 \\ 72 \end{bmatrix}$$

*Note.* The first printing of the second edition of Huitema (2011) contains alternative versions of *RW* and *l*. We recommend that the versions described in this chapter be used instead.

Both the *l* method and the recommended *RW* method can be estimated using the routines shown in the software section. The results of these analyses are shown in Table 8.4. Both methods provide estimates of the same estimand. That is, they both estimate the effect of the treatment on the treated population; the true effect is nonzero in this contrived example.

After Y is regressed (using either least-squares or Wilcoxon estimation) on the predictors (i.e., the treatment indicator, all block indicator variables, and all covariates), the treatment effect estimate is simply the coefficient associated with the treatment indicator variable. A comparison of results for *l* and *RW* reveals several important properties of the robust method.

First, the treatment effect estimate is smaller for *RW* than it is for the corresponding least-squares estimator *l*. This is because the treatment

**TABLE 8.4. Results of *l* (Least-Squares) and RW (Robust Wilcoxon) Methods Applied to Example Data Shown in Table 8.3**

| Method | Treatment effect | Standard error | t | p | 95% CI |
|---|---|---|---|---|---|
| *l* | 18.901 | 9.275 | 2.038 | 0.088 | (−3.79, 41.60) |
| RW | 17.139 | 6.851 | 2.502 | 0.046 | (0.37, 33.90) |

*Note.* Relative efficiency of RW relative to *l*: 183%.

group contains an outlier, which can be identified using Wilcoxon studentized residuals (Hettmansperger & McKean, 2011). Outliers distort the treatment effect estimate provided by the *l* method; the RW treatment estimate is affected little by these values. Second, the *t*-value for the RW method is larger than the *t*-value for the *l* method (even though the treatment effect estimate is smaller for RW). This occurred because the standard error estimate for the RW method is smaller than in the case of the least-squares analysis. The explanation for this is that the outlier in the treatment group inflated the least-squares estimate but had little effect on the standard error estimate for the RW method. Third, the relative efficiency of RW (defined as the ratio of the squared standard error for *l* over the squared standard error for RW) is (86.03/46.94), or 183%. A concomitant of this efficiency is a shorter CI for RW that does not include zero, whereas the wider *l* interval does include zero. Correspondingly, the *p*-value found using RW is less than alpha (for a 5% test), but this is not true for *l*; this is another reflection of the increased precision provided by RW. A second example, presented in the Software section of this chapter, contains additional software detail regarding input and output for RW, *l*, and two related methods.

## CONCLUSION

The matched-pairs observational study is frequently designed using the propensity score as the basis for matching. The pairs are often formed using one-to-one matching with replacement. A large simulation study was performed to evaluate the performance of 18 outcome analysis methods for this design; it clearly demonstrated the importance of incorporating the design properties into the outcome analysis. A new robust approach (the RW method) that was developed specifically for propensity-matched designs stood out as the most satisfactory among all analyses studied. RW is essentially a type of robust analysis of covariance that simultaneously incorporates blocking information, covariate information, and an approach that allows multiple-treatment units to be matched to a single control unit within any block. Advantages of this method are that (1) it provides high power, (2) it reduces bias associated with differences between treatment and matched control covariate distributions that is likely to remain after matching, and (3) it is robust to outliers and to some more general types of non-normality (such as thick-tailed distributions). Software that computes this method as well as related propensity score, matching, and outcome approaches has been developed in R and is freely available.

## SOFTWARE
### *R* Software Input and Output

We have written *R* code that computes (1) the *RW* analysis (labeled in the output as the w method), as well as (2) a "block-only" version (*W*) that includes the block columns but does not include covariates, (3) the nonrobust (least-squares) version of the *RW* analysis (*l*), and (4) a nonrobust block-only least-squares version (*L*) without covariates.

The statistical computing package R is freeware, which can run on all platforms (Windows, MAC, and linux). It can be downloaded from the Comprehensive R Archive Network (CRAN) at *http://cran.us.r-project.org*. In addition, the R package *Rfit* is needed to compute the analysis described here. This package was developed by Kloke and McKean (2012) and can be downloaded at CRAN. The current version 0.18 suffices for our outcome analysis. There are also several auxiliary R routines, which we have supplied. The driver is the *R* function *VWrfit*. The input consists of a dataset in column format of the form [Y T 1 x1 . . . xp], where the first column contains the responses Y, the second column is the treatment indicator (1 for a treated unit and 0 for a control), the third column has all entries one (the intercept column), and the fourth and subsequent columns contain the covariates.

The function *VWrfit* computes the propensity scores using the R function *glm* and then performs the matching with replacement between the treated and control units as described in the matching method section. Part of the output displays the matches within their blocks. The routine *VWrfit* then computes the Wilcoxon analyses as listed below and, for comparison, their LS counterparts. The symbol and its description of the methods computed are: W = Wilcoxon analysis of treatment effect adjusted for blocks only, w (labeled as *RW* throughout this chapter) = Wilcoxon analysis of treatment effect adjusted for blocks and covariates, L = least-squares analysis of treatment effect adjusted for blocks, and l = least-squares analysis of treatment effect adjusted for blocks and covariates. The output consists of the estimate of treatment effect, the standard error (se) of the estimate, and a (1 – alpha) CI for the treatment effect. Additional output is discussed below.

To illustrate the computation procedure, we use a dataset that is in the file example.dat. It consists of 50 observations, 20 treated and 30 control, along with four covariates. The data were generated from a null model. In particular, the true treatment effect was set at 0. We set the first two responses to be outliers.

The following code computes the analyses. This code is in the file *batWwLl*. Note that everything to the right of the symbol # is treated as a comment.

```
library(Rfit) # Download this package at CRAN
source("VWrfit.r") # Driver
source("all.r") # auxiliary R functions.
# Data must be of the form [Y T 1 x1 ... xp]
# Y is the response
# T is treatment indicator, 1 for treatment, 0 for control
# 1 is a column of ones
# x1 ... xp are the covariates
data <- matrix(scan("example.dat"),ncol=7,byrow=T)
# Reads in the data set
# Computation of the 4 procedures. 1 - alpha is the confidence
interval coefficient;
# center = "Y" will center the covariates.
# The main call
results <- VWrfit(data, alpha=.05, center="N")
results # This prints out all the output
```

The routine *VWrfit* prints out the table of estimates, standard errors, and CIs for the four procedures. For the example, this table is:

|   | est | se | lcl | ucl | length.ci |
|---|---|---|---|---|---|
| W | 0.3600939 | 4.246699 | -7.9632837 | 8.683471 | 16.64676 |
| w | 0.6228362 | 5.389197 | -9.9397959 | 11.185468 | 21.12526 |
| L | 6.8611628 | 7.290582 | -7.4281152 | 21.150441 | 28.57856 |
| l | 15.2050244 | 7.255375 | 0.9847507 | 29.425298 | 28.44055 |

Both the block-adjusted (W) and the block- and covariate-adjusted *RW* (w) Wilcoxon analyses show no treatment effect at level 0.05 because their CIs contain 0. In contrast, the two outliers impaired the LS analyses. The LS estimates of treatment effect exceed the Wilcoxon estimates by a factor of 20 and, for the block and covariate adjusted LS analysis (*I*), the CI for the treatment effect does not contain 0. The empirical measure of efficiency of the *RW* (w) relative to the *l* analysis is 1.81, so for these data the Wilcoxon analysis is 181% more efficient than the LS analysis.

Additional output is found in the attributes. These are displayed by typing:

```
results$name where name is one of these quantities:
results$s.table displays the table of above results.
```

```
results$sdata displays the blocks and the matches.
results$X1 displays the design matrix for the block
    adjusted model
results$X2 displays the design matrix for the block and
    covariate adjusted model
results$sumwilx1 displays the table of regression coefficients
    for the block adjusted model
results$sumwilx2 displays the table of regression coefficients
    for the block and covariate adjusted model
```

We have placed the code in a zip file (kmh130614.tar.gz) that users can download at *http://www.stat.wmich.edu/mckean/kmh/*. This file contains the driver *VWrfit*, the auxiliary functions, the example dataset, the file *batWwLl* which the user can run in *R* batch form to compute the analysis on the example dataset, and the output, which is in *batWwLl.Rout*. The README file is essentially this section.

## REFERENCES

Abadie, A., & Imbens, G. W. (2006). Large sample properties of matching estimators for average treatment effects. *Econometrica, 74*, 235–267.

Bang, H., & Robins, J. M. (2005). Doubly robust estimation in missing data and causal inference models. *Biometrics, 61*, 964–973.

Crump, R. K., Hotz, V. J., Imbens, G. W., & Mitnik, O. A. (2009). Dealing with limited overlap in estimation of average treatment effects. *Biometrika, 96*, 187–199.

Dehejia, R. H., & Wahba, S. (2002). Propensity score-matching methods for nonexperimental causal studies. *Review of Economics and Statistics, 84*, 151–161.

Hernan, M. A., & Robins, J. M. (2006). Estimating causal effects from epidemiological data. *Journal of Epidemiological Community Health, 60*, 578–586.

Hettmansperger, T. J., & McKean, J. W. (2011). *Robust and nonparametric statistical methods* (2nd ed.). Boca Raton, FL: CRC Press (Chapman-Hall).

Hill, J., and Reiter, J. P. (2006). Interval estimation for treatment effects using propensity score matching. *Statistics in Medicine, 25*, 2230–2256.

Huitema, B. E. (2011). *The analysis of covariance and alternatives: Statistical methods for experiments, quasi-experiments, and single-case studies*. Hoboken, NJ: Wiley.

Imbens, G. W., & Wooldridge, J. M. (2009). Recent developments in the econometrics of program evaluation. *Journal of Economic Literature, 47*, 5–86.

Kloke, J. D., & McKean, J. W. (2012). Rfit: Rank-based estimation for linear models. *The R Journal, 4*, 57–64.

Kloke, J. D., & McKean, J. W. (2013). *Nonparametric statistical methods using R*. Boca Raton, FL: CRC Press (Chapman-Hall).

Kosten, S. F. (2010). *Robust interval estimation of a treatment effect in observational* studies using propensity score matching. Unpublished doctoral dissertation, Western Michigan University, Kalamazoo.

Kosten, S. F., McKean, J. W., & Huitema, B. E. (2014). Robust outcome analysis for observational studies designed using propensity score matching. Manuscript submitted for publication.

McKean, J. W. (2004). Robust analysis of linear models. *Statistical Science, 19,* 562–570.

McKean, J. W., & Sheather, S. J. (1991). Small sample properties of robust analyses of linear models based on R-estimates: A Survey. In W. Stahel & S. Weisberg (Eds.), *Directions in robust statistics and diagnostics* (Part II, pp. 1–19). New York: Springer-Verlag.

Robins, J. M., Hernan, M. A., & Bromback, B. (2000). Marginal structural models and causal inference in epidemiology. *Epidemiology, 11,* 550–560.

Rubin, D. B. (1979). Using multivariate matched sampling and regression adjustment to control bias in observational studies. *Journal of the American Statistical Association, 74,* 318–328.

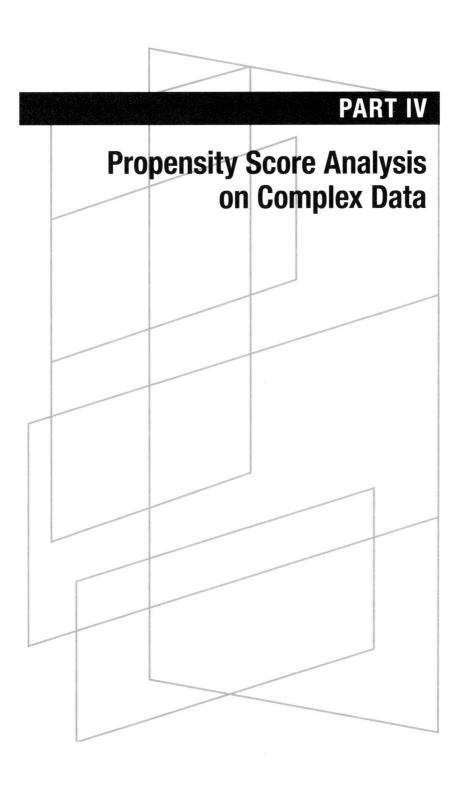

# PART IV

# Propensity Score Analysis on Complex Data

## CHAPTER 9

# Latent Growth Modeling of Longitudinal Data with Propensity-Score-Matched Groups

### Walter L. Leite

Studies of the effects of interventions commonly involve fitting latent growth models (Bollen & Curran, 2006; Duncan, Duncan, Strycker, Li, & Alpert, 2006) to secondary data from large longitudinal surveys. Datasets from longitudinal surveys are frequently used in other areas such as social, behavioral, health research, and educational studies. This chapter uses educational data to demonstrate the applications of propensity scores in latent growth modeling. Because using these secondary longitudinal datasets precludes random assignment of students to conditions, the estimates of effects of an educational intervention on growth trajectories are very vulnerable to selection bias due to prior systematic differences between groups exposed and not exposed to an intervention. In cross-sectional observational studies, commonly used propensity score methods to reduce selection bias include one-to-one matching, optimal full matching, stratification, and weighting (Austin, 2011; Stuart, 2010). The objective of this chapter is to demonstrate how to use propensity score matching with latent growth models to estimate treatment effects on individual growth trajectories. The latent growth model is a class of models within the structural equation modeling (SEM) framework that allows examination of changes in observed variables and/or latent variables (Leite, 2007) over time. In observational studies, latent growth models can be used to estimate the average treatment effect (ATE), average treatment effect on the treated (ATT) (Stuart, 2010), or other summaries of the treatment effect (Imbens, 2004).

Latent growth models have the advantage over analysis of covariance (ANCOVA), repeated-measures ANOVA, and multivariate analysis of variance (MANOVA) in estimating treatment effects in longitudinal studies because they provide greater power and allow flexible examination of the variance and covariances of the individual treatment effects (Curran & Muthén, 1999). As compared to growth curve models within the multilevel modeling framework (Goldstein, 2003; Raudenbush & Bryk, 2002; Snijders & Bosker, 2012), latent growth models have the advantage of allowing the growth trajectory in the absence of treatment to be freely estimated from the data (this will be demonstrated in the applied example in this chapter). Although this practice is exploratory as compared to testing a specific hypothesis about the growth trajectory in the absence of treatment, it minimizes model misfit due to incorrect specification of the growth trajectory, which could bias the treatment effect estimates.

In this chapter, we first overview the use of propensity score matching methods in longitudinal studies. More details about propensity score matching in general can be found in Chapters 1 and 4. Then, we present latent growth models that can be used to analyze a matched longitudinal dataset. Finally, we demonstrate the application of the models discussed with an applied example involving the examination of whether obtaining a general education diploma (GED) has an effect on the income growth of high school dropouts.

## PROPENSITY SCORE MATCHING IN LONGITUDINAL STUDIES

Propensity score matching for longitudinal studies can be accomplished by grouping individuals that received the treatment at some point during the study with similar individuals who were not exposed to the treatment at any point. The propensity score $e_{ij}(\mathbf{x}, \mathbf{v}) = pr_{ij}(z_j = 1 | x_1, \ldots, x_n, v_{1j}, \ldots, v_{nj})$ of a treatment $z$ administered at occasion $j$ to individual $i$ is estimated given time-invariant covariates $x_i, \ldots, x_n$ and time-varying covariates $v_{ij}, \ldots, v_{nj}$ measured prior to that treatment exposure. Propensity scores for each treatment occasion can be estimated with several methods such as logistic regression and data mining methods (McCaffrey, Ridgeway, & Morral, 2004; Setoguchi, Schneeweiss, Brookhart, Glynn, & Cook, 2008). (See Chapter 3 for more discussions of propensity score estimation.)

Once propensity scores are estimated, matching can be performed using different ratios (e.g., one-to-one, one-to-many) and algorithms (greedy, optimal, and genetic) (Gu & Rosenbaum, 1993; Rosenbaum, 1989; Sekhon, 2011). The analysis of matched samples may require the use of weights to account for matching with replacement, as well as weights to account for data collection with complex sampling designs, poststratification, and/or nonresponse adjustments (Hahs-Vaughn & Onwuegbuzie, 2006). With one-to-one matching without replacement, the outcomes of treated units (e.g., subjects) at each measurement occasion as well as the outcomes of matched individuals are assigned a weight of one, while the outcomes of unmatched units are assigned a weight of zero and dropped from the analysis. If one-to-one matching with replacement is performed, untreated units matched more than once receive a weight that is the inverse of the number of times matched. To use a caliper, which is a maximum distance within which matches are possible, untreated units outside of any caliper receive a weight of zero. Matching within calipers has been shown to improve matching performance, as well as enforce common support (Austin, 2009; Gu & Rosenbaum, 1993). When a caliper is used, treated units with no untreated units within their calipers as well as untreated units not within a caliper of a treated unit are dropped before weights are calculated.

The following equation can be used to obtain weights to estimate the ATT for all matching methods, including one-to-many matching with replacement:

$$w_i = z_i + (1 - z_i)\frac{n_M}{n_T}\sum_{l=1}^{n_{Ti}}\frac{1}{n_{Ml}} \tag{9.1}$$

where $z_i$ is a binary treatment indicator with a value of one if the unit $i$ was treated and zero otherwise. For treated units $w_i = 1$; for untreated units $n_{Ti}$ is the total number of treated units that untreated unit $i$ was matched to, and $n_{Ml}$ is the number of untreated units matched to treated unit $l$. $n_M$ is the total number of matched units, and $n_T$ is the total number of treated units.

In applications of propensity score methods to estimation of treatment effects in longitudinal observational studies, it is desirable to have at least one measurement of the outcome taken prior to any treatment exposure so that balance in the outcome distributions prior to treatment can be established between treated and matched groups. This is important because the outcome prior to treatment is frequently the strongest confounder in estimating the treatment effect. The following section presents three latent growth models that can be used to estimate treatment effects when a nonrandom sample of study participants is exposed to the treatment after a single measurement of the outcome is taken. Following treatment participation, multiple follow-up measurements are taken. Even though latent growth modeling has been frequently used with this research design, the use of latent growth models combined with propensity score methods to strengthen causal inference is still incipient. Extended versions of the latent growth models discussed here for observational longitudinal studies with multiple treated groups are discussed in Leite at al. (2012).

## THE MULTIPLE-GROUP LATENT GROWTH MODEL WITH A TREATMENT FACTOR

The multiple-group latent growth model with a treatment factor (MG-LGM-TF) fits latent growth models simultaneously to treated and matched groups. Muthén and Curran (1997) and Curran and Muthén (1999) proposed this model for single-treatment randomized studies, but it has not been widely applied. Tomarken and Waller (2005) discussed possible reasons for the scarcity of applications of SEM to experimental designs, and they point to sample size requirements of SEM as the most critical obstacle. Leite at al. (2012) recently extended Muthén and Curran's (1997) model to quasi-experimental designs, more specifically to propensity-score-matched designs with multiple-treatment occasions. Because quasi-experimental studies using propensity score matching commonly have large sample sizes, it is possible that Muthén and Curran's (1997) model will receive renewed interest in the academic community. Differently from Leite at al. (2012), here we discuss Muthén and Curran's (1997) model for a single treated and propensity-score-matched group, which is a more common design in the literature than designs with multiple-treatment groups.

A key component of the MG-LGM-TF is the determination of a normative growth trajectory for treatment and matched groups in the absence of treatment, which is defined by placing equality constraints on growth parameters across treatment and matched groups. The normative growth trajectory can be understood as the potential growth of the treatment group if it was not exposed to treatment. A latent factor is specified for the treatment group to capture the treatment effect, which corresponds to change in the scores over time in addition to the normative growth trajectory (Curran & Muthén, 1999; Muthén & Curran, 1997). This model falls into the class of additive growth models discussed by Hancock and Lawrence

(2006). Following Bollen and Curran's (2006) notation, the matrix form of MG-LGM-TF with two groups (i.e., treated and matched) is:

$$\begin{bmatrix} r_{1i} \\ r_{2i} \\ \vdots \\ r_{ji} \end{bmatrix} = \begin{bmatrix} 1 & 0 & \lambda_{21} \\ 1 & \lambda_{11} & \lambda_{22} \\ \vdots & \vdots & \vdots \\ 1 & \lambda_{1j} & \lambda_{2j} \end{bmatrix} \begin{bmatrix} \alpha_i \\ \beta_i \\ \delta_i \end{bmatrix} + \begin{bmatrix} \varepsilon_{1i} \\ \varepsilon_{2i} \\ \vdots \\ \varepsilon_{ji} \end{bmatrix} \quad (9.2)$$

where $i$ indexes individuals, $j$ indexes measurement waves, $r_{ji}$ are responses, $\alpha_i$ is the level factor, $\beta_i$ is the shape factor, and $\delta_i$ is the treatment effect factor. The loadings of the level factor are fixed to 1, $\lambda_{1i}$ are loadings of the shape factor, and $\lambda_{2i}$ are loadings of the treatment effect factor. The vector of means and covariance matrix of the level, shape, and treatment effect factors are

$$\mathbf{M} = \begin{bmatrix} \mu_\alpha \\ \mu_\beta \\ \mu_\delta^z \end{bmatrix}, \; \boldsymbol{\Phi} = \begin{bmatrix} \sigma_\alpha^2 & \sigma_{\alpha\beta} & \sigma_{\alpha\delta} \\ \sigma_{\alpha\beta} & \sigma_\beta^2 & \sigma_{\beta\delta} \\ \sigma_{\alpha\delta} & \sigma_{\beta\delta} & \sigma_\delta^2 \end{bmatrix} \quad (9.3)$$

To establish the normative growth trajectory, the means $\mu_\alpha$ and $\mu_\beta$, variances $\sigma_\alpha^2$ and $\sigma_\beta^2$, covariance $\sigma_{\alpha\beta}$ of the level and shape factors, and the residual variances $\sigma_{\varepsilon_i}^2$ must be constrained to equality across treatment and matched groups. The mean $\mu_\delta$ and variance $\sigma_\delta^2$ of the treatment factor should be fixed at zero for the matched group and freely estimated for the treated group. The covariances $\sigma_{\alpha\beta}$ and $\sigma_{\beta\delta}$ between the level and shape factors, respectively, as well as the treatment factor, should also be fixed at zero for the matched group.

The individual treatment effects are summarized by $\mu_\delta$, which can be the ATT, ATE, or another summary, depending on how matching was performed and observation weights were defined. $\mu_\delta$ is the mean of the treatment effect across all measurement occasions, but mean treatment effects at each specific time (e.g., ATT at wave three) can also be obtained by multiplying the factor loadings $[\lambda_{21}, \lambda_{22}, \ldots, \lambda_{2j}]$ and the treatment factor mean $\mu_\delta$.

The variance $\sigma_\delta^2$ of individual treatment effects is also an important summary because even when $\mu_\delta$ is zero, a large variance of the treatment effect could indicate that some individuals benefited from treatment, while others did not. The covariances between the treatment factor and the level and shape factor, which are freely estimated for the treated group, also have interesting interpretations: A significant $\sigma_{\alpha\delta}$ indicates whether the magnitude of the treatment effect is positively or negatively associated with the individual status of the outcome before treatment. A significant $\sigma_{\beta\delta}$ indicates that the amount of individual change during the study in the absence of treatment is related to how much they benefit from the treatment.

Latent growth models are commonly specified with a diagonal residual covariance matrix allowing heterogeneity of residual variances, but more complex residual covariance structures such as autoregressive and moving average should also be investigated (Sivo, Fan, & Witta, 2005). In the MG-LGM-TF, the residual covariance matrix should be constrained to equality across treated and matched groups to ensure that the only differences between groups are attributed to the treatment effect (see the example Mplus program in Appendices B–D).

The timing of exposure to treatment and hypotheses about change of treatment effects across time are defined by the vector of factor loadings $[\lambda_{21}, \lambda_{22}, \ldots, \lambda_{2j}]$ of the treatment factor. These loadings must be zero for outcomes measured prior to treatment exposure. Specific hypotheses about how treatment effect change over time can be tested by fixing factor loadings to specific patterns. A researcher can also freely estimate some factor loadings of the treatment factor to explore the direction of change in treatment effect over time.

## THE PARALLEL-PROCESS LATENT GROWTH MODEL WITH A TREATMENT FACTOR

Leite at al. (2012) proposed an extension of the parallel-process latent-growth model (Cheong, MacKinnon, & Khoo, 2003) or bivariate latent curve model (Bollen & Curran, 2006) to estimate the effects of multiple treatments in quasi-experimental studies using propensity score matching. Here we will discuss a special case of Leite at al.'s (2012) multiple-group parallel-process latent growth model where there is a single treated group: The parallel-process latent growth model with a treatment factor (PP-LGM-TF) is fit to a dataset where each unit is a treated/matched pair. Therefore, it requires that the dataset of outcomes is organized so that each row contains measurements of the outcome for a treated individual followed by measurements of the outcome for the corresponding matched individual. For example, if the outcome was measured in four occasions for each individual, each row will have eight values consisting of four observations for a treated individual and another four for the matched individual. The matrix form of the PP-LGM-TF is

$$\begin{bmatrix} r_{1mp} \\ r_{2mp} \\ \vdots \\ r_{jmp} \\ r_{1tp} \\ r_{2tp} \\ \vdots \\ r_{jtp} \end{bmatrix} = \begin{bmatrix} 1 & 0 & 0 & 0 & 0 \\ 1 & \lambda_{11} & 0 & 0 & 0 \\ \vdots & \vdots & \vdots & \vdots & 0 \\ 1 & \lambda_{1j} & 0 & 0 & 0 \\ 0 & 0 & 1 & 0 & \lambda_{12} \\ 0 & 0 & 1 & \lambda_{11} & \lambda_{22} \\ \vdots & \vdots & \vdots & \vdots & \vdots \\ 0 & 0 & 1 & \lambda_{1j} & \lambda_{2j} \end{bmatrix} \begin{bmatrix} \alpha_{mp} \\ \beta_{mp} \\ \alpha_{tp} \\ \beta_{tp} \\ \delta_{tp} \end{bmatrix} + \begin{bmatrix} \varepsilon_{1mp} \\ \varepsilon_{2mp} \\ \vdots \\ \varepsilon_{jmp} \\ \varepsilon_{1tp} \\ \varepsilon_{2tp} \\ \vdots \\ \varepsilon_{jtp} \end{bmatrix} \quad (9.4)$$

where $p$ indexes matched pairs, $j$ indicates measurement waves, $m$ indicates matched status, and $t$ indicates treated status. Similarly to the MG-LGM-TF, a normative growth trajectory in the absence of treatment can be established by imposing the constraints $\mu_{\alpha_m} = \mu_{\alpha_t}$, $\mu_{\beta_m} = \mu_{\beta_t}$, $\sigma^2_{\alpha_m} = \sigma^2_{\alpha_t}$, $\sigma^2_{\beta_m} = \sigma^2_{\beta_t}$, $\sigma_{\alpha_m \beta_m} = \sigma_{\alpha_{pt} \beta_{pt}}$. In addition, if a diagonal residual covariance matrix is specified, the constraints $\sigma^2_{\varepsilon_{jm}} = \sigma^2_{\varepsilon_{jt}}$ should also be imposed. Similar constraints across parameters for matched and treated observations should be applied to nonzero elements of the residual covariance matrix if a nondiagonal residual covariance matrix is specified. Similarly to the MG-LGM-TF, the treatment effect factor $\delta_{tp}$ is summarized by $\mu_\delta$ and $\sigma^2_\delta$, while the loadings $[\lambda_{12}, \lambda_{22}, \ldots, \lambda_{2j}]$ of the treatment effect factor specify the timing of initiation and hypothesized change trajectory of the treatment effect. The products of the loadings of the treatment factor and $\mu_\delta$ quantify the mean of the treatment effect (e.g., ATT, ATE) at each specific time.

## THE LATENT GROWTH MODEL WITH A DUMMY TREATMENT INDICATOR (LGM-DTI)

In the latent growth model with a dummy treatment indicator (LGM-DTI), the treatment effects for each measurement occasion are the estimates of the path coefficients from a dummy-coded treatment indicator $z_i$ to the outcomes. The normative growth trajectory is defined by a common shape factor for both treated and matched individuals. The LGM-DTI is

$$\begin{bmatrix} r_{1i} \\ r_{2i} \\ \vdots \\ r_{ji} \end{bmatrix} = \begin{bmatrix} 1 & \lambda_1 \\ 1 & \lambda_2 \\ \vdots & \vdots \\ 1 & \lambda_j \end{bmatrix} \begin{bmatrix} \alpha_i \\ \beta_i \end{bmatrix} + \begin{bmatrix} \gamma_1 \\ \gamma_2 \\ \vdots \\ \gamma_j \end{bmatrix} z_i + \begin{bmatrix} \varepsilon_{1i} \\ \varepsilon_{2i} \\ \vdots \\ \varepsilon_{ji} \end{bmatrix} \quad (9.5)$$

The coefficients $\gamma_1, \gamma_2, \ldots, \gamma_j$ capture the treatment effect (e.g., ATT, ATE) at multiple measurement waves and allow flexible changes of the treatment effect across time. These coefficients should be constrained to zero for measurements that occurred prior to treatment implementation. For example, if individuals are treated between waves one and two, then $\gamma_1$ should be constrained to zero. If the coefficients $\gamma_1, \gamma_2, \ldots, \gamma_j$ are proportional to the loadings of the shape factor $\lambda_1, \lambda_2, \ldots, \lambda_j$ for corresponding measurement waves, then the LGM-DTI can be simplified by having a single path from $z_i$ to $\beta_i$. Details about how a longitudinal growth model with a treatment effect on the slope as a special case of the model shown in Equation 9.5 are provided by Stoel, van den Wittenboer, and Hox (2004). A likelihood ratio test can be used to compare the two models. For example, if a linear latent growth model with $z_i$ predicting the slope is found to fit similarly (i.e., a nonsignificant likelihood ratio test) to a linear version of the LGM-DTI, a researcher can conclude that the treatment effect changes linearly across time.

## DEMONSTRATION

In this section, public-access data from the 1997 National Longitudinal Survey of Youth (NLSY97) will be used to estimate the ATT of obtaining the GED on earnings of high school dropouts. Simple comparison of average wages of high school dropouts and terminal GED recipients (i.e., those who did not attend college) is not appropriate because these populations differ with respect to many variables that also related to future wages (Heckman, Humphries, & Mader, 2010). Therefore, propensity score matching was used in this example to balance confounding variables across GED recipients and nonrecipients. The ATT of GED on earnings over a 4-year period was estimated with versions of the latent growth models presented above. Differently from the research reviewed by Heckman at al. (2010), we will focus on evaluating the immediate effects of the GED during the short period of four years after certification.

### Method

#### Sample

We obtained a sample of 777 high school dropouts from the NLSY97 who either did not obtain a GED or obtained a GED but never pursued higher education. Individuals who obtained the GED and then obtained an associate's degree or higher were not included in the sample. From the total sample, 175 (22.5%) obtained the GED, where 49 were certified at age 18, 59 at age 19, 45 at age 20, and 22 at age 21. The remaining 602 sample members did not obtain the GED by age 24. For this sample, we used NLSY97 data collected from 1997 to 2010. It is important to note that the NLSY97 sample was obtained by combining two complex stratified multistage area probability samples where the second sample oversampled black and Hispanic individuals (U.S. Bureau of Labor Statistics, 2014). Therefore, the use of sampling weights is recommended to adjust estimates and standard errors for the effects of oversampling, differences in response rates, and attrition. In implementations of propensity score matching to complex samples, sampling weights should be included in propensity score estimation, matching process, and treatment effect estimation. Not all implementations of matching algorithms can account for sampling weights. The genetic algorithm proposed by Sekhon (2011) used in this chapter can accommodate sampling weights.

This demonstration does not use sampling weights because the PP-LGM-TF uses matched pairs as the unit of analysis and cannot incorporate individual weights. With the MG-LGM-TF and the LGM-DTI, sampling weights can be used in model estimation using pseudo-maximum likelihood estimation for continuous outcomes and weighted least-squares estimation for categorical outcomes (Asparouhov, 2005). Both are available in the Mplus software but are not used in this example to keep consistency of estimation method across models.

## Outcomes

The outcomes of the latent growth model analyses were 5 years of income measures for each individual, collected when participants were 17 to 24 years old. For GED recipients, the five outcome measurements consist of one measurement prior to obtaining the GED and four measurements after the award. Non-GED recipients were propensity score matched to GED recipients based on their characteristics at a single year (see description of matching procedures later in this chapter), and therefore their five outcomes analyzed were from the year they were matched and the following four years.

In the NLSY97, participants were asked to report their total income. For this question, there were 11–24% of missing data across measurement waves, which included participants who provided "Don't know" responses. However, for these responses, the next question asked participants to estimate income based on seven categories: (1) $1 to $5,000, (2) $5,001 to

$10,000, (3) $10,001 to $25,000, (4) $25,001 to $50,000, (5) $50,001 to $100,000, (6) $100,001 to $250,000, and (7) More than $250,000. After categorizing the continuous income data obtained with the first question using the same thresholds of the second question, and combining with the responses to the second question, percentages of missing data across measurement waves were between 1.9 and 3.9%. Therefore, latent growth model analyses presented here used ordinal outcomes obtained from combining two questions about income. Also, Category 7 was deleted because it had no responses, and the single response in Category 6 was recoded to Category 5. The remaining 41 missing values were imputed once using the *mice* package (Van Buuren & Oudshoorn, 2000) in R. Multiple imputation has been shown to perform better than single imputation because it preserves variability in the dataset (Peugh & Enders, 2004), but in this example analysis, we chose single imputation of the outcome because of its simpler implementation (i.e., combining imputed datasets is not needed) and the percentage of missing data was small.

## Covariates

We used propensity score matching to balance differences between GED participants and non-participants in 42 time-invariant covariates and 10 time-varying covariates[1] measured in the year prior to the year when GED completion was reported. Confounding variables to be balanced were selected based on results from prior studies about differences between the population of high school dropouts and GED recipients (Heckman et al., 2010; Ou, 2008). The covariates balanced included cognitive measures such as Armed Services Vocational Aptitude Battery (ASVAB) scores and best grades in high school, demographic variables such as age, gender and ethnicity, family variables such as the index of family routines and family income, measures of delinquency behavior such as drug use, gang membership, criminal acts and arrests, high school behavior (e.g., absences, fights, suspensions), and income prior to GED certification. Missing data in the covariates were imputed once using information from all covariates with the method of multivariate imputation by chained equations implemented by the mice package (Van Buuren & Oudshoorn, 2000) in the R statistical software. We did not use multiple imputation for the covariates because its main advantage over single imputation—namely, the preservation of variability in the dataset, which in turn results in adequate estimation of standard errors (Peugh & Enders, 2004)—is not related to obtaining propensity scores. However, there has been little research comparing missing data methods for treatment effect estimation with propensity score methods (see Mitra & Reiter, 2012, for a related study). Also, see Chapter 12 for more discussions on this topic.

Propensity Score Analysis

Given that the dataset had 10 time-varying covariates, it was possible that an untreated individual was not a good match for a certain GED recipient at one age, but was the best match for that GED recipient at a different age. In order to allow for untreated individuals to be considered for matching at multiple ages, a long-format longitudinal file was created where there was one row for each GED recipient with time-invariant and time-varying covariates measured at the year prior to GED award and four rows for each non-GED recipient, each with time-invariant and time-varying covariates measured at a different age from 17 to 20 years old. Therefore, four propensity scores were estimated for each non-GED recipient, which differ due to change in time-varying covariates. This strategy created 602 × 4 = 2,408 possible matches for the 175 GED recipients. Having a large ratio of untreated to treated has been shown to be a key factor in improving matching performance (Gu & Rosenbaum, 1993). Propensity scores were obtained using a logistic regression model including 42 time-invariant and 10 time-varying covariates, with standard errors corrected for the effects of clustering (i.e., four observations per non-GED recipient), which was estimated with the *svyglm* function of the *survey* package in the R statistical software. Alternative approaches to estimate the propensity scores for these data are multilevel logistic regression (Leite, Jimenez, Kaya, Sandbach, & MacInnes, 2012, May) and a separate logistic regression model per age group (Leite et al., 2012).

One-to-one propensity score matching within a 0.25 standard deviation caliper was performed using Diamond and Sekhon's genetic matching algorithm (Diamond & Sekhon, 2005, July), implemented by the *Matching* package (Sekhon, 2011) in the R statistical software. Although the matching algorithm selected units without replacement, in this example we had four propensity scores per non-GED recipient, which allowed the same untreated individual to be used as a match to more than one treated individual, but at different measurement waves. This resulted in 23 non-GED recipients matched twice and two matched three times. The models to estimate the ATT accounted for the clustering effect produced by the matching method (see the next section). The enforcement of a caliper resulted in four treated observations being dropped due to lack of common support (i.e., there was no untreated observation within their calipers). Although dropping treated observations implies reduction of the generalizability of the ATT, in this case the loss of observations was small.

Covariate balance after matching was evaluated by obtaining the standardized differences between means (for continuous variables) or proportions (for categorical variables) between treated and matched groups on the covariates included in the propensity score model, with the *twang* package in R (Ridgeway, McCaffrey, Morral, Burgette, & Griffin, 2013). The maximum covariate difference after matching was 0.150 standard deviations, which was considered adequate for this example, but a stricter 0.1 standard deviation criterion for adequate balance has been recommended (Austin, 2011). The R code for propensity score estimation, genetic propensity score matching, and covariate balance evaluation is shown in Code A in the Software section of this chapter.

### Latent Growth Modeling

The MG-LGM-TF, PP-LGM-TF, and LGM-DTI were fit to 5 years of ordinal income data from the NLSY97 to estimate the ATT of GED certification, using Mplus 7.11 (Muthén & Muthén, 2013). We chose to fit three different models to demonstrate that they provide similar results, but specific advantages and disadvantages of each model as compared to each other are presented in the Conclusion section. Parameter estimation was performed with normal-theory robust maximum likelihood (MLR) estimation treating the ordinal outcomes as continuous, which has been shown to perform well if the number of categories is five or larger (Rhemtulla, Brosseau-Liard, & Savalei, 2012). Taylor-series linearization was used to obtain standard errors (Stapleton, 2006) in Mplus (i.e., the ANALYSIS command had TYPE = complex) to account for the clustering effects produced by allowing non-GED recipients to be matches at multiple years.

The three latent growth models were specified with the normative growth trajectory freely estimated, which was accomplished by setting the loading of the first outcome on the shape factor to zero and the loading of the last outcome to one, but freely estimating the other loadings. Setting the last loading to one has the advantage of allowing the interpretation of the other nonzero loadings as proportions of the total growth between the first and last measurement waves. This specification is the most flexible and does not test any specific hypothesis about the normative growth trajectory, such as a hypothesis that growth is linear in the absence of treatment. Alternatives to this specification would be to fix the loadings of the shape factor to values that corresponded to a hypothesized normative growth trajectory.

The models were also specified with freely estimated change trajectory of treatment effects over time. In the MG-LGM-TF and PP-LGM-TF, this was accomplished by setting the loading of the first outcome on the treatment factor to zero and the loading of the second outcome to one, but freely estimating the other loadings. This specification has the advantage of allowing the mean of the treatment factor to be interpreted as an immediate effect, while the freely estimated loadings of the treatment factor indicate how the treatment effect changes over time. In the LGM-DTI, path coefficients between the dummy treatment indicator and the outcomes were freely estimated, which allows capturing change of treatment effects across time. Alternatives to these model specifications would be to constrain or fix the loadings of the treatment factor in the MG-LGM-TF and PP-LGM-TF or constrain the path coefficients of the dummy treatment indicator in the LGM-DTI in ways that would impose a specific hypothesis about change in the treatment effect over time. For example, constraining these parameter estimates to equality for all post-treatment outcomes would allow evaluation of the hypothesis that the treatment effect is constant over time. The LGM-DTI provides ATT estimates at each postimplementation measurement wave, while with the MG-LGM-TF and PP-LGM-TF, these ATT estimates were obtained by multiplying the treatment factor loadings by the treatment factor mean with the MODEL CONSTRAINT: command in Mplus (see Codes B–D in the Software section of this chapter). Estimates of the ATT were tested for significance with a Wald test, while estimates of the variance of the treatment factor and covariances of the treatment factor with the level and shape factors were tested with the Satorra–Bentler adjusted chi-square difference test (Satorra & Bentler, 1994).

## Results

Evaluation of model fit across the multiple specifications of the MG-LGM-DTI, PP-LGM, and LGM-DTI was performed using the chi-square test at alpha = .05, and fit indices (i.e., root mean square error of approximation ≤ .08, confirmatory fit index ≥ .90, Tucker–Lewis index ≥ .90, standardized root mean square residual ≤ .10). The chi-square statistic did not support the exact fit of the MG-LGM-TF ($\chi^2$ (20) = 0.034, $p < .05$) but it is not significant for the PP-LGM-TF ($\chi^2$ (41) = 49.849, $p > .05$) and the LGM-DTI ($\chi^2$ (8) = 8.861, $p > .05$). However, all the fit indices examined indicate close fit of the three models to the data (see Table 9.1).

**TABLE 9.1. Model-Fit Information**

| Model | $\chi^2(df)$ p-value | RMSEA $p \leq .05$ | CFI | TLI | SRMR |
|---|---|---|---|---|---|
| MG-LGM-TF | 33.018 (20) 0.034 | 0.062 0.278 | 0.943 | 0.943 | 0.070 |
| PP-LGM | 49.849 (41) 0.162 | 0.036 0.749 | 0.963 | 0.959 | 0.063 |
| LGM-DTI | 8.861 (8) 0.929 | 0.018 0.817 | 0.996 | 0.993 | 0.025 |

Note. RMSEA, root mean square error of approximation; CFI, confirmatory fit index; TLI, Tucker–Lewis index; SRMR, standardized root mean square residual.

Figure 9.1 is a diagram of the model specification for the group of GED recipients in the MG-LGM-TF, with only statistically significant parameter estimates presented. In this diagram, alpha, beta, and delta are the level, shape, and treatment factors, respectively. The means of factors are indicated within the circles, and the variances are on the left side of the circles. The factor loadings of the shape factor [0.000 0.424 0.823 0.964 1.000] show that the normative growth trajectory is approximately linear until wave three, then decelerates from wave three to wave five. Figure 9.1 only shows two factor loadings of the treatment factor because the loading of $r_2$ was fixed to one and the loading of $r_3$ was statistically significant, but not the loadings of $r_4$ and $r_5$. Table 9.2 shows the estimated ATT of obtaining the GED at each measurement time. Because the treatment factor loading of $r_2$ is 1, the ATT of the second measurement (i.e., −0.193, $p < .05$) is equal to the mean of the treatment factor. The treatment effect was of similar magnitude at the third measurement (−0.208, $p < .05$) but was nonsignificant at the fourth and fifth measurements. The variance of the treatment factor and its covariances with the level and shape factors were not statistically significant ($\chi^2(3) = 3.045$, $p = 0.3847$), indicating no variability in the effect of GED across individuals.

Figure 9.2 shows the diagram for the PP-LGM-TF with statistically significant coefficients. The loadings [0.000 0.421 0.813 0.959 1.000] of the two identical-shape factors for treated and untreated observations indicate a nonlinear normative growth trajectory very similar to the one estimated with the M-LGM-TF. Table 9.2 shows that the ATT of the GED was only statistically significant at the second measurement (−0.187, $p < .05$) and third measurement (−0.200, $p < .05$). A chi-square difference test indicated that the variance of the treatment factor and its covariances with

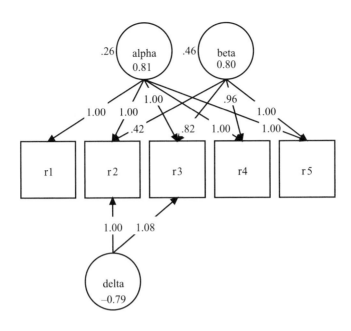

**FIGURE 9.1.** MG-LGM-TF for group of GED recipients.

**TABLE 9.2. Parameter Estimates Describing the ATT**

|  | MG-LGM-TF | PP-LGM-TF | LGM-DTI |
|---|---|---|---|
| Year 2 | **−0.193** | **−0.187** | **−0.197** |
|  | (0.086) | (0.086) | (0.093) |
| Year 3 | **−0.208** | **−0.200** | −0.173 |
|  | (0.101) | (0.095) | (0.114) |
| Year 4 | −0.041 | −0.034 | −0.044 |
|  | (0.103) | (0.094) | (0.720) |
| Year 5 | −0.55 | −0.050 | −0.032 |
|  | (0.084) | (0.089) | (0.805) |
| Mean of treatment factor | **−0.193** | **−0.187** | — |
|  | (0.086) | (0.086) |  |
| Variance of treatment factor | 0.135 | 0.129 | — |
|  | (0.142) | (0.146) |  |
| Correlation of intercept and treatment factor | −0.080 | −0.082 | — |
|  | (0.071) | (0.075) |  |
| Correlation of shape and treatment factors | −0.036 | −0.034 | — |
|  | (0.120) | (0.125) |  |

*Note.* Standard errors are in parentheses. Statistically significant coefficients at alpha = .05 are in **bold**.

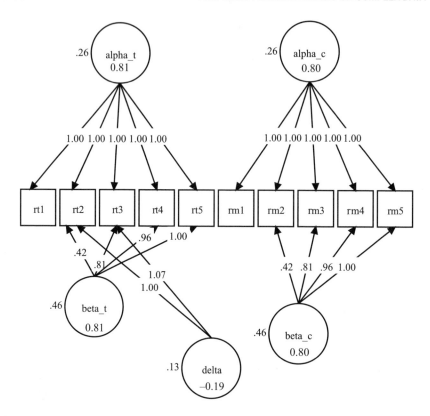

**FIGURE 9.2.** The PP-LGM-TF.

the level and shape factors of the treated group were not statistically significant ($\chi^2(3) = 3.143$, $p = 0.3701$).

Figure 9.3 presents the diagram for the LGM-DTI. The loadings of the normative growth trajectory [0.000 0.417 0.801 0.970 1.000] obtained with this model also agree closely with the other two models. However, with the LGM-DTI only the ATT at the second wave was significant ($-0.197$, $p < .05$) but not the ATT at waves 3 to 5.

With all models, there was a significant negative effect of obtaining a GED on income at the first year after award (i.e., the second measurement wave), indicating that GED recipients earned less than nonrecipients on the first year after certification. The MG-LGM-TF and the PP-LGM-TF also identified significant negative effects on income at the third measurement wave. This can be explained by job transition difficulties: GED recipients may experience a transition period after obtaining the GED where they are searching for a career opportunity, while nonrecipients maintain previous

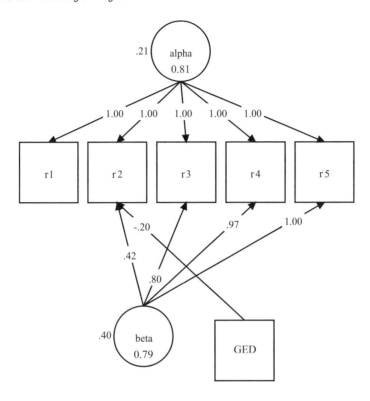

**FIGURE 9.3.** The LGM-DTI.

employment. After two years, there were no significant differences in income between GED recipients and nonrecipients with any of the models estimated.

## CONCLUSION

All three latent growth models combined with propensity score matching provide similar estimates of the treatment effect. Although this indicates that a researcher could use any of the three models, the MG-LGM-TF is the most flexible and should be preferred, for reasons that will be detailed here. The PP-LGM-TF and the LGM-DTI should only be considered in situations where the MG-LGM-TF fails to converge or results in an improper solution (e.g., negative variances or correlations of absolute value larger than one) (Chen, Bollen, Paxton, Curran, & Kirby, 2001), assuming that the requirements of these two models are met.

Because the MG-LGM-TF is a multiple-group model, it is more likely to have more convergence and improper solution problems than the PP-LGM-TF and the LGM-DTI. In a simulation study of the MG-LGM-TF with random assignment of individuals to treatments, Pitts (1999) found that improper solutions only occurred with the MG-LGM-TF but not with single-group models. Also, nonconvergence and improper solutions were more common with small sample sizes or when the ratio of the sample sizes of the two groups is small. This finding suggests that MG-LGM-TF used with one-to-one matching, as was done in this study, may be more likely to converge than with one-to-many matching, because the latter would cause imbalance in group sample sizes.

The MG-LGM-TF and the PP-LGM-TF represent the treatment effect as a latent factor, and thus allow examination of the variance of individual treatment effects and the covariances between treatment effect, level, and shape factors. These parameters can have interesting interpretations for applied researchers (Curran & Muthén, 1999). In contrast, the LGM-DTI only estimates fixed treatment effects (i.e., path coefficients corresponding to the ATT at each time). Therefore, this is a major limitation of the LGM-DTI as compared to both the MG-LGM-TF and the PP-LGM-TF. Furthermore, the LGM-DTI assumes that the treatment and control groups have equal variances of the intercept and normative growth shape, and that the treatment affects means but not variances. Using an additive latent growth model that is a special case of the LGM-DTI discussed here, Pitts (1999) showed that when this assumption is violated, the chi-square goodness-of-fit test fails to indicate any problem. The MG-LGM-TF and the PP-LGM-TF do not make this assumption. However, the PP-LGM-TF is much more limited than the MG-LGM-TF and LGM-DTI in terms of the types of propensity score methods that can be used. Because the PP-LGM-TF requires pairing of units, it is only suited for use with one-to-one matching, while the MG-LGM-TF and the LGM-DTI can be used with any type of propensity score matching, stratification, or weighting method. Given the limitations of the LGM-DTI and PP-LGM-TF, the MG-LGM-TF emerges as the recommended model to combine with propensity score matching for estimation of treatment effects in longitudinal observational studies.

Additional methodological work is needed with respect to comparing the three models discussed in this chapter with respect to power. In a simulation study of latent growth models for multiple propensity-score-matched groups, which are more general versions of the models presented here, Leite et al. (2012) found no difference in power between models. However, Pitts (1999) compared the MG-LGM-TF with a restricted version of the LGM-DTI (i.e., one that assumes that the treatment effect changes over time proportional to the change in normative growth trajectory) and found that the MG-LGM-TF allowed higher power than the LGM-DTI.

Because they define the treatment effect as a latent factor, the MG-LGM-TF and PP-LGM-TF require longitudinal studies with a larger number of measurement occasions than the LGM-DTI. With five measurement occasions, the MG-LGM-TF and PP-LGM-TF are overidentified without any constraints in the covariance matrix of the growth and treatment factors, and with a diagonal residual covariance matrix allowing heterogeneity of residual variances. With four measurement occasions, it will be necessary to impose an additional constraint to obtain model overidentification. In contrast, the LGM-DTI can be used with two measurements (i.e., pre–post designs) or three measurements (i.e., pre–post–post designs). Within the structural equation modeling framework, other models not discussed in this chapter have been proposed to estimate treatment effects in short longitudinal experimental studies. For example, Mun, von Eye, and White (2009) proposed a structural equation model for pre–post–post designs, while McArdle and Prindle (2008) presented a latent change score model for pre–post designs. These models could also be used with propensity score methods to estimate treatment effects in observational studies.

## SOFTWARE

### A. R Code for ps Estimation, Matching and Covariate Balance Evaluation

```
# Fit logistic regression model to estimate Propensity scores
ps.model.GED = glm(formula(long.data[,c(75,1:44,46,48:52,58,62,
      63)]), data = long.data, family=binomial)
#Extract propensity scores
ps = fitted(ps.model.GED)
long.data$ps = ps
# Perform 1 to 1 genetic matching without replacement
library(Matching) #Load required library
match.genetic.1.1 = GenMatch(Tr=long.data$GED, X =
      long.data$ps, fit.func = "qqmax.max", estimand = "ATT",
      M=1, pop.size = 1000, replace = F, ks = F, nboots=0,
      MemoryMatrix = F, exact = F, ties = F, verbose=T,
      paired = F, caliper = 0.25)
# Assess covariate balance
library(twang) #Load required library
balance.table = bal.stat(data=long.data[c(match.genetic.1.1
      $matches[,1], match.genetic.1.1$matches[,2]),], vars =
      names (long.data[,c(2:44,46,48:52,58,62,63)]),
      treat.var = "GED", w.all = 1, sampw = 1, estimand =
      "ATT", multinom = F)
```

```
balance.table = balance.table$results #obtain table with
    balance measures
summary(balance.table$std.eff.sz)
```

## B. Mplus code for the MG-LGM-TF

```
TITLE:
Growth model of earnings for the NLSY97;
DATA:
FILE IS data.csv;
VARIABLE:
names are group id r1-r5;
usevariables are r1-r5;
grouping is group (0=noGED 1=GED); !Identify treatment and
    control groups
cluster is id; !Some individuals were matched more than once,
    but at different years
ANALYSIS:
type=complex; !Request design based analysis to account for
    clustering effects
estimator=mlr; !Request robust maximum likelihood estimation
MODEL:
!specify the level and shape factors
!some loadings are freely estimated to allow nonlinear
    normative growth trajectory
alpha beta | r1@0 r2* r3* r4* r5@1;
!specify treatment effect factor
!labels are used for free the factor loadings to allow
    calculation of time specific effect
delta BY r1@0 r2@1
    r3(L3)*
    r4(L4)*
    r5(L5)*;
model GED: !model for GED recipients (only the parts that are
    different from overall model)
[delta](MT); !treatment factor mean
delta*; !treatment factor variance
delta with alpha* beta*; !covariance between treatment factor
    and level and
shape factors
!constraints are placed in the parameters below to enforce
    normative growth trajectory
[alpha](i1);
[beta](s1);
alpha (vi1);
beta (vs1);
alpha with beta (c1);
```

```
r1(e1);
r2(e2);
r3(e3);
r4(e4);
r5(e5);
model noGED: !model for matched group of non-recipients of GED
!treatment factor parameters are constrained to zero.
[delta@0];
delta@0;
delta with alpha@0 beta@0;
!constraints are placed in the parameters below to enforce
      normative growth trajectory
[alpha](i1);
[beta](s1);
alpha (vi1);
beta (vs1);
alpha with beta (c1);
r1(e1);
r2(e2);
r3(e3);
r4(e4);
r5(e5);
model constraint: !this section calculates the time-specific
      treatment effects for times 3, 4 and 5
!the treatment effect for time 2 is equal to the treatment
      factor mean.
new(EFF3 EFF4 EFF5);
EFF3 = L3*MT; !effect at time 3
EFF4 = L4*MT; !effect at time 4
EFF5 = L5*MT; !effect at time 5
 OUTPUT:
standardized TECH1 TECH4;
```

## C. Mplus Code for the PP-LGM-TF

```
TITLE:
parallel_process LGM analrsis with matched groups
DATA:
FILE IS parallel_process_matched_data_for_mplus.csv;
VARIABLE:
NAMES ARE idtreat idmatch agetreat agematch
      rt1-rt5
      rm1-rm5;   !there are outcomes for treatment and matched
                  pairs.
USEVARIABLES = rt1-rt5
      rm1-rm5;
cluster = idmatch; !Some individuals were matched more than
      once, but at different years
```

```
ANALYSIS:
TYPE = complex;  !request design based analysis to account for
     cluster effects estimator=mlr; !Request robust maximum
     likelihood estimation
MODEL:
!specify level and shape factors and nonlinear normative growth
     trajectory for matched units.
alpha_c beta_c | rm1@0 rm2* rm3* rm4* rm5@1;
!specify level and shape factors and nonlinear normative growth
     trajectory for treated units.
alpha_t beta_t | rt1@0 rt2* rt3* rt4* rt5@1;
!Place constrains in the shape factor loadings to define
     normative growth trajectory
beta_c by rm1@0
     rm2*(nl1)
     rm3* (nl2)
     rm4*(nl3)
     rm5@1;
beta_t by rt1@0
     rt2* (nl1)
     rt3* (nl2)
     rt4*(nl3)
     rt5@1;
!define loadings of the treatment effect factor.
delta BY rt1@0 rt2@1
     rt3* (L3)
     rt4* (L4)
     rt5* (L5);
delta; !variance of the treatment effect factor
delta with alpha_c@0 beta_c@0; !covariances of treatment effect
     factor with level and shape
[delta] (MT); !mean of the treatment effect factor
!put constraints in growth parameters to enforce normative
     growth trajectory
[alpha_c](i1);
[beta_c](s1);
[alpha_t](i1);
[beta_t](s1);
alpha_c (vi1);
beta_c (vs1);
alpha_t (vi1);
beta_t (vs1);
alpha_c with beta_c (c11);
alpha_t with beta_t (c11);
rt1 rm1 (e1);
rt2 rm2 (e2);
rt3 rm3 (e3);
rt4 rm4 (e4);
rt5 rm5 (e5);
```

```
model constraint: !calculate the treatment effect at times 3, 4
    and 5
new(EFF3 EFF4 EFF5);
EFF3 = L3*MT; !effect at time 3
EFF4 = L4*MT; !effect at time 4
EFF5 = L5*MT; !effect at time 5
OUTPUT:
standardized TECH1;
```

## D. Mplus Code for the LGM-DTI

```
TITLE:
growth model of earnings for the NLSY97;
DATA:
FILE IS multigroup_matched_data_for_mplus.csv;
VARIABLE:
names are GED id r1-r5;
usevariables are GED r1-r5;
cluster is id; !Some individuals were matched more than once,
    but at different rears
ANALYSIS:
TYPE = complex; !request design based analysis to account for
    cluster effects estimator=mlr; !Request robust maximum
    likelihood estimation
MODEL:
!specify the level and shape factors
!some loadings are freely estimated to allow nonlinear
    normative growth trajectory
alpha beta | r1@0 r2* r3* r4* r5@1;
r2-r5 on GED; !Specify treatment effects at each time
OUTPUT:
standardized TEC
```

### NOTE

1. A complete list of covariates used in this example can found at the author's website (*http://education.ufl.edu/leite*).

### REFERENCES

Asparouhov, T. (2005). Sampling weights in latent variable modeling. *Structural Equation Modeling, 13*, 411–434.

Austin, P. C. (2009). The relative ability of different propensity score methods to balance measured covariates between treated and untreated subjects in observational studies. *Medical Decision Making, 29*, 661–677.

Austin, P. C. (2011). An introduction to propensity score methods for reducing the effects of confounding in observational studies. *Multivariate Behavioral Research, 46,* 399–424.

Bollen, K. A., & Curran, P. J. (2006). *Latent curve models: A structural equation perspective.* Hoboken, NJ: Wiley.

Chen, F., Bollen, K. A., Paxton, P., Curran, P. J., & Kirby, J. B. (2001). Improper solutions in structural equation models: Causes, consequences, and strategies. *Sociological Methods and Research, 29,* 468–508.

Cheong, J., MacKinnon, D. P., & Khoo, S. T. (2003). Investigation of mediational processes using parallel process latent growth curve modeling. *Structural Equation Modeling, 10,* 238–262.

Curran, P. J., & Muthén, B. O. (1999). Application of latent curve analysis to testing developmental theories in intervention research. *American Journal of Community Psychology, 27,* 567.

Diamond, A., & Sekhon, J. S. (2005, July). *Genetic matching for estimating causal effects: A general multivariate matching method for achieving balance in observational studies.* Paper presented at the Political Methodology Summer Conference, Tallahassee, FL.

Duncan, T. E., Duncan, S. C., Strycker, L. A., Li, F., & Alpert, A. (2006). *An introduction to latent variable growth curve modeling: Concepts, issues, and applications* (2nd ed.). Mahwah, NJ: Erlbaum.

Goldstein, H. (2003). *Multilevel statistical models.* New York: Halsted.

Gu, X. S., & Rosenbaum, P. R. (1993). Comparison of multivariate matching methods: Structures, distances, and algorithms. *Journal of Computational and Graphical Statistics, 2,* 405–420.

Hahs-Vaughn, D. L., & Onwuegbuzie, A. J. (2006). Estimating and using propensity score analysis with complex samples. *Journal of Experimental Education, 75,* 31–65.

Hancock, G. R., & Lawrence, F. R. (2006). Using latent growth models to evaluate longitudinal change. In G. R. Hancock & R. O. Mueller (Eds.), *Structural equation modeling: A second course* (pp. 171–196). Greenwich, CT: Information Age Publishing.

Heckman, J. J., Humphries, J. E., & Mader, N. S. (2010). The GED. *NBER Working Paper series.* Cambridge, MA: National Bureau of Economic Research.

Imbens, G. W. (2004). Nonparametric estimation of average treatment effects under exogeneity: A review. *Review of Economics and Statistics, 86,* 4–29.

Leite, W. L. (2007). A comparison of latent growth models for constructs measured by multiple items. *Structural Equation Modeling, 14,* 581–610.

Leite, W. L., Jimenez, F., Kaya, Y., Sandbach, R., & MacInnes, J. W. (2012, May). *A comparison of propensity score methods for the estimation of treatment effects with multilevel observational data.* Paper presented at the Modern Modeling Methods Conference, Storrs, CT.

Leite, W. L., Sandbach, R., Jin, R., MacInnes, J. W., & Jackman, M. G. (2012). An evaluation of latent growth models for propensity score matched groups. *Structural Equation Modeling: A Multidisciplinary Journal, 19*, 437–456.

McArdle, J. J., & Prindle, J. J. (2008). A latent change score analysis of a randomized clinical trial in reasoning training. *Psychology and Aging, 23*, 702–719.

McCaffrey, D. F., Ridgeway, G., & Morral, A. R. (2004). Propensity score estimation with boosted regression for evaluating causal effects in observational studies. *Psychological Methods, 9*, 403–425.

Mitra, R., & Reiter, J. P. (2012). A comparison of two methods of estimating propensity scores after multiple imputation. *Statistical Methods in Medical Research*.

Mun, E. Y., von Eye, A., & White, H. R. (2009). An SEM approach for the evaluation of intervention effects using pre–post–post designs. *Structural Equation Modeling: A Multidisciplinary Journal, 16*, 315–337.

Muthén, L. K., & Muthén, B. O. (2013). Mplus (Version 7.0). Los Angeles: Muthén & Muthén.

Muthén, B. O., & Curran, P. J. (1997). General longitudinal modeling of individual differences in experimental designs: A latent variable framework for analysis and power estimation. *Psychological Methods, 2*, 371–402.

National Center for Education Statistics. (2013). Surveys and programs. Retrieved June 25, 2013, from *http://nces.ed.gov/surveys*.

Ou, S. R. (2008). Do GED recipients differ from graduates and school dropouts?: Findings from an inner-city cohort. *Urban Education, 43*, 83–117.

Peugh, J. L., & Enders, C. K. (2004). Missing data in educational research: A review of reporting practices and suggestions for improvement. *Review of Educational Research, 74*, 525–556.

Pitts, S. C. (1999). *The use of latent growth models to estimate treatment effects in longitudinal experiments*. Doctoral dissertation, Arizona State University.

Raudenbush, S. W., & Bryk, A. S. (2002). *Hierarchical linear models: Applications and data analysis methods* (2nd ed.). Thousand Oaks, CA: Sage.

Rhemtulla, M., Brosseau-Liard, P. E., & Savalei, V. (2012). When can categorical variables be treated as continuous?: A comparison of robust continuous and categorical SEM estimation methods under suboptimal conditions. *Psychological Methods, 17*, 354–373.

Ridgeway, G., McCaffrey, D., Morral, A., Burgette, L., & Griffin, B. A. (2013). Toolkit for weighting and analysis of nonequivalent groups: A tutorial for the *twang* package. Retrieved from *http://cran.r-project.org/web/packages/twang/vignettes/twang.pdf*.

Rosenbaum, P. R. (1989). Optimal matching for observational studies. *Journal of the American Statistical Association, 84*, 1024.

Satorra, A., & Bentler, P. M. (1994). Corrections to test statistics and standard errors in covariance structure analysis. In A. von Eye & C. C. Clogg (Eds.), *Latent variables analysis: Applications for developmental research* (pp. 399–419). Thousand Oaks, CA: Sage.

Sekhon, J. S. (2011). Multivariate and propensity score matching software with automated balance optimization: The matching package for r. *Journal of Statistical Software, 42*, 1–52.

Setoguchi, S., Schneeweiss, S., Brookhart, M. A., Glynn, R. J., & Cook, E. F. (2008). Evaluating uses of data mining techniques in propensity score estimation: A simulation study. *Pharmacoepidemiology and Drug Safety, 17*, 546–555.

Sivo, S. A., Fan, X., & Witta, E. L. (2005). The biasing effects of unmodeled arma time series processes on latent growth curve model estimates. *Structural Equation Modeling, 12*, 215–231.

Snijders, T. A. B., & Bosker, R. J. (2012). *Multilevel analysis: An introduction to basic and advanced multilevel modeling* (2nd ed.). Thousand Oaks, CA: Sage.

Stapleton, L. M. (2006). An assessment of practical solutions for structural equation modeling with complex sample data. *Structural Equation Modeling, 13*, 28–58.

Stoel, R. D., van den Wittenboer, G., & Hox, J. (2004). Including time-invariant covariates in the latent growth curve model [Article]. *Structural Equation Modeling, 11*, 155–167.

Stuart, E. A. (2010). Matching methods for causal inference: A review and a look forward. *Statistical Science, 25*, 1–21.

Tomarken, A. J., & Waller, N. G. (2005). Structural equation modeling: Strengths, limitations, and misconceptions. *Annual Review of Clinical Psychology, 1*, 31–65.

U.S. Bureau of Labor Statistics. (2014). National longitudinal survey of youth 1997: Sample design & screening process. Retrieved March 6, 2014, from *www.nlsinfo.org/content/cohorts/nlsy97/intro-to-the-sample/sample-design-screening-process*.

Van Buuren, S., & Oudshoorn, C. G. M. (2000). Multivariate imputation by chained equations: MICE V1.0 user's manual. *TNO Prevention and Health*. Leiden: Netherlands Organization for Applied Scientific Research (TNO).

# CHAPTER 10

# Propensity Score Matching on Multilevel Data

## Qiu Wang

In empirical studies for treatment effects, researchers often sample larger units (e.g., subjects) from a hierarchically structured or multilevel population (Cochran, 1963; Scott & Smith, 1969). Examples of larger units include clusters (Donner, 1998), groups (Cornfield, 1978; Murray, 1998; Raudenbush, 1997), communities (Freedman, Green, & Byar, 1990; Martin, Diehr, Perrin, & Koepsell, 1993; Thompson, Pyke, & Hardy, 1997), and schools (Hedges, 2007; Hong & Raudenbush, 2006; Murray et al., 1994; Raudenbush, 1997). In addition, researchers may conduct cluster-randomized trials (CRTs; Donner & Klar, 2000; Murray, 1998; Raudenbush, 1997) using clusters comprised of multiple individuals (Bloom, 2005). When clusters are assigned to the treatment, the incomparability between treatment and control groups can arise from Level-1 or Level-2 covariates (Raab & Butcher, 2001), resulting in selection bias. Indeed, selection bias occurs frequently in observational studies (Rosenbaum, 2005) and leads to an inappropriate estimate of the treatment effect (Rubin, 1973). When multilevel data are used, selection bias must be evaluated (Berger, 2005) and removed from the estimate of the treatment effect in the analysis stage (Hong & Raudenbush, 2006). The dual-matching method proposed in this chapter is used to approximate a matched cluster-randomized design to reduce bias in the estimate of the treatment effect for multilevel data.

## DUAL MATCHING

Matching, as a post-hoc sample balancing technique, has been widely used in observational studies to reduce estimation bias of the treatment effect because it can significantly improve comparability of the groups (Cochran, 1953; Rubin, 2001). Decades ago, to study treatment effects, dual matching was used in experimental studies with clusters. Pittman (1921, as cited in McCall, 1923), conducted the delaying match after the final test scores had been collected. In order to achieve comparability at both the cluster and individual levels, Pittman (McCall, 1923, p. 49) matched individuals after cluster-level covariates such as wealth and quality of population were taken into account in matching. Unfortunately, the literature has not followed up to investigate the potential of Pittman's dual matching in research and practice. Using large-scale group-randomized trial data, Griffin, McCaffrey, and Pane (2009) found that matching on different sets of Level-2 covariates resulted in different levels of statistical power. The use of propensity scores estimated from kindergarten retention data to approximate the CRT design has been studied by Hong and Raudenbush (2006). Rather than using the estimated propensity scores for matching, the researchers used them to stratify the data, then treated the propensity scores as covariates to analyze stratified data in order to thereby estimate the treatment effect using the hierarchical linear model. This chapter demonstrates the use of propensity score matching to achieve cluster-level and individual-level treatment–control group balance, which may potentially reduce selection bias when multilevel large-scale data are used to estimate the treatment effect.

Bias or error occurs when the expected value of the estimate (observed score or observed treatment effect) differs from the value being estimated (true score or true effect) through sampling (Särndal, Swensson, & Wretman, 2003). Selection bias (Heckman, 1979) can occur in two situations: (1) self-selection by objects being studied and (2) sample selection by researchers or data analysts. Using selection-biased samples results in a biased estimate of the effect of a treatment that should have been randomly assigned. The effect of selection bias causes the initial group difference that has been studied for decades. Neyman (1923) pointed out that the plot characteristic besides the treatment impacted potential yield, which implies that the plot characteristic can be a source of selection bias (in Rubin, 1990, p. 283). Similarly, Gosset ("Student," 1923, in Rubin, 1990) found that the initial differences among the groups affected the outcome besides the treatment. The initial difference can bias the treatment effect estimation and mislead one's conclusion (Campbell & Stanley, 1966). Given the multilevel nature of educational settings, for example, participants are not assigned to groups at random, initial difference can occur at the Level-1 covariates and/or at Level-2 covariates. The multilevel nature of data also exists in other settings, such as patients nested within clinics, employees nested within companies, politicians nested within states, and so on. The following two sections demonstrate how selection bias on covariates affects the estimate of the treatment effect at the individual and group level.

### Definition of Bias at Individual Level

Counterfactual Model

In an ideal case, which involves no covariates $X$, the counterfactual responses (Holland, 1986; Morgan & Winship, 2007) in treatment and control groups can be written as $r_i^z = \mu^z + u_i^z$, where $r_i^z$ is the ith counterfactual response under treatment ($z = 1$) or control ($z = 0$). $\mu^z$ represents the mean of $z$th group's responses. $u_i^z$ are the ith random errors in $z$th group. The composite equation is

$$r_i = \mu_0 + z * (\mu_1 - \mu_0) + (u_0 + z * \epsilon_i)$$

where $\epsilon_i = u_1 - u_0$ and $E(\epsilon_i) = 0$. Let the population-level treatment effect be $\delta$. Then,

$$\delta = \mathbb{E}(r^1 - r^0) = (\mu^1 - \mu^2)$$

Covariates $X$ can be added to the counterfactual model. Let $\mu^z = M^z(X)$ be a function of covariates $X$ (e.g., in Cochran & Rubin, 1973), such as a linear equation $M^z(X) = \alpha^z + (X - \mu_X^z)\beta^z$. Drop the subscript and let residual be $\epsilon = u^1 - u^0$. Write

$$r^z = a^0 + (X - \mu_X^0)\beta^0 + u^0 + z * (\alpha^1 - \alpha^0) + \\ + z^*[X(\beta^1 - \beta^0) - \mu_X^1\beta^1 + \mu_X^0\beta^0] + (u^0 + z * \epsilon)$$

Further simplify the equation to obtain the treatment effect, denoted as $\delta(X)$, and

$$\delta(X) = \mathbb{E}\{(\alpha^1 - \alpha^0) + [X(\beta^1 - \beta^0) - \mu_X^1\beta^1 + \mu_X^0\beta^0] + \epsilon\}$$

Bias occurs when the estimate of treatment effect is *not* equal to the true value, that, $\delta(X) \neq \delta$. Thus, bias is defined as $\Delta(X) = \delta(X) - \delta$.

### How Selection Bias Causes Biased Treatment Effect Estimate

The detailed decompositions below identify illustrative situations where bias may occur. Assume that there are no measurement errors on $X$ and that the expectations of the residuals $u^1$ and $u^0$ are zero; bias reduction will then focus mainly on components related to $M^z(X)$.

*Initial Difference on Covariates X.* The initial difference on covariates $X$ in treatment and control group can generate bias of the treatment effect.

Let $\Delta_X$ be a nonzero constant vector representing the treatment and control group mean difference of covariates. That is, $\mu_X^1 = \Delta_X + \mu_X^0$. The function $M^z(X)$ is linearly additive, with $z = 0, 1$. That is, $M^z(X + \Delta_X) = M^z(X) + M^z(\Delta_X)$. The treatment effect estimate is

$$\mathbb{E}[M^1(X + \Delta_X) - M^0(X)] = \mathbb{E}\{(\alpha^1 - \alpha^0) + [X(\beta^1 - \beta^0) - (\mu_X^0 + \Delta_X)\beta^1 + \mu_X^0 \beta^0]\}$$

Because the initial difference $\Delta_X$ is not equal to zero, the treatment effect is biased. If we assume the regression coefficients are the same, that is, $\beta^1 = \beta^0 = \beta$, then the bias component can be identified as $\Delta(X) = \beta \Delta_X$.

*Unequal Regression Coefficients of Treatment and Control Groups.* If the treatment and control group means are equal, that is, $\mu_X^1 = \mu_X = \mu_X^0$, the difference between the egression coefficients of treatment and control groups will bias the treatment effect estimate. In this situation, the bias component is

$$\Delta(X) = \mathbb{E}[(X - \mu_X)\Delta_\beta], \text{ with } \Delta_\beta = \beta^1 - \beta^0$$

In practice, the unequal regression coefficient of the treatment and control groups may be due to the interaction terms between covariates $X$ and treatment status variable $z$. Let $\beta_{X \times z}$ be the regression coefficient of the interaction terms. The regression coefficient of covariates $X$ in the treatment group is $\beta^1 = \beta^0 + \beta_{X \times z}$. This implies $\Delta_\beta = \beta_{X \times z}$. One can add an interaction term of a covariate $x$ and $z$ in the regression and test if this coefficient is statistically zero.

## Bias and Selection Bias in Multilevel Data

In a hierarchically structured or multilevel population (Cochran, 1963), ith individual is assumed to be nested in kth cluster. At student level (Level 1), outcome $r_i^k$ and $X_i^k$ covariates are observed. At cluster level (Level 2), $W_k$ covariates are also available. Let $z$ be a binary treatment–control indicator, with 1 representing the treatment group, 0 otherwise. The relationship between outcome variable and covariates is modified from Schmidt and Houang (1986) in a counterfactual sense:

$$r_{ik}^z = \alpha^z + \left(\mu_{X_k}^z - \mu_X\right)\beta_X + \left(W_k^z - \mu_W\right)\beta_W + u_k^z + \left(X_{X_k}^z - \mu_{X_k}^z\right)\beta +$$
$$+ \left(X_{X_k}^z - \mu_{X_k}^z\right)\beta_k^* + e_{ik}^z$$

where $z = 0, 1$ and $\beta_k^* = \beta_X - \beta$. Also, $\mu_X$ and $\mu_W$ are the population means. $\mu_{X_k}$ is the population mean of the Level-1 covariates in $k$th cluster, $\beta_X$ includes the between-Level-2-unit regression coefficients of the aggregated means of Level-1 covariates, $\beta_W$ includes the regression coefficient of the observed Level-2 covariates, $\beta$ includes the pooled within-Level-2-unit regression coefficient of the Level-1 covariates, and vector $\beta_k$ includes the within-Level-2-unit regression coefficients of the Level-1 covariates in $k$th class. The counterfactual treatment effect is

$$\mathbb{E}[r_{ik}^1 - r_{ik}^0] = \mathbb{E}(\alpha^1 - \alpha^0) + \mathbb{E}\left(\mu_{X_k}^1 - \mu_{X_k}^0\right)(\beta_X - \beta - \beta_k^*) + \mathbb{E}\left(W_k^1 - W_k^0\right)\beta_W +$$
$$+ \mathbb{E}(u_k^1 - u_k^0) + \mathbb{E}\left(X_{X_k}^1 - X_{X_k}^0\right)(\beta + \beta_k^*) + \mathbb{E}(e_{ik}^1 - e_{ik}^0)$$

In the counterfactual case,[1] $\left(X_k^1 - X_k^0\right) \equiv \left(\mu_{X_k}^1 - \mu_{X_k}^0\right) \equiv \left(W_k^1 - W_k^0\right) \equiv 0$ holds, and the expected treatment effect is

$$\mathbb{E}(\alpha^1 - \alpha^0) + \mathbb{E}(u_k^1 - u_k^0) + \mathbb{E}(e_{ik}^1 - e_{ik}^0)$$

The treatment effect is unbiased because the residual expectations are zero. However, bias can result in at least one of the three situations: $\left(X_k^1 - X_k^0\right) \neq 0$, $\left(W_k^1 - W_k^0\right) \neq 0$, and $\left(\mu_{X_k}^1 - \mu_{X_k}^0\right) \neq 0$. The three situations represent different sources of selection bias. $\left(W_k^1 - W_k^0\right) \neq 0$ indicates that treatment and control groups are not comparable at Level-2 units. $\left(X_k^1 - X_k^0\right) \neq 0$ indicates the Level-1 difference within $k$th class. $\left(\mu_{X_k}^1 - \mu_{X_k}^0\right) \neq 0$ represents the difference due to the noncomparable aggregated means of the Level-1 covariates $X$ within $k$th class.

## Level-1, Level-2, and Dual Matching

### Level-1 Matching

There is Level-1 bias within $k$th class. That is, $\left(X_k^1 - X_k^0\right) \neq 0$, implying that the counterfactual equivalence is not satisfied in practice. In other words, the $i$th student is either in the treatment group or in the control group, but not in both. For a patient, say John in the treatment group, there is no exact John-equivalent in the control group. The two groups are not equivalent. Here, Level-1 matching can be conducted using covariates $X$ to match each treated individual with one from nontreated individuals. $\left(\mu_{X_k}^1 - \mu_{X_k}^0\right) \neq 0$ occurs when the aggregated means of the Level-1 covariates $X$ within $k$th cluster are noncomparable. This type of second-level bias can be reduced when the bias on Level-1 covariates $X$ is removed. By ignoring the hierarchical structure, treated individuals are matched with control individuals to compute bias reduction rate. The analysis units for treatment effect are the outcomes of the matched individuals.

### Level-2 Matching

Treatment and control groups are not comparable at Level-2 units such as clusters; that is, $\left(W_k^1 - W_k^0\right) \neq 0$ in the counterfactual sense. Bias reduction here focuses on second-level units, and one would conduct *Level-2 matching*. By ignoring Level-1 variables, clusters are matched by using Level-2 propensity scores to compute the bias reduction rate.

### Dual Matching

When both Level-1 and Level-2 covariates are not comparable, *dual matching* is needed, including both Level-2 matching and Level-1 matching. That is, treated clusters are first matched with control clusters, then, within each matched treatment–control pair, individuals are matched. The three detailed matching procedures are discussed in the section Simulation Study.

## DEMONSTRATION

The example uses a data-driven *sampling study* (MacCallum, Roznowski, & Necowitz, 1992) to evaluate how well matching reduces selection bias.

### Data Source

The Second International Mathematics Study (SIMS; International Association for the Evaluation of Education Achievement, 1977) used longitudinal design to study the effects of the curriculum and the classroom instruction. The classroom process was "mapped" on the targeted eighth grade (Cohort 2) where the 13-year-old students were found. Two waves of mathematic achievement data were collected, with the first wave at the beginning of the school year (Time 0), and the second at the end of the school year (Time 1). In this design, Cohort 2 at Time 0 was in control condition.

After the "treatment" of one year of schooling, Cohort 2 at Time 1 data were collected to assess the schooling effect ($\delta_{C2T1-C1T0}$), defined as the "changes in mathematics achievement over the time-span of one school year at the particular grade level" (Wiley & Wolfe, 1992, p. 299). SIMS data were collected from seven countries. This chapter uses only SIMS data collected in the United States (Wolfe, 1987). The final dataset includes 2,296 students in 126 regular classes. The average class size is about 27. Tables 10.1 and 10.2 list the descriptive statistics of the outcome variables and covariates (Schmidt & Burstein, 1993).

## Designed Model

The conceptual model fitted on SIMS–USA data is displayed in Figure 10.1. It is a two-level structural equation model (Muthén, 1994). In the Level-1 model, posttest score is predicted by pretest score. Pretest score is predicted by four student characteristics and five latent variables. The latent constructs and their surrogate variables are described in Table 10.1. In the Level-2 model, the intercept of pretest ($\beta_0$) is predicted by four class/school-level variables. The intercept of posttest ($\alpha_0$) is predicted by $\beta_0$ and three class-level teacher variables. The Level-1 and Level-2 residuals are mutually independent of one another.

*Level-1 Model*

$r_{post} = \alpha_0 + \alpha_1 r_{pre} + e_{post}$
$r_{pre} = \beta_0 + \beta_1 AGE + \beta_2 EDUCEPT + \beta_3 FAMILY + \beta_4 MHWKT +$
$\quad + \beta_5 EDUINSP + \beta_6 SLFENCRG + \beta_7 FMLSUPRT + \beta_8 MTHIMPT +$
$\quad + \beta_9 SES + e_{pre}$

where $e_{post} \sim N(0, \sigma^2_{e_{post}}), e_{pre} \sim N(0, \sigma^2_{e_{pre}})$.

*Level-2 Model*

$\beta_0 = \gamma_0 + \gamma_1 OLDARITH + \gamma_2 OLDALG + \gamma_3 CLASSSIZE + \gamma_4 MONTHLY + u_{\beta_0}$
$\alpha_0 = \beta_0 + \gamma_5 NEWALG + \gamma_6 NEWGEOM + \gamma_7 TPPWEEK + u_{\alpha_0}$

where $u_{\beta_0} \sim N(0, \sigma^2_{u_{\beta_0}}), u_{\alpha_0} \sim N(0, \sigma^2_{u_{\alpha_0}})$.

**TABLE 10.1. Level-1 Descriptive Statistics of the Final Two-Level Structural Equation Model**

| Variables | Label | Description | Mean |
|---|---|---|---|
| Educational Inspiration (EDUINSP) | YPWANT | Learn more match (inverse code, 1–5[a]) | 4.73 |
| | YPWWELL | Parents want me to do well (1–5[a]) | 4.24 |
| | YPENC | Parents encourage me to do well match (inverse code, 1–5[a]) | 4.37 |
| Self-Encouragement (SLFENCRG) | YIWANT | I want to do well on math (1–5[a]) | 4.32 |
| | YMORMTH | Looking forward to taking more (1–5[a]) | 3.24 |
| | YNOMORE | Take no more math if possible (inverse code, 1–5[a]) | 3.73 |
| Family Support (FMLSUPRT) | YPINT | Parents are interested in helping math (inverse code, 1–5[a]) | 3.72 |
| | YFLIKES | Father enjoys doing math (inverse code, 1–5[a]) | 3.53 |
| | YMLIKES | Mother enjoys doing math (inverse code, 1–5[a]) | 3.25 |
| | YFABLE | Father is able to do math homework (inverse code, 1–5[a]) | 3.92 |
| | YMABLE | Mother is able to do math homework (inverse code, 1–5[a]) | 3.71 |
| Math Importance (MTHIMPT) | YMIMPT | Mother thinks math important (1–5[a]) | 4.60 |
| | YFIMPT | Father thinks math important (1–5[a]) | 4.55 |
| Socioeconomic Status (SES) | YFEDUC | Father education level (1–4[b]) | 3.38 |
| | YMEDUC | Mother education level (1–4[b]) | 3.35 |
| | YFOCCN | Father's occupation national code (1–8[c]) | 4.26 |
| | YMOCCN | Mother's occupation national code (1–8[c]) | 4.11 |
| Age | XAGE | Grand mean centered age | 0.00 |
| Parental Help | YFAMILY | How frequent family help (1–3[d]) | 1.75 |
| Education | EDUECPT | Derived from YMOREED: Years of education parents expected (1–4[e]) | 2.97 |
| Homework Time | YMHWKT | Typical week hours math homework per week | 2.98 |

*Note.* [a]1 = not at all like, 2 = somehow unlike, 3 = unsure, 4 = somehow like, 5 = exactly like.
[b]1 = little schooling, 2 = primary school, 3 = secondary school, 4 = college or university or tertiary education.
[c]1 = unskilled worker, 2 = semi-unskilled worker, 3 = skilled worker lower, 4 = skilled worker higher, 5 = clerk sales and related lower, 6 = clerk sales and related higher, 7 = professional and managerial lower, 8 = professional and managerial higher.
[d]1 = never/hardly, 2 = occasionally, 3 = regularly.
[e]1 = 1 = up to 2 years, 2 = 2 to 5 years, 3 = 5 to 8 years, 4 = more than 8 years.
N = 2,296.

**TABLE 10.2. Level-2 Descriptive Statistics of the Final Two-Level Structural Equation Model**

| Variables | Label | Description | Mean |
|---|---|---|---|
| | | Teacher/class-level covariates | |
| Class Size | CLASSIZE | Created from the number of students in class | 26.60 |
| Opportunity to Learn | OLDARITH | Prior OTL of arithmetic | 7.10 |
| | OLDALG | Prior OTL of algebra | NA |
| | OLDGEOM | Prior OTL of geometry | 3.19 |
| | NEWARITH | This year's OTL of arithmetic | NA |
| | NEWALG | This year's OTL of algebra | 59.61 |
| | NEWGEOM | This year's OTL of geometry | 41.37 |
| Class Instruction | TPPWEEK | Actual number of hours of math instructions per week | 5.09 |
| | | School-level covariates | |
| Qualified Math Teacher Rate | MTHONLY | Proportion of qualified math teachers | 0.14 |

Note. N = 126.

Mplus (Muthén & Muthén, 1998–2011) is used to fit the proposed two-level SEM to obtain factor loadings, regression coefficients, and residual variances. These model-based estimates are treated as known values to generate longitudinal data of Cohort 2 at Time 0 (e.g., grade 7 in $Year_{i-1}$) and Time 1 (e.g., grade 8 in $Year_i$). In practice, Cohort 2 at Time 0 data may not be collected. Another cohort such as Cohort 1 at Time 1 (e.g., grade 7 at $Year_i$) can be treated as the "replacement" to estimate schooling effect, denoted now as $\hat{\delta}_{C2T1-C1T1}$. This design is called the *synthetic cohort design* (SCD; Wiley & Wolfe, 1992), which has been widely used in aging and epidemiological studies. Selection bias occurs due to the difference between Cohort 1 at Time 1 and Cohort 2 at Time 0. The schooling effect estimation bias in SCD is defined as

$$\text{Bias}\left(\hat{\delta}_{C2T1-C1T1}\right) = \mathbb{E}\left(\hat{\delta}_{C2T1-C1T1}\right) - \delta_{C2T1-C1T1}$$

In the exemplary synthetic cohort design data, Cohort 1's Time 1 data are noncomparable with Cohort 2 at Time 0, so we can examine how well

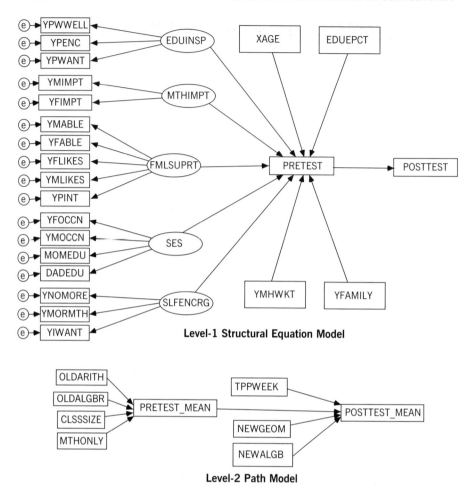

**FIGURE 10.1.** Two-level structural equation model.

matching can reduce the selection bias and increase schooling effect estimation accuracy. Five types of selection bias of exemplary data of Cohort 1 at Time 1 include (1) C1T1's Level-1 covariate means differ from C2T0's, (2) C1T1's Level-1 covariate variances differ from C2T0's, (3) C1T1's Level-2 covariate means differ from C2T0's, (4) C1T1's Level-2 covariate variances differ from C2T0's, and (5) C1T1's Level-1 and Level-2 covariate means differ from C2T0's. Individual level matching, cluster level matching, and dual matching are conducted using the R (R Development Core Team, 2007).

## Matching Evaluation

The estimation bias reduction rate (Cochran & Rubin, 1973) is computed as

$$100\left(1 - \frac{\text{treatment effect bias after matching}}{\text{treatment effect bias before matching}}\right)\%$$

A larger value of bias reduction rate indicates a better performance of matching. Table 10.3 summarizes the results.

## Three Matching Routines

Matching is conducted using the R (R Development Core Team, 2007) module *MatchIt* (Ho, Imai, King, & Stuart, 2011) and Match (Sekhon, 2007). The R codes are available in the appendices in Wang (2010).

### Level-1 Matching

By ignoring the multilevel structure, individuals are matched. The detailed matching procedures are as follows:

**TABLE 10.3. Bias Reduction Rates of the Three Types of Matching**

|  | Propensity score matching | | Mahalanobis distance matching | |
| --- | --- | --- | --- | --- |
|  | Larger caliper | Smaller caliper | Larger caliper | Smaller caliper |
| Level-1 matching | | | | |
| Noncomparable Level-1 covariate means | 72.03 | 78.44 | 16.56 | 24.03 |
| Noncomparable Level-1 covariate variances | 1.79 | 1.35 | –7.51 | –9.48 |
| Level-2 matching | | | | |
| Noncomparable Level-2 covariate means | 63.55 | 68.81 | 0.00 | 5.26 |
| Noncomparable Level-2 covariate variances | –8.20 | –167.8 | 5.34 | –21.18 |
| Dual matching | | | | |
| Noncomparable Level-2 covariate means | 37.21 | NA | NA | NA |
| Noncomparable Level-1 covariate means | 78.19 | NA | NA | NA |

1. Randomly draw 100 classes from the pseudo-population of Cohort 2 at Time 0. Let $n_j$ be the class size of $j$th class. The sample size is $n^{C2T0} = \sum_{j=1}^{100} n_j$. Randomly draw 100 classes from the pseudo-population of Cohort 1 at Time 1. Let $n_{j'}$ be the class size of $j'$th class. The sample size is $n^{C2T1} = \sum_{j=1}^{100} n_{j'}$. Let $(r, X, W)_i^{C2T0}$ be the $i$th data record of the Cohort 2 at Time 0 sample, with $i = 1, 2, \ldots, n_{C2T0}$. Vector $r$ represents the Level-1 pretest score variable. $X$ is the Level-1 variable vector including both the latent and the observed. $W$ is the Level-2 variable. Let $(r, X, W)_{i'}^{C2T1}$ be the $i'$th data record of Cohort 2 at Time 1 sample, with $i' = 1, 2, \ldots, n_{C2T1}$.

2. Pool the two random samples together to estimate the Level-1 propensity scores. The propensity score ($e^1$) represents the probability that a student belongs to focal Cohort 2, whose cohort ID is coded as 1. The logarithm of the odds, $\log[e^1/(1 - e^1)]$, is computed for each student and used for matching (Stuart & Rubin, 2008). Because the simulated bias occurs at only Level-1, the Level-2 covariates $W$ are not used to compute propensity scores. Among the total of $n_{C2T0}$ units in the sample drawn from Cohort 2 at Time 0, for the $i$th data record $(r, X, W)^{C2T0}$, find one data record $(r, X, W)^{C1T1}$ from Cohort 1 at Time 1, so that $Min[(X)^{C2T0}, (X)^{C1T1}]$ reach a preset value, which is a small number called caliper in matching literature (e.g., Stuart & Rubin, 2008). The smaller the caliper, the more comparable the two data points will be. $Min [a, b]$ is a function that computes the minimum distance between quantity $a$ and quantity $b$ in terms of log-odds or Mahalanobis distance. The matched data are used to compute the $i$th bias reduction rate.

3. Repeat 1–3 for 200 times, which are the replications. This results in 200 bias reduction rates.

4. Compute and report the average bias reduction rate across the 200 duplications to evaluate the bias reduction rate.

### Level-2 Matching

In Level-2 matching, classes are matched using Level-2 propensity scores. The analysis units are the means of the matched classes.

1. Randomly draw 100 classes from the pseudo-population of Cohort 2 at Time 0. Randomly draw 100 classes from the pseudo-population of Cohort 1 at Time 1. Let $\left(\bar{r}, \bar{X}, W\right)_k^{C2T0}$ be the $k$th data record of the sample drawn from Cohort 1 at Time 0, with $k' = 1, 2, \ldots, 100$. Let $\left(\bar{r}, \bar{X}, W\right)_{k'}^{C2T1}$ be the $k'$th data record of the sample drawn from Cohort 1 at Time 1, with $k' = 1, 2, \ldots, 100$. $\bar{r}$ represents the class mean of the pretest score. $\bar{X}$ represents the means of the Level-1 variables, including both latent and observed. $W$ represents Level-2 variables.

2. Pool the two random samples together to estimate the Level-2 propensity scores. The Level-2 propensity score ($e^2$) represents the probability that a class belongs to Cohort 2 (note: here, 2 does not mean a square), whose cohort ID is coded as 1. The logarithm of the odds, $\log[e^2/(1 - e^2)]$, is computed for each class and used for matching. Because of the hierarchical structure, Level-2 covariates $W$ play a critical role in computing propensity scores.

3. For the $i$th data record $\left(\bar{r}, \bar{X}, W\right)_k^{C2T0}$ find *one* data record $\left(\bar{r}, \bar{X}, W\right)_{k'}^{C2T1}$ from Cohort 1 at Time 1, so that $Min\left[(W)_k^{C2T0}, (W)_{k'}^{C2T1}\right]$ is less than a caliper (Stuart & Rubin, 2008). The smaller the caliper, the more comparable the two data points will be. The matched classes are used to compute the $i$th bias reduction rate.

4. Replicate 1–3 for 200 times, which results in 200 bias reduction rates.

5. Compute and report the average of the 200 bias reduction rates.

## Dual Matching

Dual matching involves two parts. First, Level-2 units such as clusters are matched. Second, within each pair of matched treatment–control clusters, individual units are matched. The detailed matching procedures are as follows:

1. Conduct the first three steps of Level-2 matching. The matched classes are used to compute the $i$th cluster-level bias reduction rate.

2. Within each pair of the matched classes from Level-2 matching, conduct Level-1 matching following the second step. The matched units are used to compute the $i$th dual-matching bias reduction rate.

3. Replicate 1–2 for 200 times, which results in 200 class-level bias reduction rates and 200 dual-matching bias reduction rates.
4. Compute and report the average class-level bias reduction rate and the average dual-matching bias reduction rate.

## Results

When the cohorts' multilevel data are different only on Level-1 covariate means, propensity score matching on Level-1 covariates reduces estimation bias by 78% (or 72%) using a caliper of 0.01 (or 0.2) standard deviations. Mahalanobis distance matching only reduces 16% (or 24%) of the estimation bias when the caliper is 0.2 (or 0.01) standard deviations. However, when the cohorts' multilevel data are different only on Level-1 covariate variances, propensity score matching on Level-1 covariates reduces estimation bias by less than 3%. Mahalanobis distance matching even increases estimation bias by more than 8%. When the cohorts' hierarchically structured data are different only on Level-2 covariate means, propensity score matching on Level-2 covariates reduces estimation bias by 63.55% (or 68.81%) when the caliper is 0.2 (or 0.01) standard deviations. Mahalanobis distance matching only reduces estimation bias by less than 6%. When the cohorts' hierarchically structured data are different only on Level-2 covariate variances, matching does not help reduce estimation bias.

When the cohorts' hierarchically structured data have different covariate means at both Level 1 and Level 2, dual matching significantly reduces the initial bias. Matching only on Level-2 covariates reduces 37.01% of the initial bias when the caliper is 0.2 standard deviations. If there is a further matching Level-1 covariates after Level-2 matching, the initial bias is reduced an extra 39.65%. Thus, the initial bias is reduced by a total of 76.66%.

## DISCUSSION AND CONCLUSION

Synthetic cohorts are commonly used in aging studies in the field of epidemiology to estimate the synthetic cohort effect (Heimberg, Stein, Hiripi, & Kessler, 2000; Kessler, Stein, & Berglund, 1998). Making causal inference from policy-based treatment is understanding "the causal effect of one of the turning point events and treatments on development trajectories" in the life course (Haviland & Nagin, 2005, p. 576). The synthetic cohort design of this chapter can be treated as a specific case of the one-time-point treatment effect estimation approach discussed in Haviland and Nagin (2005).

Compared with a longitudinal design, the synthetic cohort design involves only one set of multiple informative data during several periods. The synthetic cohort design and other one-time-point treatment effect estimation approaches are irreplaceable. Increasing data collection frequency in a longer time period can improve the quality of research given a fixed number of samples, but it can significantly increase the research cost (Bloom, Richburg-Hayes, & Black, 2007). Furthermore, most of the events during the life course are one-time occurrences, and some events can be emotionally negative and should/cannot be repeated. The use of synthetic cohort design can examine the impact of the one-time-occurrence event in the life course and help researchers understand individual development and change (Haviland & Nagin, 2005). A dummy variable can be created to represent the cohort membership index and can be used in data analysis. For example, the synthetic cohort effect is the noncomparability between two cohorts and is captured by the statistical significance of the interactions of the dummy variable and the background characteristics (Heimberg et al., 2000). This way it can reveal on which background characteristics the two cohorts are different. In turn, propensity score matching is necessary to create comparable groups in the study. Specifically, the propensity score can be used to create comparable groups through dual matching when hierarchically structured data are involved. These comparable groups created through dual matching are called synthetic cohorts that can be followed and studied across the life course in epidemiology studies (Haviland & Nagin, 2005). For example, Campbell and Hudson (1985) use rare life events of seniors to pool observed panel survey data to create synthetic cohorts, which are comparable groups to be further analyzed through the discrete time-series analysis.

Matching does not help to reduce bias when the multilevel data are different only on Level-1 or Level-2 covariate variances. This is because when covariate means, either at Level 1 or Level 2, are identical between Cohort 2 at Time 0 and Cohort 1 at Time 1, the initial bias is very small; matching helps little in reducing, or even increases, bias in this situation. When the multilevel data are different on both Level-1 covariates and Level-2 covariates, matching at only the cluster level helps reduce bias. But initial bias (about 40%) due to Level-1 covariate means between Cohort 2 at Time 0 and Cohort 1 at Time 1 still exists. Therefore, dual matching is the optimal approach.

Research has suggested that when the true propensity score model is known and sample size is large, propensity score is a better approach

(Sekhon & Diamond, 2008). In the exemplary data, each condition determines a "true" and known propensity score model. The sample size is about 2,700, which is large. Thus, Mahalanobis distance matching cannot achieve optimal results. Future studies may use smaller Level-1 and Level-2 sample sizes to examine the performances of the three proposed matching approaches on hierarchically structured data.

In most research settings, valid inferences must account for the multilevel structure of the data. Matching is an effective tool for improving precision when random assignment is achieved and for accounting for selection bias when random assignment is impossible. Different studies present different requirements for matching. This chapter demonstrated the potential of using propensity scores in dual matching to improve the accuracy of estimating treatment effect. However, matching only reduces bias in practice, but it cannot completely remove the bias involving treatment effect estimates.

## NOTE

1. If randomization is used, equivalence is at the expectation/mean Level rather than at Level-1–2 units or Level-1–1 units. The subscripts, $k$ of Level-2 units and $i$ of Level-1 units, will be dropped. Thus, holds. For the purpose of simplicity, this chapter uses the counterfactual model to define bias and demonstrates how selection bias occurs.

## REFERENCES

Berger, V. (2005). *Selection bias and covariate imbalances in randomzied clinical trials*. Chichester, UK: Wiley.

Bloom, H. S. (2005). Randomizing groups to evaluate place-based programs. In H. S. Bloom (Ed.), *Learning more from social experiments: Evolving analytic approaches*. New York: Russell Sage Foundation.

Bloom, H. S., Richburg-Hayes, L., & Black, A. R. (2007). Using covariates to improve precision for studies that randomize schools to evaluate educational interventions. *Educational Evaluation and Policy Analysis*, 29(1):30–59. Available at www.wtgrantfoundation.org/usr_doc/RSChapter4Final.pdf.

Campbell, R. T., & Hudson, C. M. (1985). Synthetic cohorts from panel surveys. *Research on Aging*, 7(1), 81–93.

Campbell, D. T., & Stanley, J. C. (1966). *Experimental and quasi-experimental designs for research*. Chicago: Rand McNally College.

Cochran, W. G. (1953). Matching in analytical studies. *American Journal of Public Health*, 43, 684–691.

Cochran, W. G. (1963). *Sampling techniques*. New York: Wiley.
Cochran, W. G., & Rubin, D. B. (1973). Controlling bias in observational studies: A review. *Indian Journal of Statistics, Series A, 35*, 417–446.
Cornfield, J. (1978). Randomization by group: A formal analysis. *American Journal of Epidemiology, 108*(2), 100–102.
Donner, A. (1998). Some aspects of the design and analysis of cluster randomization trials. *Journal of the Royal Statistical Society: Series C (Applied Statistics), 47*(1), 95–113.
Donner, A., & Klar, N. (2000). *Design and analysis of cluster randomization trials in health research*. London: Arnold.
Freedman, L. S., Green, S. B., & Byar, D. P. (1990). Assessing the gain in efficiency due to matching in a community intervention study. *Statistics in Medicine, 9*(8), 943–952.
Griffin, B. A., McCaffrey, D. F., & Pane, J. F. (2009). *Evaluating the impact of blocking on power in group-randomized trials*. Paper presented at the annual conference of the Society for Research on Educational Effectiveness (SREE), Washington, DC.
Haviland, A. M., & Nagin, D. S. (2005). Causal inferences with group-based trajectory models. *Psychometrika, 70*(3), 557–578.
Heckman, J. J. (1979). Sample selection bias as a specification error. *Econometrica: Journal of the econometric Society, 47*(1), 153–161.
Hedges, L. V. (2007). Correcting a significance test for clustering. *Journal of Educational and Behavioral Statistics, 32*(2), 151–179.
Heimberg, R. G., Stein, M. B., Hiripi, E., & Kessler, R. C. (2000). Trends in the prevalence of social phobia in the United States: A synthetic cohort analysis of changes over four decades. *European Psychiatry, 15*(1), 29–37.
Ho, D. E., Imai, K., King, G., & Stuart, E. A. (2011). MatchIt: Nonparametric preprocessing for parametric causal inference. *Journal of Statistical Software, 42*(8), 1–28. Available at http://imai.princeton.edu/research/les/matchit.pdf.
Holland, P. W. (1986). Statistics and causal inference. *Journal of the American Statistical Association, 81*(396), 945–960.
Hong, G., & Raudenbush, S. W. (2006). Evaluating kindergarten retention policy. *Journal of the American Statistical Association, 101*(475), 901–910.
International Association for the Evaluation of Educational Achievement. (1977). *The Second International Mathematics Study*. Amsterdam: Author. Available at http://www.iea.nl/sims.html.
Kessler, R. C., Stein, M. B., & Berglund, P. (1998). Social phobia subtypes in the national comorbidity survey. *American Journal of Psychiatry, 155*(5), 613–619.
Martin, D. C., Diehr, P., Perrin, E. B., & Koepsell, T. D. (1993). The effect of matching on the power of randomized community intervention studies. *Statistics in Medicine, 12*(3–4), 329–338.
MacCallum, R. C., Roznowski, M., & Necowitz, L. B. (1992). Model modications in covariance structure analysis: The problem of capitalization on chance. *Psychological Bulletin, 111*(3), 490–504.

McCall, W. A. (1923). *How to experiment in education*. New York: Macmillan.
Morgan, S. L., & Winship, C. (2007). *Counterfactuals and causal inference: Methods and principles for social research*. New York: Cambridge University Press.
Murray, D. M. (1998). *Design and analysis of group-randomized trials*. New York: Oxford University Press.
Murray, D. M., Rooney, B. L., Hannan, P. J., Peterson, A. V., Ary, D. V., Biglan, A., et al. (1994). Intraclass correlation among common measures of adolescent smoking: Estimates, correlates, and applications in smoking prevention studies. *American Journal of Epidemiology, 140*(11), 1038–1050.
Muthén, B. O. (1994). Multilevel covariance structure analysis. *Sociological Methods and Research, 22*(3), 376–398.
Muthén, L. K., & Muthén, B. O. (1998–2011). *Mplus user's guide* (6th ed.). Los Angeles: Authors.
Neyman, J. (1923). On the application of probability theory to agricultural experiments: Essay on principles, section 9 (translated in 1990). *Statistical Science, 5,* 465–480.
R Development Core Team. (2007). *R: A language and environment for statistical computing*. Vienna: R Foundation for Statistical Computing. Retrieved from www.R-project.org.
Raab, G. M., & Butcher, I. (2001). Balance in cluster randomized trials. *Statistics in Medicine, 20*(3), 351–365.
Raudenbush, S. W. (1997). Statistical analysis and optimal design for cluster randomized trials. *Psychological Methods, 2*(2), 173–185.
Rosenbaum, P. R. (2005). Observational study. In B. S. Everitt & D. C. Howell (Eds.), *Encyclopedia of statistics in behavioral science* (pp. 1451–1462). Chichester, UK: Wiley.
Rubin, D. B. (1973). Matching to remove bias in observational studies. *Biometrics, 29*(1), 159–183.
Rubin, D. B. (1990). Formal modes of statistical inference for causal effects. *Journal of Statistical Planning and Inference, 25*(3), 279–292.
Rubin, D. B. (2001). Using propensity scores to help design observational studies: Application to the tobacco litigation. *Health Services and Outcomes Research Methodology, 2*(3), 169–188.
Särndal, C. E., Swensson, B., & Wretman, J. (2003). *Model assisted survey sampling*. New York: Springer-Verlag.
Schmidt, W., & Houang, T. R. (1986). Ein vergleich von drei analyseverfahren fur hierarchist strukturierte daten. In M. v. Saldern (Ed.), *Mehrebenenanalyse* (pp. S71–S81). Weinheim: Germany: PVU.
Schmidt, W. H., & Burstein, L. (1993). Concomitants of growth in mathematics achievement during the population of a school year. In L. Burstein (Ed.), *The IEA Study of Mathematics III: Student growth and classroom processes* (pp. 309–327). Oxford, UK: Pergamon Press.
Scott, A., & Smith, T. M. F. (1969). Estimation in multi-stage surveys. *Journal of the American Statistical Association, 64*(327), 830–840.

Sekhon, J. S. (2007). Multivariate and propensity score matching software with automated balance optimization: The matching package for R. *Journal of Statistical Software, 10*(2), 1–51.

Sekhon, J. S., & Diamond, A. (2008). Genetic matching for estimating causal effects: A general multivariate matching method for achieving balance in observational studies. Retrieved July 18, 2009, from *http://sekhon.berkeley.edu/papers/GenMatch.pdf*.

Stuart, E. A., & Rubin, D. B. (2008). Matching with multiple control groups with adjustment for group differences. *Journal of Educational and Behavioral Statistics, 33*(3), 279–306.

Thompson, S. G., Pyke, S. D. M., & Hardy, R. J. (1997). The design and analysis of paired cluster randomized trials: An application of meta-analysis techniques. *Statistics in Medicine, 16*(18), 2063–2079.

Wang, Q. (2010). *Matching for bias reduction in treatment effect estimation of hierarchically structured synthetic cohort design data.* Unpublished doctoral dissertation, Michigan State University, East Lansing, MI.

Wiley, D. E., & Wolfe, R. G. (1992). Major survey design issues for the IEA Third International Mathematics and Science Study. *Prospects, 22*(3), 297–304.

Wolfe, R. G. (1987). *Second international mathematics study: Training manual for use of the databank of the longitudinal, classroom process surveys for population A in the IEA Second International Mathematics Study.* Contractor's Report, Washington, DC: Center for Education Statistics.

## CHAPTER 11

# Propensity Score Analysis with Complex Survey Samples

### Debbie L. Hahs-Vaughn

A number of organizations, for any number of reasons, collect survey data from various constituents (individuals as well as institutions). Most of the survey data are freely and publicly accessible online. For example, the National Center for Education Statistics (NCES) collects survey data on a wide variety of education-related topics, and the National Science Foundation (NSF) collects data on various science-related topics.

Given the magnitude of the type of data collected, often national or international in scope, these data are collected through probability-sampling methods other than a simple random sample and thus are referred to as *complex samples*. Complex samples are often characterized by unequal selection probability, stratification, and/or homogeneous clusters, among other survey design issues (Skinner, Holt, & Smith, 1989). Likely because much of this large-scale data is so easy to access, many users are not cognizant of the survey design—not understanding that appropriate analyses require that the complex sampling design (specifically) be accommodated in order for the results to be representative of the intended population and to ensure that variance estimates are correct.

The past few decades have brought rapid advances in the analysis of complex survey samples, and techniques for dealing with complex designs are becoming increasingly common in statistical software packages (Chambers & Skinner, 2003). However, misinformation about the impact of complex sample designs on parameter estimates from standard statistical procedures seems to prevail. Particularly for those individuals relying on comprehensive nationally representative survey databases for their research, the need to address design elements during the data analysis phase is critical for making correct interpretations. More specifically, more attention has been given to analysis of complex sampling issues using propensity score analysis (e.g., DuGoff, Schuler, & Stuart, 2014; Hahs-Vaughn, 2013; Hahs-Vaughn & Onwuegbuzie, 2006; Zanutto, Lu, & Hornik, 2005). These publications help researchers understand complex sampling issues and the rise in the application of propensity score analysis, and also suggest the timeliness of the topic in this chapter.

This chapter presents (1) a content analysis of published educational literature to provide information about the extent to which propensity score analysis has been applied to complex samples and how the sampling design has been addressed in propensity score analysis in educational studies; (2) a demonstration of the use of propensity score methods with complex samples; and (3) a quantification of the effects of ignoring the sampling design when using propensity score analysis as compared to various approaches for adjusting for complex sample designs in propensity score analysis.

## ISSUES IN ANALYZING COMPLEX SURVEY SAMPLES

Rosenbaum and Rubin (1983) are credited with introducing propensity score analysis as a technique to study observational data, allowing causal inferences to be drawn when randomization is not possible (Rubin, 1997). See Chapter 1 in this book for an overview of propensity score analysis. While propensity score analysis has been widely adopted in many research fields, its application to complex survey data is also quite common. A systematic review by Hahs-Vaughn (2013) found that 86 of the studies published between November 2009 and March 2013 had applied propensity score analysis to answer substantive research questions, and nearly one-half had done so with complex samples.

Complex samples are survey data that have been collected by means other than a simple random sample. Two primary issues related to complex samples must be addressed when analyzing the data: (1) the multistage sampling method that creates homogeneous clusters; and (2) unequal selection probabilities (e.g., oversampling or selection based on probability proportional to size sampling), adjustments for participant nonresponse, and stratification and poststratification raking that creates disproportionate sampling (Kalton, 1983; Kish, 1995).

The first issue in complex samples is that many times, because it is not possible to apply a simple random sampling procedure for collecting the data, complex samples have been collected by combining sampling methods such as cluster, stratified, or multistage-sampling methods. As an example, the Early Childhood Longitudinal Study available through NCES is a three-stage sampling design in which the primary sampling unit (PSU) consists of selection of counties or groups of counties followed by schools within those counties and then students within those schools. Stratification and probability proportional to size (PPS) are applied at the first two stages, with stratification (disproportionate to size) at the final stage.

With nesting of clusters within strata and the sampling of individual units from the clusters, complex samples often violate the assumption of random sampling. Ignoring violations of this assumption is a model misspecification that can lead to underestimation of standard errors associated with variable effects and, consequently, increased Type I error rates (Lee & Forthofer, 2006) and misinterpretation of relationships within the data (Kenny & Judd, 1986; Kish, 1995; Lumley, 2004; Murray, 1998; Raudenbush & Bryk, 2002).

The second issue in most complex samples is that there is disproportionate sampling due to unequal selection probability, nonresponse and nonconverage, and poststratification (Kalton, 1989). In complex sample data, weights are available that reflect selection probability, participant nonresponse, and poststratification raking (Lee & Forthofer, 2006). In the most basic form, weights represent the inverse of the probability of a unit being selected in the sample (Pfeffermann, 1993). Analyses that do not accommodate disproportionate sampling through the application of weights may result in poor performance of test statistics (and thereby poor performance of confidence intervals) as well as biased parameter estimates (Korn & Graubard, 1995; Pfeffermann, 1993).

Thus, analyzing complex survey data without addressing the issues of homogeneity or disproportionate sampling that occurs due to nonsimple random sampling methods tends to create parameter estimates that are biased and standard errors that are underestimated (Kaplan & Ferguson, 1999; Pfeffermann, 1993). To address these two issues, two approaches have been suggested as ways to appropriately analyze complex sample data: (1) model based and (2) design based.

## MODEL- VERSUS DESIGN-BASED APPROACH

The homogeneity that may result from the non-simple random sampling procedure can be addressed by using a model- or design-based approach (Kalton, 1983). A model-based approach, also referred to as a disaggregated approach, partitions the variance of the outcome into between and within variances and does so directly through the statistical methodology (Heck & Mahoe, 2004). Multilevel analysis is an example of a model-based approach. While a model-based approach will accommodate the homogeneity between clusters, this does not address unequal selection probability (however, most multilevel software allows for the application of weights to address disproportionate sampling) (Snijders & Bosker, 2012). Although less common in practice, a completely model-based approach does not require weights because variables used for oversampling are included as covariates in the model.

Sample weights, in their most basic form, are the inverse of selection probability (Kish, 1995) computed as $w_{Bi} = 1/\pi_i$, where $w_{Bi}$ refers to the base weight and $\pi_i$ is the selection probability for the $i$th sampled unit. A sample weight represents the number of units (e.g., individuals) in the population that the sampled unit represents (Biemer & Christ, 2008; Kish, 1995). Thus, their purpose is to make the distributions of the variables in the sampled data approximate that of variables in the population so that unbiased estimates of population characteristics from the sampled data can be obtained (Winship & Radbill, 1994). It is appropriate to introduce sample weights when there is unequal selection probability (i.e., disproportionate sampling) as well as inequalities in the sampling frame and/or sampling procedures, differences in nonresponse and/or noncoverage, and statistical adjustment of estimates (e.g., ratio estimation and poststratification adjustments) (Kish, 1995). In many instances, the sampling weight is the product of the inverse of the probability of selection for the unit (i.e., base or design weight), $w_{Bi}$, nonresponse adjustment factor, $w_{NRi}$, and poststratification adjustment factor, $w_{NCi}$; that is, $w_i = (w_{Bi})(w_{NRi})(w_{NCi})$ (Biemer & Christ, 2008). In multistage sampling, the product of the selection probability at each state of sampling equates to the probability of selection. Readers interested in other selection probabilities are referred to other sources (see Lohr, 2010).

The nonresponse weight is the inverse of the estimated probability of responding and is computed as $w_{NRi} = (\pi_{Ri})^{-1}$, where $\pi_{Ri}$ equals the probability of unit $i$ responding. The weight that thus corrects for nonresponse is the product of the base and nonresponse weights [i.e., $(w_{Bi}) \times (w_{NRi})$]. The poststratification weight is computed as

$$w_{NCh^*i^*} = \frac{N_{n^*}}{\sum_{i=1}^{n_{h^*}} w_{Bh^*i} W_{NRh^*i}}$$

where $h$ are the mutually exclusive and exhaustive cells into which the respondents have been poststratified, $N$ is the total target population size, and the noncoverage adjustment is for unit $i^*$ in a particular cell, $h^*$ (Biemer & Christ, 2008).

A design-based approach (which is the focus of this chapter), also referred to as an aggregated approach, is essentially a single-level model in which the design issues of a complex sample are appropriately addressed (Thomas & Heck, 2001). In a single-level approach, model parameters are estimated using weights and methods that adjust for standard errors given the complex nature of the sampling, and this is the most appropriate strategy for addressing the issues of disproportionate sampling and homogeneous groups (i.e., multistage sampling), respectively (Hahs-Vaughn, 2005; Thomas & Heck, 2001). Most standard statistical software now provides capabilities for analyzing complex sample data in this way, and many can accommodate different techniques for addressing variance estimation for complex sample data including linearization (e.g., Taylor-series linearization [Rust, 1985]) and replication methods (e.g., jackknife [JK] procedures and balanced repeated replication [BRR] procedures [Wolter, 1985]). In addition, crude adjustments to the standard errors based on estimated design effects are possible. The design effect is an index that measures the effect of the sampling design on the variance (Kish, 1995). In this alternative, the normalized weight (the raw base weight divided by its mean [Peng, 2000]) is divided by the design effect (Thomas & Heck, 2001) to create a design effect (DEFF) adjusted weight that is applied to the data. Computationally, this can be seen as

$$\frac{w_{Bi}/\overline{w}_{Bi}}{SE_{CS}^2/SE_{SRS}^2} = \frac{NORMWT}{DEFF}$$

Applying this design effect adjusted weight to the data adjusts the relative weight to reflect the sample rather than population (through the normalized weight) and also adjusts the relative weight down as a function of the design effect.

With Taylor-series linearization, the estimated variance is a weighted combination of variance within a stratum that is computed by the first-order derivatives across that stratum's primary sampling units (PSUs)

(Kalton, 1983). Linearization techniques are accomplished in specialized software by applying a base weight, strata, and cluster variables. With replication methods, repeated samples are taken from the observed data. Within each subsample, the desired statistic is calculated, and the variance is then estimated from the subsample data (Rust & Rao, 1996). There are different types of replication approaches based on how the subsamples are drawn. These include, for example, BRR, JK methods (JK1, JK2, and JK*n*), and bootstrapping. Replication methods are conducted within specialized software by applying a base weight and multiple replicate weights. Which replication method is selected is dependent on the sampling design and more specifically, if and/or how stratification was used and the number of PSUs within each stratum. For example, in cases when the sampling design does not involve stratification, JK1 is appropriate. In contrast, if stratification was used in the sampling design and two PSUs per stratum were selected, then JK2, BRR, or BRR with Fay's correction is appropriate. JK*n* is the correct replication method to use when more than two PSUs per stratum were selected (Rust & Rao, 1996). Bootstrapping is implemented at the PSU level with the bootstrapping performed separately within each stratum with new replicate weights produced based on the bootstrap function (Asparouhov & Muthen, 2010; Stapleton, 2008).

A substantial number of complex survey data are available to researchers, and current software is designed to more adequately analyze it. Recently, how to apply the propensity score method to improve the quality of complex sample data analysis has been given some attention (e.g., DuGoff et al., 2014; Hahs-Vaughn & Onwuegbuzie, 2006; Hahs-Vaughn, 2013; Zanutto et al., 2005). As propensity score analysis is a multi-step process, there are various points at which the sample design can be considered, the primary being at the point of propensity score estimation and post hoc propensity score estimation when estimating treatment effect (DuGoff et al., 2014). One suggestion is to include the sample weight in estimating the propensity score (DuGoff et al., 2014) and thus the estimation of the propensity score (i.e., the propensity score model) does not need to be weighted (DuGoff et al., 2014; Zanutto et al., 2005). As Zanutto and colleagues (2005) state, "estimated propensity scores are used only to form subclasses with similar background covariates in the sample data and not to make inferences about the population-level propensity score model, it is not necessary to use survey-weighted estimation for the propensity score model" (pp. 69–70). It can be argued that this approach creates imprecision in estimating the treatment effect as samples that are matched by propensity score without complex sample adjustment are not necessarily good matches in estimating treatment effects when weighted.

# PROPENSITY SCORE ANALYSIS WITH COMPLEX SAMPLES IN THE LITERATURE

## Methods

Data Source

A content analysis of applied propensity score analysis published studies was conducted to determine the extent to which complex samples are analyzed and the extent to which the sampling design was acknowledged in the propensity score analysis. To identify the studies, an electronic search without a date of publication restriction was conducted in ERIC-EBSCO Host in May 2013. The electronic search used the following keywords to identify potentially appropriate studies: "propensity score," "propensity anal*," or "propensity match*," with the asterisk identifying all terms with that prefix regardless of ending (e.g., *analysis, analyses; match, matched, matching*). These terms have also been used in similar searches (Hahs-Vaughn, 2006, 2013). From the identified studies, abstracts were reviewed to identify applied studies. Studies that were purely methodological or nonempirical (e.g., commentary) were excluded. The remaining studies were subject to full review, coding for complex sample elements.

Coding Form

Elements of the coding form developed by Thoemmes and Kim (2011) and modified by Hahs-Vaughn (2013) to include items related to complex samples were used for coding. Specifically, the following items developed by Hahs-Vaughn (2013) were coded from the articles subject to full review: (1) complex sampling design (yes, no); (2) complex survey data source; (3) accommodation of complex sampling design (yes, no); and (4) description of complex survey adjustment.

## Results

Using the search previously discussed, there were 265 publications through May 3, 2013, identified from the ERIC search. Of those, there were 179 journal publications, 86 ERIC documents, 13 reports, and 1 book. The abstracts of the 179 journal publications were reviewed; 11 studies were deemed to be solely methodological in nature, and two articles were deemed to be nonempirical. These manuscripts were excluded from further review. A full review of the remaining 168 studies was undertaken. During the full review, five additional articles were excluded (three were commentaries and did not contain empirical research, one was theoretical, and one used simulated data only), resulting in a final sample size of 163.

Of the 163 studies, 45% ($n = 74$) had analyzed complex survey data. Of the remaining studies, 44% ($n = 71$) had not used complex samples. It was not possible to determine if the data had a complex data structure in 18% ($n = 11$) of the studies. In a review of the 74 studies that had analyzed complex survey data, less than 25% ($n = 18$, 24%) had made some type of adjustment for the sampling design. However, there was clearly no consensus on how to address the design, with some studies applying a weight during the propensity score estimation, some using the weight as a covariate in the propensity score estimation, and others applying the weight after propensity score estimation. Of the 56 studies that did *not* address the sampling, a small percentage (less than 10%) acknowledged that the data were a complex survey but did not make any type of adjustment. These results illustrate the widespread use of complex survey data with propensity score analysis but the limited understanding of how to marry propensity score analysis with the data. For researchers who do understand the nuances of complex survey data, this illustrates the lack of consensus on how to approach propensity score analysis with this type of data.

## DEMONSTRATION OF PROPENSITY SCORE ANALYSIS WITH COMPLEX SAMPLES

### Methods

Using the NCES's Early Childhood Longitudinal Study—Kindergarten Class of 1998–1999 (ECLS-K), a propensity score analysis to examine eighth-grade reading as a function of public/private school attendance was used to demonstrate how to apply the propensity score method to a complex sample. Analysis was conducted with and without addressing complex sample issues. While the empirical example employs an example from education, readers are reminded that the process and implications are applicable across complex surveys in general regardless of discipline.

### Data Source

ECLS-K provides data on children at entry into school and ultimately through eighth grade (NCES, n.d.). Variables are available in the ECLS-K on the child, parent, teacher, and school. During the base year of data collection (1998–1999), a multistage probability sample was used to select a nationally representative sample of children attending kindergarten during the base year. Geographic areas (counties or groups of counties) were the PSUs and were selected with probability proportional to size. Of the 100 PSUs selected, the 24 largest were included with certainty. The remaining 76 PSUs were further partitioned into strata, and two PSUs from each stratum were selected without replacement. Public and private schools that offered kindergarten programs and that were located in the PSUs were the secondary sampling unit. The students within the school selected were the third sampling unit. Asian/Pacific Islanders were oversampled during the base-year data collection. More detailed information on the survey methodology can be found in the technical report (Tourangeau et al., 2004).

### Delimitations

The sample was delimited to children who met the following criteria: (1) nonzero longitudinal child base weight (C1_7SC0 [$n$ = 2,369]); (2) did not change school type between rounds (i.e., did not move from public to private school or vice versa) ($n$ = 2,121)[1]; (3) first-time kindergartener in the base year ($n$ = 1,919) (P1FIRKDG = 1); and (4) complete data on the outcome, eighth-grade reading IRT scale score ($n$ = 1901) (C7R4RSCL).

### Missing Data

A total of 60 variables were ultimately used to estimate the propensity score. Of these, there were 40 continuous and 20 categorical variables. There were minimal missing data on the continuous variables used to estimate the propensity score. The range of units (e.g., subjects) with missing data was 0 to 432. Of the continuous variables, 12 of the 45 continuous variables had between 5 and 10% missing, and 5 of the 45 had between 10 and 17% missing. Replacement of missing values for the continuous variables was dealt with using expectation maximization (EM) in SPSS Missing Value Analysis v. 21. There were also minimal missing data on the categorical variables, with only one of the 19 categorical variables having more than 10% missing (specifically 11%) and three with 1 to 5% missing. For the variable with 11% missing, the missing was included as a category in the propensity score estimation. For all other categorical variables, the missing was not estimated but included in the reference category (i.e., "0").

### Complex Sample Adjustment

As indicated previously, propensity score analysis software does not currently allow for direct adjustment for complex samples. Thus, "best available" adjustments were done throughout the propensity score analysis process: two are a priori adjustments made prior to propensity score estimation, and two are post-hoc adjustments made after the propensity score has been estimated.

The a priori and post-hoc adjustment included linearization in the propensity score estimation. This first and best case scenario (of those illustrated) when estimating the propensity scores uses Taylor-series linearization as the analytic approach to address the complex sampling design, applying the child base (C1_C7SC0), strata (C17SCSTR), and cluster (C17SCPSU) weights using SPSS v. 21 Complex Samples. Linearization was followed through in the analyses to estimate the treatment effect (and thus provide post-hoc adjustment as well). This is referred to as the *linearization adjustment*. The a priori adjustment included the survey weight as a covariate in the propensity score estimation. The estimation of treatment effect was conducted with no weight applied. This is referred to as the *weight as covariate adjustment*.

Two complex sample (CS) adjustments conducted post hoc to estimation of the propensity score are demonstrated. The first CS post-hoc adjustment applies the design effect adjusted weight (Thomas, Heck, & Bauer, 2005) which may be an option in cases when it was not possible to apply linearization, for example, in the event that researchers do not have access to software that allows linearization or replication (e.g., SPSS base package users that do not have the Complex Samples package add-on). The design effect adjusted weight was estimated as the product of the inverse design effect (DEFF) and the normalized weight (i.e., the base weight divided by the mean weight). The DEFF for the reading scale score was 6.449 (Tourangeau, Nord, Le, & Sorongon, 2009). Treatment effect was estimated with the DEFF adjusted weight applied. In this demonstration, the DEFF adjusted weight was applied to the unweighted propensity score when estimating the treatment effect only (i.e., the propensity score was estimated without acknowledgment of the complex sample design). This is referred to as the *DEFF adjustment*.

The second post-hoc CS adjustment demonstration applies a multiplicative weight that combines the survey weight and the propensity score (i.e., survey weight multiplied by the inverse of the unweighted propensity score) (Zanutto et al., 2005), which is related to weighting by the inverse of the probability of receiving the treatment (IPTW) (Rosenbaum, 1987). This application is conducted at the stage of estimating the treatment effect. Thus, in this multiplicative weight illustration, the propensity score was created without CS adjustment, and recognition of the complex design comes after estimating the propensity score when computing the treatment effects. This is referred to as the *multiplicative adjustment*.

The unweighted propensity score was estimated without acknowledging the complex survey design at any stage of the analyses (estimation of propensity score or conditioning on propensity score). Hereinafter, this is termed *unweighted*.

## Results

An illustration of propensity score analysis with the ECLS-K was conducted examining eighth-grade reading as a function of public/private school attendance. The demonstration includes four different approaches to analyzing complex survey data, which are compared to analyses that do not acknowledge the complex sampling design.

### Defining Variables

The first step in the propensity analysis is to define the variables in the model, including the dependent (i.e., response) variable $(r)$, the causal variable $(z)$, and the propensity score $(e(x))$. For this demonstration, the dependent variable $(r)$ is reading performance, measured by reading IRT scale score (C7R4RSCL), which was collected during the spring of the student's eighth-grade year. The causal variable of interest is attendance in public (coded as "1") versus private school (coded as "0"). Since the data are delimited to children who did not change school type, this causal variable represents public or private school attendance from kindergarten through eighth grade.

When examining variables appropriate for estimating the propensity score, it is important to consider variables that are measured prior to the causal variable to prevent the influence of the treatment (i.e., attending public school vs. private school) on the measure. The covariates in the analyses presented here were measured during the first wave of the ECLS-K data collection (i.e., fall of the child's kindergarten year). Some of the items measured (e.g., number of nonparental hours in PreK and has the child ever attended Head Start) required the parent to recall the information. Because propensity score analysis requires covariates to be measured prior to treatment so that the covariate is unaffected by the treatment (Joffe & Rosenbaum, 1999), it is assumed that the covariates were unaffected by the child being in kindergarten at the time the parent reported the information. In other words, while these covariates were measured after treatment had commenced (i.e., in the fall semester of the year in which the child was enrolled in public or private school), it was assumed that the values reported by the parents are those that would have been measured prior to treatment.

The covariates included in the model represent a mix of variables that have been identified through previous research to be related to public or private school attendance as well as variables that were hypothesized to be related to decision on school type. These included demographic types of variables (e.g., age at kindergarten entry, socioeconomic level, gender, race, disability status, biological mother's age at first birth, non-English, Census region) as well as cognitive-related variables (e.g., reading performance, mathematics performance, general knowledge), motor skills (fine and gross), and parent and teacher reports on the child (e.g., self-control, approaches to learning, interpersonal, externalizing problem behaviors, internalizing problem behaviors). Given that parsimony is not a requirement of propensity matching, including additional variables to assist in matching is appropriate.

## Propensity Score Estimation

To estimate the propensity score, attendance at public school (i.e., the causal variable, $z$) was modeled as the outcome given the covariates ($x$) in a binary logistic regression model. There were 20 covariates initially assessed. Standardized mean differences and graphs suggested that balance was not achieved overall nor within stratum for both the weighted and unweighted models. Forty-five additional covariates (for a total of 65 covariates) were assessed. Of the 65 covariates, 5 were not included in the final propensity score estimation as they were statistically nonsignificant ($p > .20$) when correlated to both the outcome (eighth-grade reading) and treatment (public/private school attendance). The propensity score was thus estimated with 60 covariates (40 continuous, 20 categorical; for brevity, the list is not presented here but is available from the author upon request).

Logistic regression was selected as the estimation method because other options, such as probit, while available in standard statistical software, are not available in SPSS Complex Samples. The propensity score was created by saving the predicted probabilities when generating the logistic regression model. Comparisons of the aggregated weighted propensity scores to the unweighted propensity scores are presented in Table 11.1, three of which are presented graphically in Figure 11.1. Note that the propensity scores weighted by the DEFF adjustment and multiplicative adjustment are not included in the graph as both are methods performed after propensity score estimation. In aggregate, the propensity score estimated using the linearization adjustment had a higher average, decreased variability, and larger range as compared to the unweighted propensity score and any other a priori or post-hoc CS adjustment. This pattern was

**TABLE 11.1. Weighted and Unweighted Propensity Score Statistics**

| | No CS adjustment | | | CS adjustment post hoc PS estimation | | | | | | CS adjustment at PS estimation | | | | | |
| | Unweighted | | | Weighted (DEFF adjusted weight applied to unweighted PS) | | | Weight included as covariate in PS estimation | | | Weighted (linearization)[a] | | | | | |
| | All | Private | Public | All | Private | Public | All | Private | Public | All | Private | Public |
|---|---|---|---|---|---|---|---|---|---|---|---|---|
| Mean | .827 | .590 | .877 | .872 | .586 | .895 | .827 | .545 | .886 | .926 | .605 | .951 |
| Standard deviation | .203 | .248 | .152 | .174 | .243 | .146 | .216 | .257 | .150 | .151 | .293 | .093 |
| Variance | .041 | .061 | .023 | .030 | .059 | .021 | .047 | .066 | .023 | .022 | .086 | .009 |
| Range | .983 | .981 | .893 | .983 | .981 | .893 | .987 | .987 | .889 | .998 | .998 | .865 |
| Min. | .017 | .017 | .107 | .017 | .017 | .107 | .013 | .013 | .111 | .002 | .002 | .135 |
| Max. | 1.000 | .997 | 1.000 | 1.000 | .997 | 1.000 | 1.000 | 1.000 | 1.000 | 1.000 | 1.000 | 1.000 |
| 25th percentile | .756 | .401 | .826 | .833 | .414 | .864 | .753 | .345 | .839 | | | |
| 50th percentile | .910 | .603 | .937 | .946 | .590 | .956 | .921 | .545 | .945 | | | |
| 75th percentile | .976 | .790 | .983 | .988 | .798 | .990 | .986 | .756 | .991 | | | |
| n | 1,901 | 328 | 1,573 | 294 | 22 | 273 | 1,901 | 328 | 1,573 | 2,797,847 | 208,433 | 2,589,414 |
| Absolute d | .642 | | | .700 | | | .756 | | | .788 | | |

[a] Linearization estimates use linearization with AM software (calculation of percentiles was not possible in AM).

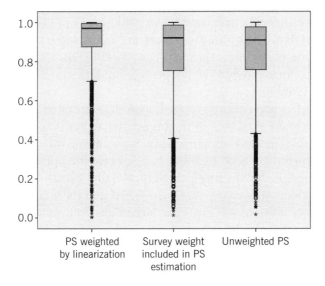

**FIGURE 11.1.** Distribution of estimated propensity score by weighting adjustment.

generally reflected when disaggregated by school type, with exceptions being a larger propensity score variation for the linearization adjustment private school students and smaller range for the linearization adjustment public school students as compared to the unweighted and other CS adjustments. Though not presented, when the propensity score was estimated with the DEFF adjustment, the results were within 1/1,000 of those of the linearization results.

Model Adequacy

After propensity score estimation, model adequacy was examined by checking balance. Balanced propensity scores ensure comparable treatment groups such that the distributions of the covariates are similar. Rosenbaum and Rubin (1983) proposed significance tests as one type of balance check, where each covariate is modeled as the outcome and the treatment group is modeled as the independent variable. Criticisms of null hypothesis significance tests, including results that are driven by sample size, have led researchers to suggest alternatives to significance tests as balance checks (Austin, Grootendorst, & Anderson, 2007; Imai, King, & Stuart, 2008), including standardized difference (i.e., effect size) (Austin, 2009b; Rubin, 2001) and graphs (Austin, 2009a). There remains, however, a lack of consensus on standards for selecting balance indices, and thus this continues to be a challenge (Fraser et al., 2011). For this illustration, absolute standardized mean differences are examined (calculated as the absolute value of the mean propensity score difference of public to private school students divided by the pooled standard deviation (Rosnow & Rosenthal, 1996).

Table 11.1 presents aggregated and disaggregated (by treatment group) descriptive statistics for the propensity scores based on approach. The absolute standardized propensity score mean difference between public and private school students in aggregate (i.e., prior to stratification) was the least for the unweighted results ($d = 0.642$), followed by the DEFF adjustment propensity score ($d = 0.701$) and the weight as a covariate propensity score ($d = 0.756$). The largest absolute standardized mean difference was for the linearization adjustment ($d = 0.789$). In comparison, the absolute standardized mean difference was less than 0.50 after stratification in all strata with the exception of one (the exception being stratum 1 for the DEFF adjustment) (see Table 11.2). Per Rubin (2001), the difference in propensity score means between the treated and control groups after matching should be less than one-half standard deviation. In cases exceeding that value, this may prevent effective matching of treated and control students. In this demonstration, there is generally evidence of overlap after stratification. Adhering to the minima and maxima comparison for overlap or common support, where the propensity score minimum and maximum values for both the treated and control groups should ensure range that each student should have a close match (Guo & Fraser, 2010), the following overlap regions and number of units excluded in the common support region are observed: unweighted, 0.107, 0.997, $n = 151$ or 8% nonoverlap; DEFF adjustment, 0.107, 0.997, $n = 151$ or 8% nonoverlap; weight as covariate adjustment, 0.111, 1.00, $n = 17$ or less than 1% nonoverlap; linearization adjustment, 0.135, 1.00, $n = 16$ or less than 1% nonoverlap. This indicates that the most overlap in common support regions resulted from the a priori complex sample adjustments (i.e., weight as covariate adjustment and linearization adjustment).

Also per Rubin (2001), the ratio of the propensity score variances after matching should be near one with variance ratios of 0.50 or 2.0 too extreme. In this demonstration, prior to stratification, all examples have ratios greater than one with the unweighted propensity score having the lowest ratio (2.662) (see Table 11.1). This is followed closely by the DEFF adjustment propensity score and the weight as a covariate adjustment (2.771 and 2.936, respectively). The largest ratio was for propensity score variances estimated by the linearization adjustment (9.926). These results also suggest evidence of nonoverlap prior to stratification, the most severe

TABLE 11.2. Mean Weighted and Unweighted Propensity Score Statistics by Subclassification

| | Unweighted | | | Weighted (DEFF adjusted weight applied to unweighted PS) | | | Weight included as covariate in PS estimation (no weight applied after) | | | Weighted (linearization) | | |
|---|---|---|---|---|---|---|---|---|---|---|---|---|
| Strata | Abs $d$ | Private | Public | Abs $d$ | Private | Public | Abs $d$ | Private | Public | Abs $d$ | Private | Public |
| 1 | 0.29 | 0.42 (0.17) $n = 194$ | 0.54 (0.14) $n = 186$ | 0.62 | 0.50 (0.19) $n = 17$ | 0.61 (0.15) $n = 42$ | 0.36 | 0.40 (0.18) $n = 216$ | 0.53 (0.13) $n = 164$ | 0.45 | 0.50 (0.55) $n = 225$ | 0.78 (0.21) $n = 337$ |
| 2 | 0.11 | 0.77 (0.05) $n = 79$ | 0.80 (0.04) $n = 301$ | 0.04 | 0.87 (0.05) $n = 3$ | 0.86 (0.03) $n = 56$ | 0.07 | 0.78 (0.06) $n = 75$ | 0.80 (0.05) $n = 305$ | 0.03 | 0.94 (0.01) $n = 63$ | 0.95 (0.04) $n = 365$ |
| 3 | 0.02 | 0.91 (0.02) $n = 44$ | 0.91 (0.02) $n = 337$ | NA | 0.94 (NA) $n = 2$ | 0.95 (0.02) $n = 57$ | 0.08 | 0.91 (0.02) $n = 24$ | 0.92 (0.02) $n = 357$ | 0.02 | 0.98 (<.01) $n = 29$ | 0.98 (0.01) $n = 339$ |
| 4 | 0.04 | 0.96 (0.01) $n = 10$ | 0.97 (0.01) $n = 370$ | NA | NA | 0.98 (<.01) $n = 59$ | 0.05 | 0.97 (0.01) $n = 5$ | 0.97 (0.01) $n = 375$ | 0.02 | 1.00 (<.01) $n = 10$ | 1.00 (<.01) $n = 301$ |
| 5 | NA | 1.00 $n = 1$ | 0.99 (.00) $n = 379$ | NA | NA | 1.00 (<.01) $n = 58$ | 0.02 | 1.00 (0.003) $n = 8$ | 1.00 (0.002) $n = 372$ | NA | 1.00 (NA) $n = 1$ | 1.00 (<.001) $n = 231$ |

*Note.* Standard deviations are in parentheses. Unweighted counts. $n = 1,901$. Stratum 5 represents the highest probability of attending a public school; stratum 1 represents the lowest probability of attending public school. Abs $d$, absolute standardized mean difference using the pooled standard deviation in the denominator.

being for linearization. After stratification, the ratios were greatly reduced with the strata within the DEFF adjustment propensity score being close to one (ranging from 0.79 to 1.06) and thus generally meeting Rubin's standards (see Table 11.2 for standard deviation values by strata), with variances outside Rubin's range only seen in the higher strata (i.e., higher probability of attending public school). The largest ratios were seen within the strata for the linearization adjustment (ranging from 0.48 to 3.67) with strata 3 (3.67) and 4 (2.55) both falling outside Rubin's range. The ratio of the variances within the strata of the unweighted model ranged from 1.22 to 2.50, with only the ratio of variances for stratum 3 falling outside Rubin's standard. Similarly, for the weight as covariate adjustment and multiplicative adjustment, there was only one ratio falling outside Rubin's recommendation, specifically for stratum 5 and stratum 3, respectively.

### Conditioning on Propensity Score

After computing the propensity score, units were then matched based on their propensity score. There are a number of different algorithms to accomplish this, two of the most commonly used being stratification and matching (Hahs-Vaughn, 2013; Thoemmes & Kim, 2011). Five strata of roughly equivalent size remove about 90% of the bias (Cochran, 1968). Because propensity score matching software that directly allows for complex sample adjustment is not available, stratification based on the propensity score is one of the best available options as at least some accommodation for the design can be included in this process (e.g., application of a weight). As stated by Zanutto et al. (2005) "subclassification provides a framework that extends naturally to incorporate survey weights from complex survey designs" (p. 60). Additionally, stratification is a good fit in this particular situation given the unbalanced treatment design—one private school student (unweighted $n$ = 328) for approximately every five public school students (unweighted $n$ = 1,573). As evidenced in the balance check presented previously, propensity scores of public school students were considerably higher (and this was the case for both weighted and unweighted data), which suggests potential difficulty in finding adequate matches even though the common support region was quite large in all cases.

To create the strata, children were sorted based on propensity score, and five strata (or subclasses) with relatively equal sample sizes per strata (unweighted $n \approx 380$) were created based on the propensity score. In creating the strata for the weighted propensity score estimates (linearization adjustment and DEFF adjustment), the same process was followed, with the additional step of applying the weight. For this example, sorting was conducted such that stratum 1 represents the lowest probability of attending public school and stratum 5 represents the highest probability of attending public school.

As seen in Table 11.2, the proportions of children by school type within strata differed by whether the complex sampling design was addressed, particularly in the strata representing the highest probability of attending public school. For example, of children with the lowest probability of attending public school (stratum 1), approximately 78% based on linearization adjustment and 54% unweighted were actually attending public school. The stratum reflecting the higher probabilities of attending public school were particularly imbalanced, with none to very few private school children in subclasses four and five; this was evident for all weighting schema as well as the unweighted model. For illustrative purposes, we will continue with this example. However, in applications of propensity score analysis, the researcher should stop at this point because of failure of the propensity score to balance treatment/control group differences and reconsider the model to achieve better balance in the higher strata.

### Estimating Treatment Effects on Reading Performance

Different types of treatment effects can be estimated. Guo and Fraser (2010) provide information on seven types of treatment effects often estimated by researchers. The two most commonly estimated in the realm of propensity score analysis are the average treatment effect (ATE), which is akin to intent-to-treat (Shadish, Cook, & Campbell, 2002), and the average treatment effect for the treated (ATT). (See Chapter 1 in this book for a more detailed description of ATT and ATE.) For purposes of this chapter, ATE has been computed as the weighted average within stratum across strata (Steiner & Cook, 2013):

$$ATE_q = \sum_{q=1}^{Q} W_q \tau_q$$

where $\tau_q$ is computed as the simple difference in means between the control and treated units, and $W_q$ equals the sum of the number control and treatment units in stratum $q$ divided by the total number of control and treatment units across all strata. ATT has been computed as the weighted average within stratum and across strata as follows (Steiner & Cook, 2013):

$$ATT_q = \sum_{q=1}^{Q} W_{Tq} \tau_q$$

where $W_{T_q}$ equals the sum of the treatment units in stratum $q$ divided by the total number of control and treatment units across all strata. Thus, ATE weights reflect the distribution of both control and treated units across strata, wherein ATT weights reflect only the treated units (Steiner & Cook, 2013). Table 11.3 presents the ATE and ATT results. Because of the substantial differences in sizes of the treatment units in the upper strata, ATT is much more consistent between the different CS adjustments as compared to ATE. The DEFF adjustment provides the lowest ATT (0.39) and the multiplicative adjustment the largest ATT (1.00). If only strata 1–3 (those strata that were more balanced across all CS adjustments) are considered in the ATT, as compared to the ATT for all strata, there are no marked differences in the pattern of results. Looking only at strata 1–3 for the ATE, however, we find that the DEFF adjustment and linearization adjustment produced similar and higher (up to five times higher) average treatment effects as compared to the ATE for strata 1–3 for the unweighted model or other CS adjustment models.

Figures 11.2 and 11.3 visually illustrate the group differences (i.e., public or private school attendance) on mean reading performance by strata for the unweighted relative to CS adjusted propensity score analysis results (see Table 11.3). As seen here, attending public school (as compared to private school) generally resulted in lower mean reading performance in grade 8. The differences in reading performance between CS adjustments were most pronounced in strata 3 and 4, which reflect higher probabilities of attending public school. In examining both public and private school students, mean reading performances for the DEFF adjustment and the linearization adjustment were nearly identical. In both cases, the mean reading performance of public school students by strata was lower as compared to the unweighted and other CS adjustments. For private school students, the unweighted and CS adjustments were more similar with the exception of the weight as covariate adjustment. In that case, the weight as covariate adjustment model contrasted substantially with a smaller mean reading gap between public and private school students in stratum 3 and a much greater reading gap in stratum 5. The results for stratum 5 become less interpretable for private school students given the small $n$, however.

The results of the independent $t$-tests are summarized in Table 11.3. The tests of inference vary quite dramatically depending on the CS adjustment. The reading performance differences between public and private school students were statistically different in all strata for the weight as a covariate adjustment and the multiplicative weight adjustment. In comparison, reading performance differences between public and private school students were not statistically different for all strata in the DEFF

**TABLE 11.3. Mean Group Differences by Subclassification and CS Adjustment**

| CS adjustment | Public M (SD) | Private M (SD) | t | p | 95% CI of the difference |
|---|---|---|---|---|---|
| Unweighted | | | | | |
| Stratum 1 | 184.83 (18.82) | 188.90 (15.54) | 2.30 | .022 | 0.58, 7.56[1] |
| Stratum 2 | 180.10 (22.85) | 180.65 (20.70) | 0.19 | 0.846 | −5.02, 6.12 |
| Stratum 3 | 174.87 (24.66) | 184.78 (15.59) | 3.66 | <.001 | 4.51, 15.30[1] |
| Stratum 4 | 166.96 (26.59) | 181.52 (20.40) | 1.72 | .087 | −2.11, 31.23 |
| Stratum 5 | 153.94 (29.56) | 130.37 (NA) | −.80 | .426 | −81.77, 34.63 |
| | | | | | |
| ATE[a] | 1.11 | | | | |
| ATE (strata 1–3)[b] | 2.91 | | | | |
| ATT[a] | 0.73 | | | | |
| ATT (strata 1–3)[b] | 0.67 | | | | |
| | | | | | |
| Weight included as covariate (a priori) | | | | | |
| Stratum 1 | 182.55 (20.25) | 187.56 (14.40) | 45.90 | <.001 | 4.80, 5.22[2] |
| Stratum 2 | 179.76 (23.19) | 180.93 (20.61) | 9.26 | <.001 | 0.92, 1.42 |
| Stratum 3 | 173.91 (25.01) | 173.84 (31.34) | −0.24 | <.001 | −0.56, 0.44[1,2,3] |
| Stratum 4 | 168.25 (25.67) | 175.16 (20.15) | 28.84 | <.001 | 6.44, 7.38[1] |
| Stratum 5 | 158.12 (28.65) | 183.59 (18.40) | 232.08 | <.001 | 25.26, 25.69[1,2] |
| | | | | | |
| ATE[a] | 7.69 | | | | |
| ATE (strata 1–3)[b] | 1.22 | | | | |
| ATT[a] | 0.74 | | | | |
| ATT (strata 1–3)[b] | 0.61 | | | | |
| | | | | | |
| DEFF adjusted weight (post hoc) | | | | | |
| Stratum 1 | 182.79 (20.44) | 185.02 (19.82) | 0.38 | 0.704 | −9.44, 13.88 |
| Stratum 2 | 172.82 (22.93) | 177.20 (24.45) | 0.32 | 0.748 | −22.73, 31.47 |
| Stratum 3 | 165.95 (28.54) | 189.23 (32.06) | 0.93 | 0.359 | −27.10, 73.65 |
| Stratum 4 | 161.83 (26.42) | NA | NA | | |
| Stratum 5 | 151.83 (26.41) | NA | NA | | |
| | | | | | |
| ATE[a] | 9.33 | | | | |
| ATE (strata 1–3)[b] | 5.98 | | | | |
| ATT[a] | 0.39 | | | | |
| ATT (strata 1–3)[b] | 0.33 | | | | |

(continued)

**TABLE 11.3.** *(continued)*

| CS adjustment | Public M (SD) | Private M (SD) | t | p | 95% CI of the difference |
|---|---|---|---|---|---|
| Weighted linearization (a priori) | | | | | |
| Stratum 1 | 182.66 (31.76) | 185.02 (45.90) | 0.71 | 0.479 | −4.13, 8.85 |
| Stratum 2 | 173.34 (38.97) | 177.32 (32.46) | 0.85 | 0.397 | −5.17, 13.13 |
| Stratum 3 | 164.96 (47.69) | 189.60 (24.88) | 4.61 | <.001 | 14.16, 35.12[2] |
| Stratum 4 | 162.45 (35.74) | 175.95 (22.36) | 1.97 | 0.057 | −3.23, 23.69 |
| Stratum 5 | 151.79 (39.21) | 130.37 (NA) | −8.29 | <.001 | 18.89, 23.95[1,3] |
| ATE[a] | 5.96 | | | | |
| ATE (strata 1–3)[b] | 6.37 | | | | |
| ATT[a] | 0.85 | | | | |
| ATT (strata 1–3)[b] | 0.77 | | | | |
| Weighted multiplicative (by unweighted strata) (post hoc) | | | | | |
| Stratum 1 | 178.90 (20.82) | 187.19 (17.32) | 92.115 | <.001 | 8.12, 8.47[1,2] |
| Stratum 2 | 178.00 (25.06) | 175.85 (27.18) | −13.54 | <.001 | −2.47, −1.84 |
| Stratum 3 | 173.33 (23.62) | 180.24 (14.55) | 72.09 | <.001 | 6.72, 7.10[3] |
| Stratum 4 | 165.72 (24.82) | 182.95 (19.51) | 67.62 | <.001 | 16.74, 17.74[1] |
| Stratum 5 | 151.27 (29.60) | 130.37 (NA) | −628.96 | <.001 | −20.97, −20.84[2,3] |
| ATE[a] | 1.88 | | | | |
| ATE (strata 1–3)[b] | 2.61 | | | | |
| ATT[a] | 1.00 | | | | |
| ATT (strata 1–3)[b] | 0.92 | | | | |
| Weighted multiplicative (aggregate) | | | | | |
| | 168.11 (27.46) | 186.86 (18.11) | 627.15 | <.001 | 18.69, 18.81 |

*Note.* Numerical superscripts denote nonoverlapping confidence intervals.
[a]ATE and ATT reflect the weighted average of individual stratum across all strata.
[b]ATE and ATT reflect the weighted average of individual stratum across strata 1–3.

Propensity Score Analysis with Complex Survey Samples 257

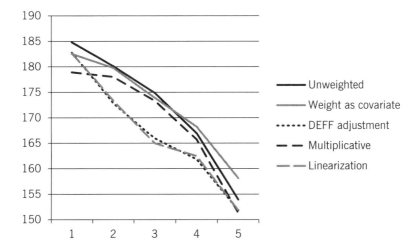

**FIGURE 11.2.** Public school student mean eighth-grade reading performance by strata and complex sample adjustment.

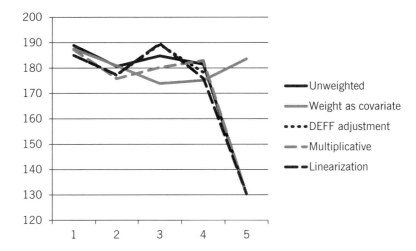

**FIGURE 11.3.** Private school student mean eighth-grade reading performance by strata and complex sample adjustment.

adjustment. Mixed results were seen for the strata in the unweighted model and linearization adjustment, with stratum 3 showing consistent statistically significant differences in both and strata 2 and 4 showing nonsignificance in both. Taking students with the lowest probability of attending public school (stratum 1) as an example, there were not statistically significant differences in mean reading performance between groups only for the DEFF adjustment and linearization adjustment models. The unweighted and other CS adjustments suggested that private school students in this stratum were performing statistically significantly higher than public school students.

To determine statistically significant differences between the unweighted results and the results for models with CS adjustments, confidence intervals of mean differences by strata were reviewed, with nonoverlapping confidence intervals suggesting statistically significant mean reading differences between groups (Schenker & Gentleman, 2001). The unweighted results resulted in nonoverlapping confidence intervals, with CS adjusted results in only two units: within stratum 1 with the multiplicative adjustment results and within stratum 3 with the weight as covariate adjustment. The most nonoverlapping confidence intervals were seen for the weight as covariate adjustment, with 7, and the multiplicative adjustment, with 6.

The nonoverlapping confidence intervals were as follows: For stratum 1, specifically between the (1) unweighted and multiplicative adjustment; and (2) weight as a covariate adjustment and multiplicative adjustment. For stratum 3, non-overlapping confidence intervals were evident for: (1) unweighted and weight as a covariate adjustment; (2) weight as a covariate adjustment and linearization adjustment; and (3) weight as a covariate adjustment and multiplicative adjustment. For stratum 4, only the weight as a covariate adjustment and multiplicative adjustment had nonoverlapping confidence intervals. For stratum 5, nonoverlapping confidence intervals were evident for: (1) weight as a covariate adjustment and linearization adjustment; (2) weight as covariate adjustment and multiplicative adjustment; and (3) linearization adjustment and multiplicative adjustment.

## CONCLUSION AND RECOMMENDATIONS

This chapter shows mixed results for the propensity score analysis based on the type of complex sample adjustment. There were consistently statistically significant differences in reading performance between public and private school students in the strata for models where the propensity score had been estimated by weight as a covariate adjustment and multiplicative adjustment. In comparison, there were no statistically significant differences in reading between public and private school students for the DEFF adjustment. Mixed results in strata in relation to differences in reading between public and private school students were seen for the unweighted and linearization adjustment models. In examining Figures 11.2 and 11.3, reading performance for DEFF adjustment and linearization adjustment was nearly identical.

Nonoverlapping confidence intervals, suggesting statistically significant differences by CS adjustment, were most evident between strata for the models with the weight as a covariate adjustment and the multiplicative adjustment. There was a slight pattern of fewer nonoverlapping confidence intervals for mean differences in reading in the lower strata (i.e., those reflecting the lowest probability of attending public school). In reviewing the ATT, the DEFF adjustment produced the lowest ATT, about one-half the size of the ATT of the unweighted, weight as covariate adjustment, and linearization adjustment models and about 40% the size of the ATT of the multiplicative adjustment.

Some patterns were evident with both the weight as covariate adjustment and multiplicative adjustment results. In both of these cases, it is important to note that there is greater direct impact of the value of the weight in either estimating the propensity score (as in the case for the weight as covariate adjustment) or weighting the data (as in the case of the multiplicative adjustment). For the ECLS-K data used in this demonstration, the average child base weight was 1,471.78 ($SD$ = 2,111.66) with a range of 14,481.85 (ranging from a minimum of 79.85 to a maximum of 14,561.70). The magnitude of these values when estimating the propensity score or when weighting the data in the multiplicative adjustment cannot be discounted, and it is not surprising that both adjustments produced statistically significant mean reading performance differences between groups and both also had the largest number of nonoverlapping mean difference confidence intervals. It seems reasonable that the results are likely an artifact of the way in which the weight was applied in the CS adjustment.

Problems were encountered when applying the DEFF adjustment after estimating the (unweighted) propensity score in that the sizes of the groups decreased dramatically, particularly for the private school students creating upper strata that were unusable. Although the distribution of private school students was minimized in the upper strata for all methods examined, it was most particularly problematic for the DEFF adjustment.

Methodologically, the results are interesting; however, substantively (in terms of evidence to support theory, research informing practice, and policy implications), the results of this study suggest great ramifications. More specifically, the ECLS-K data (and other complex survey data) are designed so that, when the sampling design is acknowledged through the analysis, the variances are estimated correctly (i.e., there is an adjustment for nonindependence) and the results are representative of all children who attended kindergarten at a particular point in time (i.e., there is an adjustment for disproportionate sampling). The analyses presented herein were weighted in various capacities to address the inherent design issues. If the weight is not applied, as stated by Kalton (1989), the sample becomes simply "a collection of individuals that represents no meaningful population" (p. 583), which likewise suggests meaningless interpretations. Failing to address correct variance estimation results in biased standard errors and thus overestimated test statistics, which leads to differences in tests of inference.

Analysis of complex samples with propensity score analysis has added complexity given the multistep propensity score analysis process. "At what point the survey weights should be incorporated, or whether they are needed at all, may still be up for debate" (Hahs-Vaughn & Onwuegbuzie, 2006, p. 55).

There are additional ramifications based on the results in this chapter. Differences in school type that *were not* important when the sampling design was considered *were* important when unweighted (and vice versa), and this varied not just based on *whether* the complex design was acknowledged but *how* it was accommodated in the propensity score analysis. The conclusions this leads to, in terms of effectiveness of programs and initiatives (such as public vs. private school attendance) and stakeholders (e.g., parents and teachers), can then fluctuate quite wildly. One may swing (depending on the complex sample adjustment) from concluding that attending a private school is important to concluding that there is not a relationship between the type of school attended (public vs. private) and reading outcomes.

It is recommended that analysis of complex samples incorporate measures to accommodate the complex survey design to allow inference to the intended population. More specifically, it is recommended that the highest level of recognition of the sample design be incorporated throughout the propensity score analysis process. This includes the use of linearization or replicate weights when estimating the propensity score as well as following through with linearization or replication in conditioning on the propensity score and estimating the treatment effects. Of the examples presented, only this method of CS adjustment recognizes the survey design at both the a priori and post-hoc stages of propensity score estimation. Thus, both the estimation of the propensity score *and* the estimate of the treatment effect are based on the intended sample with correct variance adjustment. The following reporting practices are also recommended:

1. Be transparent in presentation of the complex sample to ensure easy replication of the data. This includes specifying to the readers the name and wave of the survey (referencing appropriately so that interested readers can easily access the data source), whether public or restricted data were used, variable names (as defined in the data file), and original response scales and recoding.

2. Provide comprehensive, clear, and transparent description of the steps taken to adjust the propensity score analysis for the survey design. This includes specifying the point at which adjustment was made and how it was made, as well as being specific in defining the variables used to make the CS adjustment. Including programming language for replication is helpful.

### NOTE

1. Variables in the ECLS-K that were used to delimit change of school type were as follows: FKCHGSCH = 0 (did not change school); R3R2SCHG = 1 (did not change school) or 2 (transferred from public to public) or 3 (transferred from private to private); R4R2SCHG = 1 or 2 or 3; R4R3SCHG = 1 or 2 or 3; R5R4SCHG = 1 or 2 or 3; R6R5SCHG = 1 or 2 or 3; R7R6SCHG = 1 or 2 or 3.

### REFERENCES

Asparouhov, T., & Muthen, B. O. (2010). Resampling methods in Mplus for complex survey data. Available at *www.statmodel.com/download/Resampling_Methods5.pdf*.

Austin, P. C. (2009a). Balance diagnostics for comparing the distribution of baseline covariates between treatment groups in propensity-score matched samples. *Statistics in Medicine, 28*, 3083–3107.

Austin, P. C. (2009b). The relative ability of different propensity score methods to balance measured covariates between treated and untreated subjects in observational studies. *Medical Decision Making, 29*(6), 661–677.

Austin, P. C., Grootendorst, P., & Anderson, G. M. (2007). A comparison of the ability of different propensity score models to balance measured variables between treated and untreated subjects: A Monte Carlo study. *Statistics in Medicine, 26,* 734–753.

Biemer, P. P., & Christ, S. L. (2008). Weighting survey data. In E. D. DeLeeuw (Ed.), *International handbook of survey methodology* (pp. 317–341). New York: Erlbaum.

Chambers, R. L., & Skinner, C. J. (2003). *Analysis of survey data.* Hoboken, NJ: Wiley.

Cochran, W. G. (1968). The effectiveness of adjustment by subclassification in removing bias in observational studies. *Biometrics, 24*(2), 295–313.

DuGoff, E. H., Schuler, M., & Stuart, E. A. (2014). Generalizing observational study results: Applying propensity score methods to complex surveys. *Health Services Research, 49*(1), 284–303.

Fraser, M. W., Guo, S., Ellis, A. R., Thompson, A. M., Wike, T. L., et al. (2011). Outcome studies of social, behavioral, and educational interventions: Emerging issues and challenges. *Research on Social Work Practice, 21*(6), 619–635.

Guo, S., & Fraser, M. W. (2010). *Propensity score analysis: Statistical methods and applications.* Thousand Oaks, CA: Sage.

Hahs-Vaughn, D. L. (2005). A primer for using and understanding weights with national datasets. *Journal of Experimental Education, 73*(3), 221–248.

Hahs-Vaughn, D. L. (2006). Analysis of data from complex samples. *International Journal of Research and Method in Education, 29*(2), 163–181.

Hahs-Vaughn, D. L. (2013). *A systematic literature review of the application of propensity score analysis in the social sciences.* Paper presented at the American Educational Research Association annual meeting, San Francisco, CA.

Hahs-Vaughn, D. L., McWayne, C. M., Bulotskey-Shearer, R. J., Wen, X., & Faria, A. (2011). Methodological considerations in using complex survey data: An applied example with the Head Start Family and Child Experiences Survey. *Evaluation Review, 35*(3), 269–303.

Hahs-Vaughn, D. L., & Onwuegbuzie, A. J. (2006). Estimating and using propensity score analysis with complex samples. *Journal of Experimental Education, 75*(1), 31–65.

Heck, R. H., & Mahoe, R. (2004, April). *An example of the impact of sample weights and centering on multilevel SEM models.* Paper presented at the annual meeting of the American Educational Research Association, San Diego, CA.

Imai, K., King, G., & Stuart, E. A. (2008). Misunderstandings among experimentalists and observationalists about causal inference. *Journal of the Royal Statistical Society A, 177,* 481–502.

Joffe, M. M., & Rosenbaum, P. R. (1999). Invited commentary: Propensity scores. *American Journal of Epidemiology, 150*(4), 327–333.

Kalton, G. (1983). Models in the practice of survey sampling. *International Statistical Review, 51,* 175–188.

Kalton, G. (1989). Modeling considerations: Discussion from a survey sampling perspective. In D. Kasprzyk, G. Duncan, G. Kalton, & M. Singh (Eds.), *Panel surveys* (pp. 575–585). New York: Wiley.

Kaplan, D., & Ferguson, A. J. (1999). On the utilization of sample weights in latent variable models. *Structural Equation Modeling, 6*(4), 305–321.

Kenny, D. A., & Judd, C. M. (1986). Consequences of violating the independence assumption in analysis of variance. *Psychological Bulletin, 99*(3), 422–431.

Kish, L. (1995). *Survey sampling.* New York: Wiley.

Korn, E. L., & Graubard, B. I. (1995). Analysis of large health surveys: Accounting for the sampling design. *Journal of the Royal Statistical Society. Series A (Statistics in Society), 158*(2), 263–295.

Lee, E. S., & Forthofer, R. N. (2006). *Analyzing complex survey data* (2nd ed.). Thousand Oaks, CA: Sage.

Lohr, S. (2010). *Sampling: Design and analysis* (2nd ed.). Boston: Brooks/Cole.

Lumley, T. (2004). Analysis of complex survey samples. *Journal of Statistical Software, 9*(8), 1–19.

Manski, C. F. (1999). Choice as an alternative to control in observational studies: Comment. *Statistical Science, 14*(3), 279–281.

Murray, D. M. (1998). *Design and analysis of group-randomized trials.* New York: Oxford University Press.

National Center for Education Statistics. (n.d.). Early Childhood Longitudinal Program (ECLS). Retrieved July 14, 2008, from *http://nces.ed.gov/ecls/kindergarten.asp.*

Peng, S. S. (2000). *Technical issues in using NCES data.* Paper presented at the AIR/NCES National Data Institute on the Use of Postsecondary Databases, Gaithersburg, MD.

Pfeffermann, D. (1993). The role of sampling weights when modeling survey data. *International Statistical Review, 61*(2), 317–337.

Raudenbush, S. W., & Bryk, A. S. (2002). *Hierarchical linear models: Applications and data analysis methods* (2nd ed.). Thousand Oaks, CA: Sage.

Rosenbaum, P. R. (1987). Model-based direct adjustment. *Journal of the American Statistical Association, 82*(398), 387–394.

Rosenbaum, P. R., & Rubin, D. B. (1983). The central role of the propensity score in observational studies for causal effects. *Biometrika, 70*(1), 41–55.

Rosnow, R. L., & Rosenthal, R. (1996). Computing contrasts, effect sizes, and counternulls on other people's published data: General procedures for research consumers. *Psychological Methods, 1*(4), 331–340.

Rubin, D. B. (1997). Estimating causal effects from large data sets using propensity scores. *Annal of Internal Medicine, 127,* 757–763.

Rubin, D. B. (2001). Using propensity scores to help design observational studies: Application to the tobacco litigation. *Health Services and Outcomes Research Methodology, 2*(3–4), 169–188.

Rust, K. F. (1985). Variance estimation for complex estimation in sample surveys. *Journal of Official Statistics, 1,* 381–397.

Rust, K. F., & Rao, J. N. K. (1996). Variance estimation for complex surveys using replication techniques. *Statistical Methods in Medical Research, 5,* 283–310.

Schenker, N., & Gentleman, J. F. (2001). On judging the significance of differences by examining the overlap between confidence intervals. *American Statistician, 55*(3), 182–187.

Shadish, W. R., Cook, T. D., & Campbell, D. T. (2002). *Experimental and quasi-experimental designs for generalized causal inference.* Boston: Houghton Mifflin.

Skinner, C. J., Holt, D., & Smith, T. M. F. (Eds.). (1989). *Analysis of complex samples.* New York: Wiley.

Snijders, T. A. B., & Bosker, R. J. (2012). *Multilevel analysis: An introduction to basic and advanced multilevel modeling* (2nd ed.). Thousand Oaks, CA: Sage.

Stapleton, L. M. (2008). Variance estimation using replication methods in structural equation modeling with complex sample data. *Structural Equation Modeling: A Multidisciplinary Journal, 15*(2), 183–210.

Steiner, P. M., & Cook, D. (2013). Matching and propensity scores. In T. D. Little (Ed.), *Oxford handbook of quantitative methods.* New York: Oxford University Press.

Thoemmes, F. J., & Kim, E. S. (2011). A systematic review of propensity score methods in the social sciences. *Multivariate Behavioral Research, 46*(1), 90–118.

Thomas, S. L., & Heck, R. H. (2001). Analysis of large-scale secondary data in higher education research: Potential perils associated with complex sampling designs. *Research in Higher Education, 42*(5), 517–540.

Thomas, S. L., Heck, R. H., & Bauer, K. W. (2005). Weighting and adjusting for design effects in secondary data analyses. *New Directions for Institutional Research, 2005*(127), 51–72.

Tourangeau, K., Brick, M., Byrne, L., Le, T., Nord, C., West, J., & Germino Hausken, E. (2004). *Early Childhood Longitudinal Study, Kindergarten Class of 1998–99 (ECLS-K): Third grade methodology report.* Washington, DC: National Center for Education Statistics, U.S. Department of Education.

Tourangeau, K., Nord, C., Le, T., & Sorongon, A. (2009). *Early Childhood Longitudinal Study, Kindergarten class of 1998–99 (ECLS-K), combined user's manual for the ECLS-K eighth-grade and K–8 full sample data files and electronic codebooks.* Washington, DC: National Center for Education Statistics, Institute of Education Sciences, U.S. Department of Education.

Winship, C., & Radbill, L. (1994). Sampling weights and regression analysis. *Sociological Methods and Research, 23,* 230–257.

Wolter, K. M. (1985). *Introduction to variance estimation.* New York: Springer-Verlag.

Zanutto, E., Lu, B., & Hornik, R. (2005). Using propensity score subclassification for multiple treatment doses to evaluate a national antidrug media campaign. *Journal of Educational and Behavioral Statistics, 30*(1), 59–73.

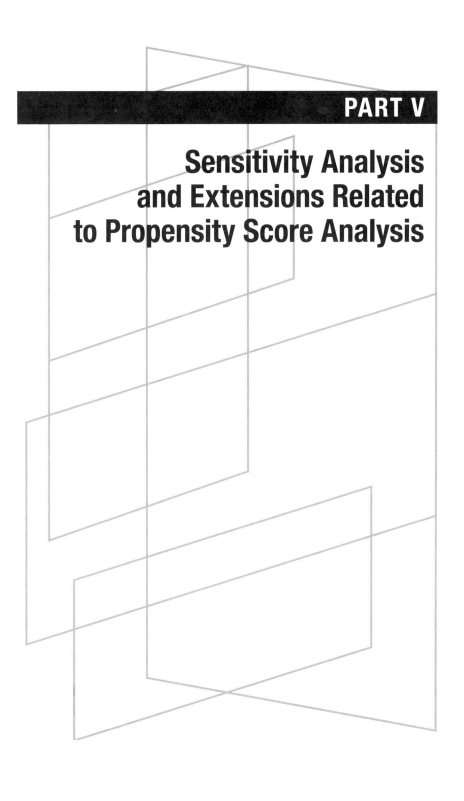

# PART V

# Sensitivity Analysis and Extensions Related to Propensity Score Analysis

# CHAPTER 12

# Missing Data in Propensity Scores

## Robin Mitra

Missing data is a fairly common occurrence when trying to proceed with a propensity score analysis. This is because propensity score analysis is typically used with observational data, and as the data collection procedure for obtaining such data is out of the analyst's control, the presence of missing values is more likely than with other types of data such as randomized controlled trials. It is thus relevant to consider how best we can handle this problem while proceeding with a propensity score analysis and obtaining appropriate inferences. It is important to first recognize the important impact of missing values. Missing data causes several complications when trying to proceed with a propensity score analysis.

First, the obvious problem is that estimating propensity scores is now not straightforward; standard regression models need to be modified to account for the missing values. A standard approach would be to use a complete case analysis, but the usual problems with such an approach of a reduced sample size and potential for bias apply here.

Second, the type of missing data can affect how to proceed with the analysis. If the missingness is present in only the covariates, then the analyst might just deal with the missing data first and then proceed with an appropriate propensity score analysis. However, if missing values are present in the outcome, $r$, then the analyst may wish to consider how best to employ a propensity score analysis, for example, by removing missing outcome values from the dataset so as to ensure treatment effects are only made using observed outcome values. In addition, as with any statistical analysis, the missing data mechanism can influence how we might best proceed. For example, missingness in the covariates might depend on the outcome values that introduce complications into how the causal path should be modeled. This complication can be seen even if the mechanism is missing at random (so if the outcome was fully observed, for example); then an appropriate strategy would take account of $r$ when dealing with the missing covariates, when in fact we typically assume the covariates are observed before the outcome. We would then be faced with a choice of either specifying what appears to be the appropriate strategy, which makes conjectures concerning the missing covariates conditional on $r$, or preserving the causal path, where covariates are observed before treatment and treatment is administered before observing the outcome.

Third, the assessment of any inferences made is problematic as traditional measures of assessing covariate balance are not applicable with missing covariate values. Assessment of balance may look appropriate using the observed covariate values, or covariate values with missing values imputed (more detail is given on that later), but if we possessed the actual true values of all the covariates, then it is possible the balance may not be so good. Hence we may unwittingly introduce bias into estimates of the treatment effect.

Here we focus on dealing with the first complication and on covariate missing values. We assume that missing data is either not present in the outcome variable or, if it was present then the analyst has removed it before proceeding with the propensity score analysis. Some references on methods proposed to handle missing outcome values are given at the end of this chapter, but this is very much an open area for research. We also assume that the missingness is missing at random (Rubin, 1976), which means that the missing data only depend on observed values in the dataset. More details are given in the next section, but in general this is the most commonly used assumption in missing data problems and in many situations it may be a reasonable assumption to make (Schafer & Graham, 2002). We also discuss some strategies for addressing the third complication that involves developing robust procedures to handle the missing values.

In this chapter we assume that treatment effects are estimated using nearest neighbor matching by taking the difference in means of the responses in the treatment and matched control groups. Of course, other uses of propensity scores to estimate treatment effects could be considered such as subclassifying on the propensity scores (Hullsiek & Louis, 2002; Rosenbaum & Rubin, 1984) or using the propensity scores for inverse probability weighted estimation (Lunceford & Davidian, 2004; Robins,

Hernan, & Brumback, 2000) but the focus of this chapter is on how to deal with the missing values in estimating propensity scores. Once the missing data problem is addressed, any propensity score method may be used. Focusing on matching is reasonable given its wide use in the literature (Austin, 2008, 2009; Cho et al., 2007; da Veiga & Wilder, 2008). Implicitly assuming propensity score matching to estimate treatment effects also makes it more compatible with the illustrations given later in the chapter.

In this chapter, we start with a description of the framework, followed by a discussion of the traditional approaches that have been proposed to address the problem. Then we focus on imputation-based approaches to handle this problem. Imputation approaches are perhaps the most appealing approach to handle the problem of missing values. We discuss this approach in more depth in the next section. Then, we illustrate how the methods can be performed in a simulation study, followed by an application of the methods to a genuine breastfeeding study. We conclude with some remarks on these approaches and discussion on some future areas for research.

## MISSING DATA WITH PROPENSITY SCORES

Suppose we have $n$ units measured on $p$ covariates, we can represent this with a $n \times p$ covariate dataset $\mathbf{X}$ with element in the $i$th row and $j$th column $x_{ij}$ corresponding to the covariate value for the $i$th unit on the $j$th covariate. We can also define a $n \times p$ missing data indicator matrix $\mathbf{M}$, where $m_{ij} = 1$ indicates $x_{ij}$ is missing and $m_{ij} = 0$ indicates $x_{ij}$ is observed, for $i = 1, \ldots, n$ and $j = 1, \ldots, p$. We can then denote the observed and missing portions of $\mathbf{X}$ by $\mathbf{X}_{obs} = \{x_{ij} : m_{ij} = 0\}$ and $\mathbf{X}_{mis} = \{x_{ij} : m_{ij} = 1\}$, respectively. We also define a response variable $\mathbf{r} = (r_1, \ldots, r_n)$ and a treatment variable $\mathbf{Z} = (Z_1, \ldots, Z_n)$. We only concern ourselves with fully observed $\mathbf{r}$ and $\mathbf{Z}$ here.

When modeling the missing data process, we consider the conditional distribution $p(\mathbf{M}|\mathbf{X}, \varphi)$, where $\varphi$ are the parameters of this distribution. If this distribution only depends on observed covariate values, that is, $p(\mathbf{M}|\mathbf{X}, \varphi) = p(\mathbf{M}|\mathbf{X}_{obs}, \varphi)$ then we say the missing values are missing at random (MAR; Rubin, 1976). This is the assumption we will be making throughout this chapter. If this assumption cannot be made, then the data are said to be not missing at random (NMAR); this is a very challenging problem to overcome in practice as the distribution governing the missing data process itself depends on values that are not known. Strategies have been proposed to address this issue (Little & Rubin, 2002) but it is not the objective of this chapter. Often a MAR assumption is plausible (Schafer & Graham, 2002) and is the most commonly accepted scenario when dealing with missing value problems.

Propensity scores are estimated using the covariate data, typically with some type of regression model. As the treatment effect is binary, the most commonly used regression model to estimate propensity scores is a logistic regression model, but any appropriate statistical model could be used to estimate propensity scores (Hanley & Dendukuri, 2009; McCaffrey, Ridgeway, & Morral, 2004; Setoguchi, Schneeweiss, Brookhart, Glynn, & Cook, 2008; Westreich, Lessler, & Funk, 2010; Woo, Reiter, & Karr, 2008). Denote the propensity scores estimated in this way by $e(x_i)$ for each unit $i$ in the data.

Now, when missing values are present in the data, rather than having $x_i$, we have $x_{obs,i}$, and so we need to determine how best to use this incomplete covariate dataset to estimate propensity scores and then proceed to make appropriate inferences. In the next section we discuss nonimputation-based approaches that address this problem, before moving on to describing the approaches based on imputation of the missing covariates.

## NONIMPUTATION APPROACHES

### Generalized Propensity Score

The earliest mention of how to deal with the problem of covariate missing values within a propensity score analysis is by Rosenbaum and Rubin (1984). They suggest the construction of a generalized propensity score that estimates propensity scores within each pattern of missing data. By doing so, they show that this will achieve balance on the observed covariates for the treated and control groups as well as balancing the distribution of missing data patterns between the two groups. This can be seen intuitively, as what we are effectively doing here is including an indicator of each unit's missing data pattern as a covariate in the model used to estimate propensity scores. So, as with other covariates included in the model, we would seek to balance this distribution for treatment and control groups, and hence balance the distribution of missing data patterns across both groups. However, as noted by Rosenbaum and Rubin (1984), there is no guarantee that the generalized propensity score will achieve balance on the true (unobserved) covariate values. Also, in some datasets the number of missing data patterns may make this approach impractical (D'Agostino, Lang, Walkup, Morgan & Karter, 2001).

## E-M Algorithm

Application of a principled model-based approach to deal with missing values here was first proposed by D'Agostino Jr. and Rubin (2000) who used an E-M algorithm (Dempster, Laird, & Rubin, 1977) that would estimate parameters from the data subject to missing values with an iterative algorithm, the last step of which estimated the propensity scores. The approach works by modeling the missing covariate data using a general location model (Olkin & Tate, 1961) for the complete data. This is a convenient model for many types of data, as it allows data comprising variables measured on a categorical scale (e.g., sex or race) as well as a continuous scale (e.g., income) to be jointly modeled.

The general location model first models the categorical variables jointly and then, conditional on the categorical data, models the continuous data. The categorical variables are cross-classified to form a contingency table, and the resulting cell counts of the table are assumed to follow a multinomial distribution. The continuous variables are then modeled with a multivariate normal distribution with a cell specific mean. With this model, missing values in the data can be handled with an E-M algorithm developed by Schafer (1997).

D'Agostino Jr. and Rubin (2000) made use of this E-M algorithm to estimate propensity scores. By treating the treatment variable $Z$ as just one extra categorical variable in the data, the E-M algorithm can be applied as before, now with an augmented contingency table that contains an extra margin due to the inclusion of $Z$. The final step in D'Agostino Jr. and Rubin (2000) is to make the $Z$ variable completely unobserved so that the E-step in the E-M algorithm will estimate fitted probabilities of being assigned to $Z = 1$, that is, the propensity scores. These propensity scores can be used to estimate treatment effects in the usual way.

The approach performed well in analysis of March of Dimes data. The approach has since been extensively referred to, in an array of fields (D'Agostino et al., 2001; Harder, Stuart, & Anthony, 2010; Tannen, Weiner, & Xie, 2009) illustrating how fundamental an issue it was for applied researchers.

While approaches based on E-M algorithms have benefits, a drawback is that the estimation of propensity scores is tied to the treatment and modeling of the missing data. We might like to use a different model for estimating propensity scores from the one we used to model the missing data. For this reason, the rest of this chapter will concentrate on more recent developments that handle the missing values through imputation.

## IMPUTATION APPROACHES

Imputation is a commonly used approach to deal with missing data, and the basic idea is that missing values in the data are "filled in" with imputations. The missing values could be imputed using a simple strategy such as by resampling observed values in each variable or by using hot deck procedures (Little & Rubin, 2002). Alternatively, a more principled model-based method could be used where missing values are imputed from their posterior predictive distribution $p(X_{mis}|X_{obs}, Z)$; in this way relationships between variables in the data, and thus statistical properties, should be preserved in the imputed data. Note that although we include the treatment variable in the imputation model we do not include the response variable $r$. It is debatable as to whether it is appropriate to use $r$ for imputation. D'Agostino Jr. and Rubin (2000) do not include the response in the modeling of missing covariate data, or indeed any variable measured post-treatment. The argument is that by doing so we may violate the causal path. If we use $r$ in our imputation model for $X_{mis}$, then we would be conjecturing values for the missing covariate values, having already observed the response values. Nevertheless, it is worth noting that others have suggested it is beneficial to include the response variable in the imputation model (Little, 1992; Moons, Donders, Stijnen, & Harrell, 2006) as it does contain important information about the distribution of the missing values. Deciding when and where it might be appropriate to include the response in the imputation model is still an open area for discussion.

Imputation as a strategy to handle missing values is quite appealing with propensity score analysis, as it allows analysts to proceed with using their usual complete data methods to estimate propensity scores and make causal inferences. So, for example, analysts can fit the usual logistic regression model to estimate propensity scores with the imputed data. Analysts can also easily pursue further modeling with the imputed data, such as subdomain/subgroup comparisons or regression adjustment to reduce residual imbalances (Hill, 2004; Hill, Reiter, & Zanutto, 2004).

In addition, unlike the case with approaches based on the E-M algorithm, the imputation and analysis are performed in two different distinct stages. This allows the models used to impute the missing values and estimate propensity scores to be independently constructed and fitted. For example, an imputation model might include all three-way interaction terms, but the model to estimate the propensity scores might only include at most two-way interactions. Essentially, by separating the process into two distinct stages, the analyst can explore various models to fit to the imputed data to best estimate the propensity scores and achieve good covariate balance, before proceeding to make inferences about the treatment effect. This would not be possible if the missing data problem and propensity score estimation were being dealt with simultaneously.

An approach proposed by Haviland, Nagin, and Rosenbaum (2007) suggested using a simple imputation strategy that fills in the missing values in a variable with their observed sample mean and then estimate propensity scores using the imputed data, but with the addition of a missing data indicator variable for each imputed variable. This is similar to the idea of generalized propensity scores proposed by Rosenbaum and Rubin (1984) and ensures that the estimated propensity score for a unit is not affected by its imputed values. While this does allow incorporation of the missing data to enter into the estimation of the propensity scores in some way, it does not always result in plausible treatment effect estimates. If the distribution of missing data patterns in the treatment group is different from that in the control group, matched controls might be selected not because of their similarity in covariate distribution, but rather because of their similarity of missing data patterns. This was illustrated in an extreme case in Mitra and Reiter (2011).

## Multiple Imputation

Multiple imputation (Rubin, 1987) is a convenient and appealing method to handle the problem of missing values. Like single imputation methods, it retains many of the benefits in the simplicity of analysis with imputed data. So, analysts can still use the same complete data method for analysis of the imputed data. In addition, multiple imputation allows the uncertainty due to the presence of missing values to be taken into account, something that single imputation does not do, at least not without complex adjustment methods. This is because, by generating multiple complete datasets and analyzing each separately, we are incorporating uncertainty into our analysis through each imputation of the missing data. We can actually consider two different ways to estimate propensity scores and treatment effects here, which have been called the Across and Within approaches in the literature (Hill, 2004; Mitra & Reiter, 2012).

Multiple imputation works by repeatedly filling in values of $X_{mis}$ $m$ times with draws from the predictive distribution, $p(X_{mis}|X_{obs}, Z)$. The analyst can then use the $m$ completed datasets $X_{com}^{(1)}, \ldots, X_{com}^{(m)}$ to estimate corresponding $m$ sets of propensity scores. Following notation outlined in Mitra and Reiter (2012), in the $k$th imputed dataset, $e(x_{i,com}^{(k)})$ denotes the estimated propensity score for unit $i$, where $i = 1, \ldots, n$ and $k = 1, \ldots, m$. The propensity scores estimated in the $k$th imputed dataset are estimated in the same way that they would have been estimated if the data were complete, for example, with a logistic regression of $Z$ on some function of the variables in $\mathbf{X}_{\text{com}}^{(k)}$.

As we now have multiple ($m$) propensity score estimates for each unit, we can consider two different ways to proceed in estimating treatment effects. Following the terminology introduced in Mitra and Reiter (2012), the first method is defined to be the Across method. In this method, we first create one propensity score estimate for each unit (denoted by $e^{A,m}(x_i)$) by averaging the $m$ propensity scores $e(x_{i,\text{com}}^{(k)})$, specifically,

$$e^{A,m}(x_i) = \frac{\sum_{k=1}^{m} e(x_{i,\text{com}}^{(k)})}{m} \qquad (12.1)$$

We thus have now only one set of propensity scores for all the units denoted by $e^{A,m} = (e^{A,m}(x_1), \ldots, e^{A,m}(x_n))'$, and analysts can use these in the usual way to find a matched control set. We assume that matching is performed with a one-to-one nearest neighbor matching scheme without replacement, although alternative ways to create the matched control set such as matching with replacement could also be implemented. The analyst then estimates the treatment effect $\tau$ in the Across approach with

$$\hat{\tau}^{A,m} = \overline{r}_T - \overline{r}_{mc}^{A,m} \qquad (12.2)$$

which is the difference in means of the outcome values in the treatment group and matched control set (selected using the averaged propensity scores $e^{A,m}$), respectively.

The second method is defined in Mitra and Reiter (2012) to be the Within method. This method uses the $m$ sets of propensity scores to create $m$ matched control sets, so matching is performed in each imputed dataset, $X_{\text{com}}^{(k)}$, using the corresponding set of propensity scores, $e(X_{\text{com}}^{(k)}) = (e(x_{1,\text{com}}^{(k)}), \ldots, e(x_{n,\text{com}}^{(k)}))'$, $k = 1, \ldots, m$. The analyst can then estimate a treatment effect within the $k$th imputed dataset, denoted by $\hat{\tau}^{W,m,k} = \overline{r}_T - \overline{r}_{mc}^{(k)}$, where $\overline{r}_{mc}^{(k)}$ is the average of the outcome values for the matched controls in the $k$th imputed dataset. The Within method then estimates a treatment effect by averaging these $m$ estimates, that is, by using

$$\hat{\tau}^{W,m} = \sum_{k=1}^{m} \hat{\tau}^{W,m,k} / m \qquad (12.3)$$

In the next section, we evaluate the performance of these two different approaches in a simulation study. It should be noted that both types of approach have been implemented in the literature. The Within method has been implemented in Song, Belin, Lee, Gao, and Rotheram-Borus (2001) and Qu and Lipkovich (2009), while the Across method has been implemented in Mitra and Reiter (2011).

An approach that can be thought to essentially build upon a single imputation approach like that proposed by Haviland et al. (2007) was developed by Qu and Lipkovich (2009) who suggest instead to multiply impute the missing values in the data and then estimate propensity scores with the addition of indicator variables for the missing data patterns as predictors in the propensity score model. Specifically, missing values are imputed from their posterior predictive distribution, $p(X_{mis}|X_{obs}, Z)$, $m$ times. Propensity scores are estimated from each imputed dataset in the manner described above, and $m$ treatment effect estimates obtained. The average of these $m$ estimates can then be used to estimate a treatment effect. Qu and Lipkovich (2009) thus implemented the Within method from their multiply imputed propensity scores.

We have not specified specific methods here for creating multiply imputed datasets. In this chapter, we assume that imputations are drawn from the posterior predictive distribution of a model fit to the data, with more details of the models considered given in the later sections. In general, we could consider there to be two broad groups of multiple imputation modeling strategies: joint modeling imputation (Ibrahim, Chen, Lipsitz, & Herring, 2005; Schafer, 1997), which involves formally drawing imputations from their posterior distributions but can be quite computational; and chained equations imputation (Raghunathan, Lepkowski, van Hoewyk, & Solenberger, 2001; Van Buuren, 2007), which is fairly quick and simple to implement but does not correspond to a formal modeling strategy.

Nowadays many software packages do allow users to multiply impute missing values using either strategy. For example the "mix" package in R (*www.r-project.org*) implements the joint modeling imputation model described in Schafer (1997), while the "MICE" package in R implements the chained equations approach described in Van Buuren (2007). In this chapter, we draw imputations from joint modeling strategies, at times making use of the "mix" package in R.

## Imputation Model Misspecification

While model-based imputation methods are appealing because they impute missing values in a more principled way than ad hoc imputation methods, they do diverge from one of the original motivating reasons for developing propensity score analysis. An appealing feature of propensity score analysis is that it relies less on a model-based approach for causal inference, as a model is not required for the response variable. While a model is often needed to estimate propensity scores, it has been argued that the exact model specification is not critical as the goal is to achieve good covariate balance; this can be readily assessed, at least if there were no missing data, using simple graphical summaries and other diagnostic tools. However, as multiple imputation is heavily dependent on a model for the data, it is possible that the estimation of propensity scores, and hence estimates of the treatment effect, are now sensitive to model misspecification, with respect to the imputation model for the missing values.

This problem was illustrated in Mitra and Reiter (2011) and is demonstrated in the next section. The solution proposed in Mitra and Reiter (2011) was to develop an imputation model for missing covariates in observational studies that is robust to model misspecification, using the fact that analysis was to be made using propensity score matching.

Similar to how D'Agostino Jr. and Rubin (2000) proceeds, Mitra and Reiter (2011) model the covariate data using a general location model, although treatment does not necessarily need to be included in the model. Rather than use an E-M algorithm, Mitra and Reiter (2011) imputed missing values from their posterior predictive distribution. This is possible with the construction of a data augmentation algorithm based on that described in Schafer (1997), and can be implemented using the "mix" package in R, but with an extension. The extension is to introduce a latent class indicator. Let us denote this by $W$, where $W_i = 1$ implies that the covariates for unit $i$ come from the same distribution as that of the treated units' covariate distribution, while $W_i = 0$ implies that the covariates for unit $i$ come from some other distribution. Although control units will not have observed values of $W_i$, by definition all treated units will possess (or be constrained to) values of $W_i = 1$. This will enable there to be sufficient information to impute/estimate the distribution of these binary latent class indicators. (As each unit will have at least some observed covariate information, there is enough information in the data to proceed with this model.) Mitra and Reiter (2011) thus propose a constrained general location latent class mixture model to impute missing covariate values.

In order to draw imputations from this method, Mitra and Reiter (2011) construct a Gibbs sampler that imputes missing values through data augmentation. The steps to impute missing covariate values are related to the Bayesian imputation procedures described in Schafer (1997). Indeed, this approach can be viewed as a mixture of general location imputation models. Some sample code to implement this method is available at the following website: *www.soton.ac.uk/~rm1s07*, and the derivation of the

Gibbs sampler is given in Mitra and Reiter (2011). In general, one can view this multiple imputation procedure as splitting the data into two (random) groups defined by those units with $W_i = 1$ and $W_i = 0$, respectively. One group corresponds to those units that have covariate distributions similar to the treated units' covariate distribution, and the other group corresponds to those units that have some other covariate distribution. Missing covariates in both groups are imputed from separate general location models using Bayesian procedures, and the latent class indicators for the controls are imputed with probability given by essentially how "close" their (possibly imputed) covariates are to the distribution of the covariates of one group relative to the other group. When there are only continuous covariates, this probability is calculated using the usual linear discriminant.

The idea behind this method is to realize that typically we are interested in finding the set of control units that have covariates similar in distribution to the treated units' covariate distribution. So when we impute missing values, we should be concerned first and foremost with generating plausible imputations for those control units. The latent class indicator allows us to deal with control units that have covariates far removed from the treated units' covariate space separately from the other units; they are thus less likely to impact upon imputations for missing covariate values in the treated units' covariate space. The essential motivation for this latent class imputation model is to allow imputations to be drawn for missing covariates in the covariate space of the treated units that are robust to the effect of outlying controls. While, by separating the data into two parts like this, we could possibly generate implausible imputations for units' covariates in the group $W_i = 0$, these units would not have been selected in the matched control set for estimating treatment effects in the first place. Thus, generating implausible imputations for this group is unlikely to have a big impact on treatment effect estimation.

## SIMULATION STUDY

Mitra and Reiter (2012) illustrate the performance of the Across and Within methods through simulations. In each simulation, they generate $n = 1{,}100$ units each with two covariates $(x_{i1}, x_{i2})' \sim N(\mu, \Sigma)$, $i = 1, \ldots, 1{,}100$, where $\mu = (10, 10)'$, and $\Sigma$ has variances equal to 5 with correlation 0.5. A response surface is also generated so that for all $i$,

$$r_i = x_{i1} + x_{i2} + \varepsilon_i, \varepsilon_i \sim N(0, 1) \tag{12.4}$$

So the true treatment effect is $\tau = 0$ for all simulations. Missing values are only introduced into $x_2$ using MAR mechanisms, so there are no missing values in $x_1$ and $r$. This is done to keep the simulations relatively simple; the missingness pattern will be monotone, and so it is relatively easy to impute the missing values.

Three treatment assignment mechanisms are investigated:

1. Assignment only depends on $x_1$. Specifically, treatment is assigned with a Bernoulli distribution given by

$$\text{logit}(P(Z_i = 1|x_i)) = -7.8 + 0.5x_{i1} \tag{12.5}$$

so that we would expect units with larger values of $x_1$ to be more likely to be allocated to the treatment group.

2. Assignment only depends on $x_2$. Specifically, treatment is assigned with a Bernoulli distribution given by

$$\text{logit}(P(Z_i = 1|x_i)) = -7.8 + 0.5x_{i2} \tag{12.6}$$

so that we would expect units with larger values of $x_2$ to be more likely to be allocated to the treatment group.

3. Assignment depends equally on $x_1$ and $x_2$. Specifically, treatment is assigned with a Bernoulli distribution given by

$$\text{logit}(P(Z_i = 1|x_i)) = -7.8 + 0.255x_{i1} + 0.255x_{i2} \tag{12.7}$$

so that we would expect units with larger values of both $x_1$ and $x_2$ to be more likely to be allocated to the treatment group.

With the distribution of $(x_{i1}, x_{i2})$ described above, a typical simulated dataset from each of the above assignment mechanisms would have approximately 100 treated units and 1,000 control units.

Two scenarios are investigated for introducing missing values in $x_2$. The first scenario uses a MAR mechanism to introduce missing values into some proportion of the control units' $x_2$ values, specifically,

$$\text{logit}(P(m_{i2} = 1|Z_i = 0, x_i)) = -10.1 + 0.9x_{i1} \tag{12.8}$$

so control units with larger $x_1$ values are more likely to be missing their $x_2$ values. An incomplete dataset generated in this way would typically have approximately 30% missing values in control units' $x_2$ values. In the second scenario, the missing data mechanism for the control units remains the same, but there is also a missing completely at random (MCAR) mechanism to introduce missing values into 30% of the treated units' $x_2$. An MCAR mechanism is used here because the treated units' covariate space is defined on a much smaller region than that of the control units' covariate space.

As the covariate data are multivariate normal and the missingness is monotone, missing $x_2$ are multiply imputed from a normal linear regression model of $x_2$ on $(x_1, Z)$ fit to the complete case data; there was no interaction term included in the model. The usual noninformative priors for linear regression are used to draw imputations from the appropriate Bayesian posterior predictive distribution. As mentioned earlier, $r$ is not included in the imputations. This has been recommended in the literature so that handling of the missing covariates and resulting creation of matched control sets is done without being affected by values of the outcome variable (D'Agostino Jr., & Rubin, 2000). There are different opinions, however, about whether this is the correct way to proceed; for example, others have shown that it can be advantageous to include the outcome variable in imputation models (Little, 1992; Moons et al., 2006).

In each of the $m$ imputed datasets, propensity scores, $e(x_{i,com}^{(k)})$, are estimated for each unit $i$ in each of $k = 1, \ldots, m$ completed datasets using a logistic regression of $Z$ on $(x_1, x_2)$. We can then compute $\hat{\tau}^{A,m}$ and $\hat{\tau}^{W,m}$ as is described in the Multiple Imputation section above and compare how close they are to the true treatment effect of 0. Mitra and Reiter (2012) implemented these simulation designs and empirically evaluated the two methods by repeating this process 1,000 times for each treatment assignment and missing mechanism scenario described above, each time using new values of $(X, Z, r, M)$. The true variance of the estimators $\hat{\tau}^{A,m}$ and $\hat{\tau}^{W,m}$ could then be empirically estimated by taking the sample variance of the 1,000 estimates. The findings from their simulations are given below.

## Simulation 1: Treatment Depends on $x_1$

Table 12.1 summarizes the point estimates and variances of $\hat{\tau}^{A,m}$ and $\hat{\tau}^{W,m}$ across the 1,000 simulations for different numbers of imputations $m$. The biases in estimates from the Across and Within methods are all quite small, with estimates of the treatment effect, $\tau$, close to the true value of

**TABLE 12.1. Properties of Treatment Effect Estimates from the Across and Within Approaches in the Simulation Where Treatment Assignment Depends Only on $x_1$**

| m | Across Pt. est. | Across variance | Across MSE | Within Pt. est. | Within variance | Within MSE |
|---|---|---|---|---|---|---|
| | | | Only control units missing $x_2$ | | | |
| 5  | 0.055 | 0.077 | 0.080 | 0.080 | 0.050 | 0.056 |
| 10 | 0.057 | 0.083 | 0.086 | 0.078 | 0.046 | 0.052 |
| 15 | 0.065 | 0.075 | 0.079 | 0.079 | 0.044 | 0.050 |
| 20 | 0.065 | 0.077 | 0.081 | 0.079 | 0.043 | 0.050 |
| 50 | 0.058 | 0.081 | 0.085 | 0.077 | 0.042 | 0.048 |
| | | | Treatment and control units missing $x_2$ | | | |
| 5  | 0.030 | 0.080 | 0.081 | 0.072 | 0.053 | 0.058 |
| 10 | 0.032 | 0.083 | 0.084 | 0.072 | 0.049 | 0.055 |
| 15 | 0.031 | 0.080 | 0.081 | 0.074 | 0.048 | 0.054 |
| 20 | 0.035 | 0.078 | 0.080 | 0.075 | 0.046 | 0.052 |
| 50 | 0.029 | 0.081 | 0.081 | 0.074 | 0.045 | 0.050 |

*Note.* The average treatment effect estimate from the fully observed data, that is, the data before introducing missing values is 0.0738. The true treatment effect is 0. When only control units are missing $x_2$, the average treatment effect estimates based on only the complete cases is 1.118. When both treated and control units are missing $x_2$, the average treatment effect estimate based on only the complete cases is 0.8961.

0. $\hat{\tau}^{A,m}$ tends to have a smaller bias compared to $\hat{\tau}^{W,m}$, but its variance tends to be a bit larger. The variance of $\hat{\tau}^{W,m}$ appears to decrease with $m$, while there is no clear relationship in the variances of $\hat{\tau}^{A,m}$ with $m$. The Within method has a smaller mean-squared error for these values of $m$ due to the bias being small with both methods' estimators.

## Simulation 2: Treatment Depends on $x_2$

Table 12.2 summarizes the results for different $m$ here. We see that there is a difference in bias between the two methods' estimators; $\hat{\tau}^{A,m}$ has substantially smaller bias than $\hat{\tau}^{W,m}$. When both treated and control units are missing $x_2$, the bias in $\hat{\tau}^{A,m}$ tends to decrease with $m$, whereas no such profile is observed for $\hat{\tau}^{W,m}$. The variance of $\hat{\tau}^{W,m}$ is still lower than $\hat{\tau}^{A,m}$ and decreases with $m$, whereas the variance of $\hat{\tau}^{A,m}$ does not show any discernible relationship with $m$. In this scenario, unlike the previous scenario, the Across

**TABLE 12.2. Properties of Treatment Effect Estimates from the Across and Within Approaches in the Simulation Where Treatment Assignment Depends on $x_2$**

| | | Across | | | Within | |
|---|---|---|---|---|---|---|
| $m$ | Pt. est. | variance | MSE | Pt. est. | variance | MSE |
| | | Only control units missing $x_2$ | | | | |
| 5  | 0.565 | 0.084 | 0.403 | 0.825 | 0.045 | 0.725 |
| 10 | 0.532 | 0.088 | 0.371 | 0.826 | 0.041 | 0.723 |
| 15 | 0.541 | 0.092 | 0.385 | 0.826 | 0.039 | 0.721 |
| 20 | 0.538 | 0.090 | 0.380 | 0.826 | 0.038 | 0.721 |
| 50 | 0.548 | 0.100 | 0.400 | 0.826 | 0.036 | 0.718 |
| | | Treatment and control units missing $x_2$ | | | | |
| 5  | 0.311 | 0.097 | 0.194 | 0.840 | 0.054 | 0.760 |
| 10 | 0.221 | 0.094 | 0.143 | 0.842 | 0.045 | 0.754 |
| 15 | 0.182 | 0.088 | 0.121 | 0.844 | 0.043 | 0.755 |
| 20 | 0.174 | 0.093 | 0.123 | 0.845 | 0.042 | 0.756 |
| 50 | 0.156 | 0.096 | 0.120 | 0.845 | 0.039 | 0.753 |

*Note.* The average treatment effect estimate from the fully observed data, that is, the data before introducing missing values is 0.0614. The true treatment effect is 0. When only control units are missing $x_2$, the average treatment effect estimate based on only the complete cases is 0.7653. When both treated and control units are missing $x_2$, the average treatment effect estimate based on only the complete cases is 0.5580.

approach dominates on mean-squared error. This is because of lower bias in estimates produced by $\hat{\tau}^{A,m}$.

## Simulation 3: Treatment Assignment Depends on Both $x_1$ and $x_2$

Table 12.3 summarizes the results for different $m$. As with the previous simulation, $\hat{\tau}^{A,m}$ again has smaller bias than $\hat{\tau}^{W,m}$. The differences in bias between the two point estimators are smaller than those observed in Table 12.2 but are still larger than those observed in Table 12.1. This is to be expected given the fact that treatment assignment now depends partly on $x_1$ and partly on $x_2$. As was the case in Table 12.2, the bias in $\hat{\tau}^{A,m}$ decreases with $m$, whereas the bias in $\hat{\tau}^{W,m}$ appears not to depend on $m$. The variance of $\hat{\tau}^{W,m}$ remains smaller than the variance of $\hat{\tau}^{A,m}$, and it still appears to decrease with $m$. In this simulation, the Across approach dominates on mean-squared error as the differences in biases between the two methods are relatively high compared to the differences in the variances.

**TABLE 12.3. Treatment Effect Estimates from the Across and Within Approaches in the Simulation Design Where Treatment Assignment Depends Equally on $x_1$ and $x_2$**

| | Across | | | Within | | |
|---|---|---|---|---|---|---|
| $m$ | Pt. est. | variance | MSE | Pt. est. | variance | MSE |
| | | | Only control units missing $x_2$ | | | |
| 5 | 0.370 | 0.059 | 0.196 | 0.548 | 0.042 | 0.343 |
| 10 | 0.338 | 0.056 | 0.170 | 0.551 | 0.039 | 0.343 |
| 15 | 0.323 | 0.053 | 0.158 | 0.550 | 0.038 | 0.341 |
| 20 | 0.319 | 0.056 | 0.158 | 0.549 | 0.038 | 0.339 |
| 50 | 0.316 | 0.056 | 0.156 | 0.550 | 0.036 | 0.338 |
| | | | Treatment and control units missing $x_2$ | | | |
| 5 | 0.275 | 0.080 | 0.155 | 0.550 | 0.046 | 0.349 |
| 10 | 0.236 | 0.077 | 0.133 | 0.551 | 0.042 | 0.345 |
| 15 | 0.209 | 0.079 | 0.122 | 0.553 | 0.040 | 0.346 |
| 20 | 0.204 | 0.079 | 0.120 | 0.553 | 0.039 | 0.345 |
| 50 | 0.196 | 0.081 | 0.120 | 0.551 | 0.038 | 0.342 |

*Note.* The average treatment effect estimates based on the covariates from the fully observed data, that is, the data before introducing missing values is 0.0467. The true treatment effect is 0. The average treatment effect estimates based on the complete cases when missing data is only introduced into control units' $x_2$ value is 0.8917. The average treatment effect estimates based on the complete cases when missing data is introduced into both treatment and control units' $x_2$ value is 0.6973.

## Reasons for Differences in Point Estimates

Mitra and Reiter (2012) considered why we observe differences between both the Across and Within methods, as both seem reasonable ways to proceed with multiply imputed data. We can see that, in terms of bias reduction, both approaches perform similarly when treatment assignment does not depend on any of the variables that have missing data, that is, $x_1$, whereas the Across approach shows greater reductions when assignment depends, at least partly, on variables with missing data, $x_2$ in our case. So from this it appears that the importance of variables with missing data in treatment assignment is key to these differences, as we now explain more fully.

In the first scenario, treatment assignment only depends on the fully observed $x_1$, and so the true propensity scores for the Across and Within methods should be the same. However, as we estimate propensity scores, the coefficient on $x_2$ in the logistic regression may well be nonzero, so that

$x_2$ may play a role when selecting controls to be in a matched control set. Nevertheless, provided we generate plausible imputations, that is, imputations are generated from the posterior predictive distribution of an appropriate model fit to the data, this role is likely to be minor, and matching should be largely driven by the $x_1$ values for treated and control units. This is why we see that Across and Within propensity scores, and hence treatment effect estimates, are generally similar here, with low biases.

In the first scenario, it may also at first seem surprising to see that the treatment effects from the Across method are slightly closer to the true treatment effect of 0 than the treatment effects estimated from the fully observed data (prior to the introduction of missing data). This is because the Across method averages propensity scores across imputations, and so effectively averages over the conditional distribution of $x_2|x_1$ when estimating propensity scores for units with missing $x_2$ values. This means that propensity scores estimated for records with missing $x_2$ are essentially determined by their $x_1$ value alone and would be closer to the true propensity score model in this scenario (where treatment is assigned using only $x_1$) than the propensity scores estimated from using both the observed $x_1$ and (unnecessary) $x_2$ values. For this reason the estimates from the Across method have a slightly smaller bias compared to the complete data estimates.

In scenarios 2 and 3, biases increase for both approaches. This is because treatment assignment now depends, at least partially, on the incomplete variable $x_2$, and so matching is partly driven with imputed $x_2$ values. As would be expected, the Within method would achieve good balance on $x_1$ and on the imputed version of $x_2$ for any given imputed dataset, as the method treats this dataset as if it were fully observed. However, as alluded to at the beginning of this chapter, it may appear that the imputed $x_2$ is well balanced but the actual $x_2$ values are imbalanced; more details on this are given later in the Model Misspecification section below. In these scenarios, it was observed that the Within method tended to select records for the matched control set with true (not imputed) $x_2$ values that were smaller than the true $x_2$ values for the treated units. This explains the positive bias in the Within estimates. The Across method actually selected matched controls with imputed values similar in distribution to the corresponding true values, but these tended to be smaller than the true $x_2$ values in the treatment group. There was a smaller difference between the true $x_2$ values in the treated and matched control groups in the Across method as compared to the Within method, which explains the smaller biases associated with the Across method. Ideally, it would be nice to illustrate these concepts with box plots of the covariate distributions in the treatment and matched control groups, but unfortunately this becomes complicated as the Within method produces $m$ sets of propensity scores, and thus $m$ sets of balance summaries, and so is not considered here.

Mitra and Reiter (2012) also noted that the Across method would tend to include fewer imputed $x_2$ values in the matched control set as compared to the matched control sets created with the Within method. As an illustration, the simulations run by Mitra and Reiter (2012) in Simulation 2 found that imputed $x_2$ values appear in the matched control sets approximately 12% more often when implementing the Within method as compared to the Across method. This is also why the Across method did not suffer as badly as the Within method from the noted imbalances based on the true $x_2$ values. This may be the case because, as noted before, the Across method estimates propensity scores for units with missing $x_2$ values using essentially only $x_1$ (averaging over the conditional distribution of $x_2|x_1$), and so they may be less likely to be picked for the matched control set when implementing the Across method.

The bias in the Within method did not seem to be affected by $m$ in all the scenarios considered in Mitra and Reiter (2012). This happens because we can view the treatment effects produced by the Within method as being independent and identically distributed due to the fact that the imputations are independently and identically distributed. We did see that the bias in the Across method decreased as $m$ increased (unless the bias was already quite small as in scenario 1). This is because propensity scores are averaged across imputations in the Across method and so would converge to their values based on the observed data. Thus in the Across method, as $m$ increases, a matched control set would be selected using propensity scores that are converging to fixed values.

The simulation results also noted various profiles in the variances of the estimates with $m$. The variances of the estimates from the Across method did not appear to show any discernible relationship with $m$. This is because the Across method averages the propensity scores across imputations to result in only one set of scores for the units. As noted above, increasing $m$ results in propensity score estimates that approach their values based on the observed data, but the impact this has reduces the bias in the estimates as opposed to the variance. Variances from the Within method, however, do exhibit a decreasing trend as $m$ increases. This is because the treatment effect estimate from the Within method is a sample mean of treatment effects estimated over multiple imputed datasets that were drawn independently, and standard results tell us that the variability in the sample mean should decrease as $m$ increases.

## Model Misspecification

To illustrate the impact of misspecified imputation models on estimates of the treatment effect, we consider the illustration from Mitra and Reiter (2012). Mitra and Reiter (2012) simulate two continuous covariates, $x_1$ and $x_2$ for $n = 1{,}200$ units that have a nonlinear relationship; in fact, the relationship is cubic in nature. This relationship is shown in Figure 12.1 which is a scatter plot of $x_2$ values against corresponding $x_1$ for each of the 1,200 units. The treatment assignment mechanism is such that the 200 treated units tend to have larger values of $x_1$ and $x_2$ than the majority of the 1,000 control units.

Missing values are then introduced in the control units' $x_2$ values with a MAR mechanism that depends on $x_1$. Specifically, the probability of $x_2$ being missing increases with $x_1$. This ensures that many missing $x_2$ values in control units share the same covariate space as the treated units' covariate space. With this design, a typical simulated dataset would have approximately 40% missing data in the control units' $x_2$ values.

Mitra and Reiter (2011) then impute missing $x_2$ using data augmentation (Tanner & Wong, 1987) via the usual multivariate normal model. This is actually just a simplification of the general location model when there are no categorical data. To distinguish this from the latent class mixture model Mitra and Reiter (2012) propose for imputation, this imputation

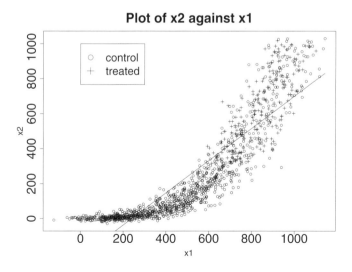

**FIGURE 12.1.** Scatter plot of $x_2$ against $x_1$ when a cubic relationship is present, illustrating the effects of using a poor imputation model.

model is denoted the one class imputation model. The model used is $(x_{i1}, x_{i2})' \sim N(\mu, \Sigma)$, with the default noninformative prior distribution $p(\mu, \Sigma) \propto |\Sigma|^{-(\frac{p+1}{2})}$. We have a monotone pattern of missing values (as only $x_2$ is missing here), and so missing values can be multiply imputed with imputations drawn from their posterior predictive distribution through a linear regression model of $x_2$ on $x_1$ fit to the complete case data.

Mitra and Reiter (2011) create $m = 100{,}000$ imputations and estimate propensity scores within each dataset using a logistic regression of treatment on $x_1$ and $x_2$ without any interactions, thus creating $m$ sets of propensity scores. As noted earlier, using any one of these sets of scores for matching should result in good balance for the treated units and control units (that might comprise a mix of observed and imputed values). Mitra and Reiter (2011) then estimate a treatment effect using the Across method performing (nearest neighbor) matching both with and without replacement to find a matched control set.

Mitra and Reiter (2011) present box plots summarizing balance from these simulations in Figure 12.2. Each of the four panels presents box plots of the true values for the treated and matched control units after applying the Across method with the one class imputation model, as well as the matched controls selected from the original complete data (before any introduction of missing data). When treatment effects are estimated using matching without replacement, the Across method has smaller lower quartiles compared to those for the treated units and matched controls selected from the fully complete data for both $x_1$ and $x_2$. When treatment effects are estimated using matching with replacement, the imbalances between the box plots of the covariate distributions of the treatment group and the matched control group selected using the Across (one class) method are more severe. The poor imputations generated mean controls that normally would not be included in the matched control set possess imputed $x_2$ values that result in them being repeatedly selected to the matched control set, exacerbating the problem of covariate imbalance.

Mitra and Reiter (2011) consider reasons for the inadequacies in balances noted in the simulation. The imputation model used assumes a linear relationship between the covariates, but we can see from Figure 12.1 that this is not a plausible assumption. The application of this imputation model can then impact the matched set selected and the resulting covariate balance. From Figure 12.1 we can see that many controls that lie above the fitted regression line (which represents the imputation model used) are likely to be included in the matched control set, but if they are missing in $x_2$, then they might receive a much lower imputed value than their

# Missing Data in Propensity Scores

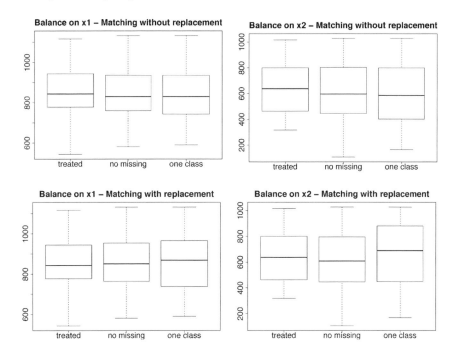

**FIGURE 12.2.** Box plots of $x_1$ and $x_2$ for the treated units, matched control units selected from the original complete data (before introduction of missing values in $x_2$), and matched control units from the (Across) one-class method in the model misspeciation simulation design. Matching is performed both without and with replacement.

true value and so no longer be selected in the matched control set (as propensity scores are estimated using the imputed data). There are also many controls that lie below the fitted regression with similar $x_1$ values to the treated units. These units would not normally be selected as matched controls, but if they were missing in $x_2$ they are likely to receive larger imputed values than their true values, and thus potentially be selected as matches. Both of these problems contribute to the covariate imbalance seen in Figure 12.1. Essentially, the problem stems from balance appearing to be acceptable on the imputed covariates while in fact being imbalanced based on the true covariate values.

While the key should of course be to design a plausible imputation model, it is not always possible to detect model inadequacies, particularly when covariates are stretched out over a large multivariate space (Hill & Reiter, 2006). Also, many analysts often use readily available routines in standard software packages to impute the missing values, similar to the one-class imputation model described in this section.

Mitra and Reiter (2011) apply their proposed latent class model to impute missing covariates and estimate propensity scores using the Across method here. We can see that a linear relationship, while clearly inappropriate over the whole covariate space, might not be so appropriate over a large covariate space, over the region where the treated units' covariates lie. This is the intuitive idea behind the latent class modeling approach. Linear (or other similar standard) modeling assumptions might not be so over a large covariate space, but might be appropriate over a smaller region. Furthermore, if we estimate treatment effects with propensity score matching, then it is in that region that we would like to generate plausible imputations, as we would be selecting matches from controls in that part of the covariate space. The latent class model works by reducing the impact that control records, far removed from the treated units' covariate space, can have on imputations of missing covariate values for control records lying in the treated units' covariate space.

Mitra and Reiter (2011) apply the latent class model to multiply impute the missing values $m = 100,000$ times with propensity scores estimated from the imputed data in the same way as before. Their results are displayed in Figure 12.3, which summarizes the true covariate balance on $x_1$ and $x_2$ for the latent class and one-class multiple imputation modeling strategies. For both matching with and without replacement, the latent class imputation model results in some improvements in the covariate balance compared to using the one-class imputation model. In addition, Mitra and Reiter (2011) generate a response surface similar to the generation process described above and show that using the latent class model can result in a reduction in the bias of the treatment effect estimates over using the one-class model for imputations. Also, Mitra and Reiter (2011) consider a scenario where the one-class imputation model is appropriately specified and compare performances of the latent class and one-class imputation models. They note that there is not much penalty in using the latent class imputation model in this scenario to estimate treatment effects (where it is not necessarily needed).

While the benefits of using the latent class imputation model have been shown explicitly for treatment effects estimated with propensity score matching, other propensity score treatment effect estimates can be used with the multiply imputed data—for example, subclassification or inverse weighting. Benefits for subclassification using the latent class model might be possible due to the similarities with matching, but it is not clear that benefits will exist to the same extent with inverse weighting. This is a topic for future investigation: whether the latent class model will act as an all-purpose improvement regardless of the method used to estimate treatment effects with the propensity scores.

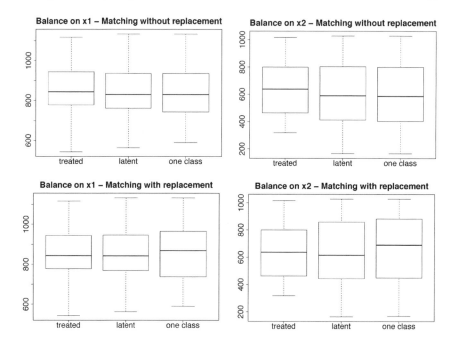

**FIGURE 12.3.** Box plots for $x_1$ and $x_2$ for treated and matched control units in the model misspecification simulation. Here, "latent" indicates controls selected via the general location latent class mixture model, and "one class" indicates controls selected via the one-class model.

## AN APPLICATION TO A BREASTFEEDING STUDY

We now return to an illustration of the Across and Within method to estimate propensity scores and treatment effects in a genuine data example. The data are taken from a subsample of the 1979 National Longitudinal Survey of Youth (NLSY79). The next section gives a brief description of the data. It is followed by an illustration taken from Mitra and Reiter (2012) that uses a simulation based on the complete cases, and the results from Mitra and Reiter (2012) that apply both methods to the full (incomplete) dataset.

### NLSY Dataset

The NLSY interviewed a sample of 12,686 youths, ages 14–22, on an annual basis from 1979. In 1986, a separate survey began to measure variables for children born to female respondents in NLSY79 known as the NLSY79 Children and Young Adults. The dataset we consider here is a subsample of the NLSY79 Children and Young Adults, which specifically looked at the effect of breastfeeding on children's cognitive development.

The study recorded the Peabody individual assessment math score (PIATM) administered at 5 or 6 years of age, which is used as the measure of a child's cognitive development. Mitra and Reiter (2011, 2012) dichomotize the variable that measures duration of breastfeeding so as to split units into two groups; the first group, which is the control group, comprises those units breastfed for less than 24 weeks, while the second group, which is the treatment group, comprises those units breastfed for 24 weeks or more. The analysis of interest is assumed to be in determining the relationship between PIATM and the effect of treatment after adjusting for relevant pretreatment variables. Mitra and Reiter (2011, 2012) use 14 pretreatment background covariates to adjust for potential confounding variables. There were seven continuous covariates: mother's age at the child's birth minus her age in 1979, mother's intelligence measured by an armed forces qualification test, mother's highest educational attainment, child's birthweight, number of weeks that the child spent in hospital, number of weeks the mother spent in hospital, and family income. There were seven categorical covariates: child's race (Hispanic, black, or other), mother's race (Hispanic, black, Asian, white, Hawaiian/Pacific Islander/American Indian, or other), child's sex, two variables indicating whether the spouse or grandparents were present at birth, number of weeks the child was born premature (0 weeks, 1 to 4 weeks, and 5 or more weeks with cut points determined from guidelines of the March of Dimes), and number of weeks that the mother worked in the year prior to giving birth (not worked at all, worked between 1 and 47 weeks, worked 48–51 weeks, and worked all 52 weeks).

Mitra and Reiter (2011, 2012) only include the first-born children in the analysis to avoid complications arising from family nesting. In addition, units with missing breastfeeding duration or PIATM scores are discarded. Several covariates in the study were not fully observed, only three covariates were completely observed, nine had missing data rates of less than 10%, family income had 22.4% of its values missing, while the number of weeks that the mother worked in the year prior to giving birth had 23.1% missing data.

## Simulation Involving the Complete Cases

Mitra and Reiter (2012) empirically compare the Across and Within methods with a simulation involving the complete cases. Missing values are reintroduced into the complete case records so that the missing data patterns are distributed in the same way that they were distributed in the original data, and missing values are imputed with the general location (one-class) model (Schafer, 1997). Missing values can be conveniently imputed from this model using the "mix" library in the statistical software package R. Then from each imputed dataset they estimate propensity scores with a main effects logistic regression, including all 14 covariates in the model. Treatment effects are then estimated with the Across and Within methods.

Mitra and Reiter (2012) simulate 100 incomplete datasets, created by repeatedly drawing from the missing data patterns, and box plots of the treatment effect estimates they obtain are given in Figure 12.4. Treatment effects were estimated using $m = 30$ imputed datasets. We can see that point estimates from both methods are similar on average, but estimates

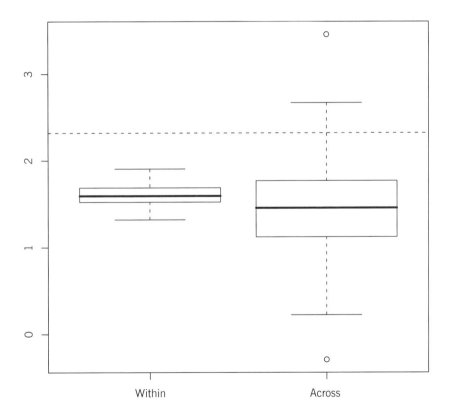

**FIGURE 12.4.** Box plots of the Within and Across treatment effect estimates in the simulation involving NLSY79 data and $m = 30$. The dotted line represents the treatment effect based on the 1,306 complete records.

from the Across method are more variable. Mitra and Reiter (2012) note that this could be because treatment assignment here does not appear to be related to variables with large amounts of missing data, so point estimates from both Across and Within methods should be similar but with less variability in the Within estimates. It was also noted that both Across and Within estimates were somewhat different compared to the treatment effect estimated prior to the introduction of missing values, which was 2.32.

## CONCLUSION

We have seen that there are principled ways to handle the problem of missing covariate values within observational studies. We focused on model-based approaches to deal with the missing values problem, and in particular the approach of multiple imputation. The sensitivity of treatment effects to implausible modeling assumptions when dealing with the missing data is a cause for concern, but that is where robust imputation models such as the latent class model can provide analysts with some protection. It should be noted that weighting-based approaches exist to deal with the missing values problem here as well. For example, Williamson, Forbes, and Wolfe (2012) construct an augmented inverse probability weighted estimator for the treatment effect that can handle the problem of incomplete covariates.

We have not dealt with the problem of missing outcome values or treatment indicators here. One might argue that we should impute these values as well and use them to make inferences about the treatment effect. However, given that we never observed these values, is it appropriate to use conjectured/simulated values that can influence our inferences, or only rely on observed values? At this point it is not clear which course of action should be taken, and indeed in some situations one approach may be better than the other. The problem of missing outcomes has been looked at by Davidian, Tsiatis, and Leon (2005) who propose an augmented inverse probability weighted estimator to handle the problem, while the estimator proposed in Williamson et al. (2012) can also handle missing outcome values and treatment indicators. More work is needed to determine how best to proceed in the presence of missing outcome and treatment values, so as to maximize the information present in the data without introducing bias into estimates of the treatment effect.

## REFERENCES

Austin, P. C. (2008). A critical appraisal of propensity-score matching in the medical literature between 1996 and 2003. *Statistics in Medicine, 27*(12), 2037–2049.

Austin, P. C. (2009). Balance diagnostics for comparing the distribution of baseline covariates between treatment group in propensity-score matched samples. *Statistics in Medicine, 28*(25), 3083–3107.

Cho, Y. B., Lee, K., Suh, K., Kim, Y., Yoon, J., Lee, H. S. H., et al. (2007). Hepatic resection compared to percutaneous ethanol injection for small hepatocellular carcinoma using propensity score matching. *Journal of Gastroenterology and Hepatology, 22*(10), 1643–1649.

da Veiga, P. V., & Wilder, R. P. (2008). Maternal smoking during pregnancy and birthweight: A propensity score matching approach. *Maternal and Child Health Journal, 12*(2), 194–203.

D'Agostino, Jr., R. B., Lang, W., Walkup, M., Morgan, T., & Karter, A. (2001). Examining the impact of missing data on propensity score estimation in determining the effectiveness of self-monitoring of blood glucose (smbg). *Health Services and Outcomes Research Methodology, 2*(3–4), 291–315.

D'Agostino Jr., R. B., & Rubin, D. B. (2000). Estimating and using propensity scores with partially missing data. *Journal of the American Statistical Association, 95*(451), 749–759.

Davidian, M., Tsiatis, A. A., & Leon, S. (2005). Semiparametric estimation of treatment effect in a pretest-posttest study with missing data (with comments and rejoinder). *Statistical Science, 20*(3), 261–301.

Dempster, A. P., Laird, N. M., & Rubin, D. B. (1977). Maximum likelihood from incomplete data via the EM algorithm. *Journal of the Royal Statistical Society. Series B (Methodological), 39*(1), 1–38.

Geda, Y. E., Roberts, R. O., Knopman, D. S., Petersen, E. C., Christianson, T. J., Pankratz, V. S., et al. (2008). Prevalence of neuropsychiatric symptoms in mild cognitive impairment and normal cognitive aging: Population-based study. *Archives of General Psychiatry, 65*(10), 1193–1198.

Hanley, J. A., & Dendukuri, N. (2009). Efficient sampling approaches to address confounding in database studies. *Statistical Methods in Medical Research, 18*(1), 81–105.

Harder, V. S., Stuart, E. A., & Anthony, J. C. (2010). Propensity score techniques and the assessment of measured covariate balance to test causal associations in psychological research. *Psychological Methods, 15*(3), 234–249.

Haviland, A., Nagin, D., & Rosenbaum, P. (2007). Combining propensity score matching and group-based trajectory analysis in an observational study. *Psychological Methods, 12*(3), 247–267.

Hill, J. (2004). Reducing bias in treatment effect estimation in observational studies suffering from missing data. *Columbia University Institute for Social and Economic Research and Policy (ISERP)*, Working Paper 04–01.

Hill, J., & Reiter, J. P. (2006). Interval estimation for treatment effects using propensity score matching. *Statistics in Medicine, 25*, 2230–2256.

Hill, J. L., Reiter, J. P., & Zanutto, E. L. (2004). A comparison of experimental and observational data analyses. In A. Gelman & X. L. Meng (Eds.), *Applied Bayesian modeling and causal inference from an incomplete-data perspective*. Hoboken, NJ: Wiley.

Hullsiek, K. H., & Louis, T. A. (2002). Propensity score modeling strategies for the causal analysis of observational data. *Biostatistics (Oxford), 3*(2), 179–193.

Ibrahim, J. G., Chen, M.-H., Lipsitz, S. R., & Herring, A. H. (2005). Missing data methods for generalized linear models: A comparative review. *Journal of the American Statistical Association, 100*(469), 332–346.

Little, R. J. A. (1992). Regression with missing X's: A review. *Journal of the American Statistical Association, 87*, 1227–1237.

Little, R. J. A., & Rubin, D. B. (2002). *Statistical analysis with missing data* (2nd ed.). New York: Wiley.

Luneceford, J. K., & Davidian, M. (2004). Stratification and weighting via the propensity score in estimation of causal treatment effects: A comparative study. *Statistics in Medicine, 23*(19), 2937–2960.

McCaffrey, D. F., Ridgeway, G., & Morral, A. R. (2004). Propensity score estimation with boosted regression for evaluating causal effects in observational studies. *Psychological Methods, 9*(4), 403.

Mitra, R., & Reiter, J. P. (2011). Estimating propensity scores with missing covariate data using general location mixture models. *Statistics in Medicine, 30*(6), 627–641.

Mitra, R., & Reiter, J. P. (2012). A comparison of two methods of estimating propensity scores after multiple imputation. *Statistical Methods in Medical Research* (online early).

Moons, K. G. M., Donders, R. A. R. T., Stijnen, T., & Harrell Jr., F. E. (2006). Using the outcome for imputation of missing predictor values was preferred. *Journal of Clinical Epidemiology, 59*(10), 1092–1101.

Olkin, I., & Tate, R. F. (1961). Multivariate correlation models with mixed discrete and continuous variables. *Annals of Mathematical Statistics, 32*(2), 448–465.

Qu, Y., & Lipkovich, I. (2009). Propensity score estimation with missing values using a multiple imputation missingness pattern (MIMP) approach. *Statistics in Medicine, 28*(9), 1402–1414.

Raghunathan, T. E., Lepkowski, J. M., van Hoewyk, J., & Solenberger, P. (2001). A multivariate technique for multiply imputing missing values using a sequence of regression models. *Survey Methodology, 27*(1), 85–95.

Robins, J. M., Hernan, M. A., & Brumback, B. (2000). Marginal structural models and causal inference in epidemiology. *Epidemiology, 11*(5), 550–560.

Rosenbaum, P. R., & Rubin, D. B. (1984). Reducing bias in observational studies using subclassification on the propensity score. *Journal of the American Statistical Association, 79*, 516–524.

Rubin, D. (1976). Inference and missing data. *Biometrika, 63*(3), 581–592.

Rubin, D. B. (1987). *Multiple imputation for nonresponse in surveys.* New York: Wiley.

Schafer, J. L. (1997). *Analysis of incomplete multivariate data.* London: Chapman & Hall.

Schafer, J. L., & Graham, J. W. (2002). Missing data: Our view of the state of the art. *Psychological Methods, 7,* 147–177.

Setoguchi, S., Schneeweiss, S., Brookhart, M. A., Glynn, R. J., & Cook, E. F. (2008). Evaluating uses of data mining techniques in propensity score estimation: A simulation study. *Pharmacoepidemiology and Drug Safety, 17,* 546–555.

Song, J., Belin, T., Lee, M., Gao, X., & Rotheram-Borus, M. (2001). Handling baseline differences and missing items in a longitudinal study of HIV risk among runaway youths. *Health Services and Outcomes Research Methodology, 2*(3–4), 317–329.

Tannen, R. L., Weiner, M. G., & Xie, D. (2009). Use of primary care electronic medical record database in drug efficacy research on cardiovascular outcomes: Comparison of database and randomised controlled trial findings. *British Medical Journal, 338,* b81.

Tanner, M. A., & Wong, W. H. (1987). The calculation of posterior distributions by data augmentation. *Journal of the American Statistical Association, 82,* 528–540.

Van Buuren, S. (2007). Multiple imputation of discrete and continuous data by fully conditional specification. *Statistical Methods in Medical Research, 16*(3), 219–242.

Westreich, D., Lessler, J., & Funk, M. J. (2010). Propensity score estimation: Neural networks, support vector machines, decision trees (cart), and meta-classifiers as alternatives to logistic regression. *Journal of Clinical Epidemiology, 63,* 826–833.

Williamson, E., Forbes, A., & Wolfe, R. (2012). Doubly robust estimators of causal exposure effects with missing data in the outcome, exposure or a confounder. *Statistics in Medicine, 31*(30), 4382–4400.

Woo, M.-J., Reiter, J. P., & Karr, A. F. (2008). Estimation of propensity scores using generalized additive models. *Statistics in Medicine, 27*(19), 3805–3816.

# CHAPTER 13

# Unobserved Confounding in Propensity Score Analysis

Rolf H. H. Groenwold
Olaf H. Klungel

Propensity score analysis is one of many statistical methods that aim to control for confounding in observational research (Rosenbaum & Rubin, 1983). These methods include matching, stratification (or subclassification), weighting, and controlling for confounding in regression analysis. What these methods have in common is that they control for *observed* confounders (Klungel et al., 2004); confounders that are not observed cannot be controlled for by these methods (Groenwold, Hak, & Hoes, 2009). Since propensity score methods do not control for unobserved confounders, results from propensity score analysis are potentially biased by unobserved confounding (Rosenbaum & Rubin, 1983; Rosenbaum & Rubin, 1984). Nonetheless, propensity score adjustment may control indirectly for unobserved confounding.

In this chapter, we focus on unobserved confounding in propensity score analysis. We particularly consider unobserved confounding due to confounders that are not measured at all, although the methods that are discussed also apply to confounders that are measured, but without sufficient detail (e.g., obesity yes/no instead of body mass index (BMI), or smoking yes/no instead of number of pack-years smoked) or with error (misclassification). The latter is sometimes referred to as residual confounding (Groenwold, Hak, & Hoes, 2009).

Unobserved confounding in medical research—in particular on the effects of medical interventions—is the key example in this chapter, but we stress that the thinking about unobserved confounding and the methods to address unobserved confounding apply to other observational research areas as well.

We start this chapter with a brief discussion of unobserved confounding in medical research. Second, a method that directly controls for unobserved confounding, propensity score calibration, is discussed in detail. Next, we discuss to what extent propensity score methods may control for unobserved confounding. Then, we explore whether the propensity score can be used as a diagnostic for unobserved confounding. Finally, we give an overview of methods to quantify the impact of unobserved confounding on results from propensity score analysis through sensitivity analysis.

## UNOBSERVED CONFOUNDING IN MEDICAL RESEARCH

It seems obvious that in daily medical practice treatments are prescribed for a reason, that is, there is a medical indication for initiating or refraining (contraindications) from a particular medical treatment. Consequently, medical treatments are predominantly prescribed to those who need the treatment the most. The treatment allocation process is therefore a selective process, and, hence, studies of intended effects of medical interventions have a large potential for confounding (also referred to as confounding by indication) when simply comparing groups of treated units (e.g., subjects) with groups of untreated units (Grobbee & Hoes, 2008).

An example of a study on an intended effect of a medical treatment is a study of influenza vaccination and the risk of mortality among elderly (Groenwold, Hoes, & Hak, 2009). Given that influenza vaccination is part of routine care, and the incidence of mortality among the elderly during an influenza epidemic is low (approximately 1%), a randomized trial is considered unethical and unfeasible. However, in an observational study, a direct comparison of mortality rates among vaccinated and unvaccinated subjects is probably confounded because particularly those subjects who have the highest risk of dying (for example, because of a high age or presence of comorbidity) are likely to take the vaccine. In observational studies on influenza vaccination, researchers therefore typically control for confounding by age, comorbidity status, and medication use (as a proxy for severity of comorbidity). The low mortality rates among the elderly during influenza epidemics requires large cohorts to study the effects of influenza vaccination. These large cohorts are often based on health care registries of routinely collected health care information, including demographics, comorbidity status, and medication use. However, these registries typically do not have detailed information on biomarkers and life-style factors (smoking, exercise levels, dietary habits, etc.). And even if information on, for example, BMI is collected, it is likely to be registered selectively and not uniformly for all subjects in such a registry (i.e., there is a reason for registering BMI, for example, because of severe obesity). Consequently, observational studies of the effects of influenza vaccination among the elderly using routinely collected health care data have the potential to be biased by unobserved confounding by, for example, life style factors.

When medical treatments are selectively nonprescribed to those who have the largest risk of an adverse event, this will increase the potential for confounding in studies of the unintended effects of such treatments. For example, consider the study of the possible increased risk of myocardial infarction by inhaled beta-2 agonist use among patients with chronic obstructive pulmonary disease (COPD) (Groenwold et al., 2011). Particularly those patients who have the most severe forms of COPD are likely to be prescribed inhalation beta-2 agonists. Since severity of COPD is not routinely registered in the health care databases, a direct comparison between users and nonusers is potentially confounded by severity of disease.

Clinical endpoints such as mortality and adverse events are usually rare in clinical studies. Because medical research on rare health outcomes requires large numbers of subjects, such research is often conducted using large health care registries. However, in such registries there is typically no information on life-style factors or biomarkers (blood pressure, cholesterol levels, heart rate, etc.). Hence, in observational research on the effects of medical treatments, researchers have to make a trade-off between the size of the dataset and the number and quality of confounders that are observed. In both of these examples, observed confounders are controllable by means of the propensity score. Obviously, the propensity score model could only include confounders that were *observed*, and, hence, propensity score analysis could not control for confounders that were not observed ("unobserved confounding").

It is important to recognize that studies of unintended effects of medical treatment do not necessarily suffer from confounding. When adverse events cannot be anticipated, for example, the development of angioedema when using angiotensin-converting enzyme (ACE) inhibitors, the perceived risk of an adverse event will not differ between patients and hence not guide clinical decision making regarding initiation of therapy. Hence, in studies of unanticipated unintended effect, confounding will likely not play an important role (Miettinen, 1983; Vandenbroucke, 2004).

Applications of propensity score methods are obviously not restricted to medical research. For example, in a study of a program for men who batter women, propensity score analysis (i.e., propensity score stratification) was used to assess the effect of program completion on re-assault (Jones, D'Agostino, Gondolf, & Heckert, 2004). Another example is a study that aimed to evaluate a multi-intervention school improvement program in Jamaica using propensity score matching to control for differences between schools enrolled in the program and control schools (Lockheed, Harris, & Jayasundera, 2010). In the latter study, variables included in the propensity score model were either related to enrollment in the program or determinants of student achievement (outcome of the study). In parallel to the aforementioned examples from the field of medical research, propensity score methods are used to control for differences between groups other than the causal factor of interest. Also in these examples, potential confounders may be unobserved, potentially invalidating the results of the study.

## PROPENSITY SCORE CALIBRATION

An obvious way to control for unobserved confounding is to collect information on the unmeasured confounder. However, this appears impractical for studies using large health care registries. A practical approach would be to control for unobserved confounding in propensity score analysis by obtaining information on unobserved confounders in a subset of the study population. For example, in a health care registry-based study of influenza vaccination, no information was available on the potential confounder smoking (Groenwold, Hoes, Nichol, & Hak, 2008). Rather than collecting information on smoking among all units in the study, questionnaires were sent out to a subset of approximately 1% of the total cohort size. The information of the unobserved confounders collected from the subset can be incorporated in the propensity score analysis using propensity score calibration (Stürmer, Schneeweiss, Avorn, & Glynn, 2005; Stürmer, Schneeweiss, Rothman, Avorn, & Glynn, 2007).

The basic idea of propensity score calibration is that a propensity score analysis of the full dataset yields precise (due to the size of the dataset), yet potentially biased, estimates of the exposure–outcome relation (due to unobserved confounding). Additional confounder information from a subset of the full study population can be used to correct for the bias, while maintaining the advantage of the size of the full dataset.

In propensity score calibration, two propensity score models are fitted within the subset. The first is a propensity score model including the observed confounders that are observed in the full dataset; this model is referred to as the error-prone model and is defined as

$$PS_{ep} = \text{prob}(z = 1|\mathbf{x}_{ep}) \tag{13.1}$$

where $z$ indicates the treatment status and $\mathbf{x}_{ep}$ is a vector of values of the confounders that are observed in the full dataset. The second propensity score model includes confounders that are observed in the full dataset as well as the additional set of confounders that are only observed within the subset (i.e., the "unobserved confounders"); this model is referred to as the gold standard model and is defined as:

$$PS_{gs} = \text{prob}(z = 1|\mathbf{x}_{gs}) \tag{13.2}$$

where $z$ indicates the treatment status and $\mathbf{x}_{gs}$ is a vector of values of the confounders that are observed in the full dataset as well as the additional set of confounders that are only observed within the subset. Obviously, the $PS_{gs}$ can only be estimated for the subset of units for whom the additional confounders are observed. Within the full dataset, only the error-prone propensity score model can be used to control for confounding. For example, if the treatment–outcome association is modeled using a logistic model, one could include the (continuous) propensity score as a covariate in the model to control for confounding:

$$\text{prob}(r = 1|z, PS_{ep}) = (1 + \exp[-(\alpha_0 + \alpha_z z + \alpha_x PS_{ep})])^{-1} \tag{13.3}$$

where $r$ indicates the binary response (e.g., clinical outcome of interest), $\alpha_0$ is the intercept of the model, and $\alpha_z$ and $\alpha_x$ indicate the regression coefficients of the relation between treatment and outcome and $PS_{ep}$ and outcomes, respectively. If indeed important confounders are missing from the error-prone propensity score model, the treatment effect (estimated by the coefficient $\alpha_z$) is biased by unobserved confounding because $PS_{ep}$ inadequately controls for confounding, due to the missing confounders. The bias in the estimated treatment effect can be controlled for by first relating the gold standard propensity score to the error-prone propensity score using a linear model:

$$E[PS_{gs}|z, PS_{ep}] = \gamma_0 + \gamma_z z + \gamma_x PS_{ep} \qquad (13.4)$$

where $\gamma_0$ is the intercept of the model, and $\gamma_z$ and $\gamma_x$ indicate the regression coefficients of the relation between treatment and $PS_{gs}$ and $PS_{ep}$ and $PS_{gs}$, respectively. Equation 13.4 is referred to as the measurement error model, which quantifies the measurement error in the error-prone propensity score model compared to the gold standard propensity score model. The key notion of propensity score calibration is that the discrepancy between these two models is due to the unobserved confounders that are included in the gold standard model, which can therefore be applied in the full dataset in order to control for unobserved confounding (by those confounders that were additionally observed in the subset).

If the treatment–outcome relation were expressed as an odds ratio (OR), the relation between the treatment and outcome that is observed in the full dataset ($OR^* = \exp(\alpha_z)$) and the true (unbiased) treatment–outcome relation (OR) is

$$OR = OR^*/A \qquad (13.5)$$

where $A$ is a correction factor to control for unobserved confounding. The value of $A$ depends on the discrepancy between the error-prone and the gold standard propensity score models:

$$A = \gamma_z \alpha_x / \gamma_x \qquad (13.6)$$

Instead of controlling the observed relation between the treatment and outcome (i.e., applying Equation 13.5), one could also impute the predicted value of the $PS_{gs}$ based on Equation 13.4 in the full dataset, for those units that are not in the subset (Stürmer et al., 2007). After imputing the predicted $PS_{gs}$ values for those units for whom certain confounders were unobserved, the (imputed) gold standard propensity score can be used to control for confounding using all available data.

In propensity score calibration, the error-prone propensity score is considered a surrogate for the gold standard propensity score. This implies that the error-prone propensity score is independent of the outcome, given the gold standard propensity score and treatment. This assumption is referred to as surrogacy and can be formally assessed in the subset of data, for which information on treatment, outcome, gold standard propensity score, and error-prone propensity score is available. If this assumption cannot be evaluated in the data, surrogacy can be assumed if the direction of confounding (i.e., direction of associations with treatment and outcome) is the same for the observed and unobserved confounders (Lunt, Glynn, Rothman, Avorn, & Stürmer, 2012).

Obviously, propensity score calibration only controls for "unobserved" confounders that are observed in the subset. Hence, in observational research, estimated treatment effects may still be biased by unobserved confounders that were not in the subset even after conducting propensity score calibration. A cautionary note is needed about inference of the estimated treatment effects. It is recommended that bootstrapping be used to obtain the correct standard errors of the estimates of treatment effect (Stürmer et al., 2007). Furthermore, misspecification of the model relating the error-prone propensity score to the gold standard propensity score (Equation 13.4) may incompletely control for the additional confounders in the gold standard propensity score model (Stürmer et al., 2007).

## INDIRECT CONTROL FOR UNOBSERVED CONFOUNDING

Although propensity score methods do not directly control for unobserved confounding, controlling for unobserved confounding may be achieved indirectly by controlling for the observed confounders that are included in the propensity score model. Consider, as an analogy, the example study of influenza vaccination mentioned above. A potential confounder that was unobserved in that study was smoking: smoking is a risk factor for mortality, and possibly those who smoke are more likely to receive the vaccine. Smoking status is likely to be related to COPD status (a disease that is often the result of smoking). Therefore, if you have information about COPD status, to some extent you also have information about smoking status, and thus controlling for COPD status is expected to control (at least partially) for smoking status as well. Or, to put it differently, after controlling for COPD, the confounding effect of smoking will probably be small. Indirect control of unobserved confounding by controlling for the observed confounders is sometimes referred to as "adjustment by proxy." In the example, one does not control for smoking directly, but only indirectly by adjusting for a proxy of smoking, that is, COPD status.

The key assumption underlying indirect control of unobserved confounding by controlling for the observed confounders is that there is some correlation between observed and unobserved confounders (Fewell, Davey Smith, & Sterne, 2007). We illustrate this assumption by simulations (for details see Endnote 1). Results from these simulations, presented in Figure 13.1, show that the bias of treatment effect estimates due to confounding

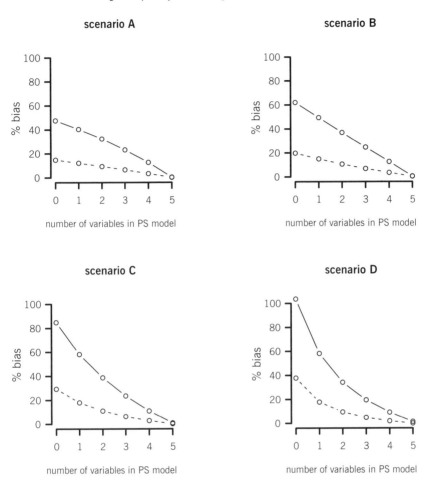

**FIGURE 13.1.** Relation between the number of confounders included in the propensity score (PS) model and the bias of treatment effect estimates from PS analysis. *Note*: Figures are based on simulated datasets of 100,000 units that included five standard normally distributed confounders (sampled from a multivariate normal distribution with a predefined mutual correlation). Correlations between confounders were set at 0.0 (scenario A), 0.1 (scenario B), 0.3 (scenario C), and 0.5 (scenario D), respectively. The log(odds) of binary treatment increased by 0.2 (solid line) or 0.1 (dashed line) per standard deviation (*SD*) increase of the confounders. The value of the continuous outcome increased by 0.2 (solid line) or 0.1 (dashed line) per *SD* increase of the five confounders and by 1.0 if the treatment was present. Propensity scores were estimated using logistic regression, and treatment effect estimates were adjusted for confounding by including the PS as a covariate in the linear outcome model, in which the outcome was regressed on the treatment and the continuous PS.

reduces with an increasing number of confounders included in the propensity score model. This does not come as a surprise. However, it is interesting to note the impact of the correlation between the confounders. Let's compare the scenarios where the confounders have a mutual correlation of 0.0 (i.e., the confounders are independent of each other, Scenario A) and 0.5 (i.e., the confounders are strongly correlated, Scenario D). After inclusion of three of the five confounders, for example, the magnitude of the remaining bias is smaller when the confounders are correlated compared to the situation where the confounders are independent. Stated differently, due to the correlation between the confounders (i.e., shared information), controlling for a number of confounders will already control for the largest part of the confounding that was present. One could say that in Scenario D controlling for three out of five confounders already controls for part of the unobserved confounding by the two confounders that are omitted from the propensity score model. This observed pattern would be even more pronounced in situations where the correlation even exceeds 0.5. In the event of two perfectly correlated confounders, adding the second confounder to the propensity score model that already includes the first confounder will not add to the validity of treatment effect estimates (if we simply ignore multicollinearity).

## Correlated Confounders

In empirical data on British women ages 60–79 years, the age-adjusted pairwise correlations between nongenetic characteristics (e.g., demographics, comorbidity status, medication use, life-style factors, biomarkers) ranged between 0.0 and approximately 0.5, with a skew distribution (median 0.08, IQR 0.06 – 0.13) (Smith et al., 2007). Hence, although correlations in empirical data are less extreme than in the simulations presented in Figure 13.1, one could argue that after including a substantial set (e.g., > 20) of confounders to the propensity score model, adding even more confounders is likely to have limited impact on the treatment effect estimates (Toh, García Rodríguez, & Hernán, 2011). Obviously, this only holds true for unobserved confounders that are correlated to the observed confounders. We note that including confounders that are independent (i.e., not correlated) of confounders already included in the propensity score model obviously increases the validity of the propensity score analysis. In the above-mentioned example of the observational study of the effects of influenza vaccination, potential confounders were added consecutively to the propensity score model, and it was indeed observed that after adjustment for demographics and comorbidity status, additional inclusion of information on medication use in the propensity score model did not materially affect the influenza vaccine effect estimate (Groenwold, Hoes, et al., 2009).

## Example: Indirect Control for Unobserved Confounding

As an example of indirect control for confounding in empirical research, consider an observational study of the effect of nonsteroidal antiinflammatory drugs (NSAIDs) and the risk of upper gastrointestinal bleeding, in which confounding was controlled for by propensity score adjustment (Toh, García Rodríguez, & Hernán, 2012). In this study, the propensity score model incorporated 18 confounders, including information on demographics, comorbidity, and medication use. The unadjusted odds ratio of the effect of the NSAID use on upper gastrointestinal bleeding was 1.50, which gradually decreased after adjustment for observed confounders to an OR of 0.81. Additional to these 18 confounders, three additional confounders were considered: smoking, alcohol consumption, and body mass index. For only in 78% of the study population, information on all confounders was available. Confounding adjustment for those three additional confounders was achieved by propensity score calibration, which yielded an OR of 0.80.

In a separate analysis, the high-dimensional propensity score (hd-PS) algorithm was applied to select 500 covariates, which were included in a propensity score model in addition to age and sex. The hd-PS methods try to maximize indirect control for unobserved confounding by including a large number (typically hundreds) of variables in the propensity score model (Schneeweiss et al., 2009). Variables are selected using an automated algorithm that focuses on the prevalence of confounders, the magnitude of the association between potential confounders and treatment, and the association between potential confounders and outcome. Including hundreds of confounders in the hd-PS leaves little room for unobserved confounding by variables that are correlated to the observed confounders. Still, hd-PS methods do not control (directly nor indirectly) for variables that are independent of the observed confounders. The hd-PS analysis yielded an OR of the effect of NSAID use of 0.78 (Toh, García Rodríguez, & Hernán, 2011). Hence, in this particular example, additional information on a large number of confounders that were likely correlated to the observed confounders did not materially change the observed effects of treatment.

# THE PROPENSITY SCORES AS A DIAGNOSTIC FOR UNOBSERVED CONFOUNDING

It has been argued that certain characteristics of the propensity score can be used to identify the presence (or absence) of unobserved confounding. We will review several of these aspects and explicate which assumptions underly these claims.

## Balance Measures for Propensity Scores

In their seminal papers, Rosenbaum and Rubin called the propensity score a "balancing score" (Rosenbaum & Rubin, 1983; Rosenbaum & Rubin, 1984): conditional on the propensity score, covariates (i.e., confounders) tend to be balanced between the treatment groups. It is good practice to evaluate the actual balance obtained by the propensity score model by comparing treated and untreated units, conditional on the propensity score (e.g., within quintiles of the propensity score).

Several statistical measures to evaluate the balance of covariates between treatment groups have been proposed. Examples include the standardized difference (Austin, 2009), the postmatching $c$-statistic (Franklin, Rassen, Ackermann, Bartels, & Schneeweiss, 2014), the Kolmogorov–Smirnov distance, and the overlapping coefficient (Belitser et al., 2011). The standardized difference is commonly used in observational medical research. It is the difference in means (or proportions) between two treatment groups, standardized by the pooled standard deviation (Austin, 2009). Thus, a small value of the standardized difference for a certain confounder indicates that the particular confounder is balanced between the treatment groups, whereas large values indicate imbalance.

Obviously, researchers can only assess balance of confounders that are actually observed. Balance of unobserved confounders cannot be determined in the observed data. Nevertheless, if observed and unobserved confounders are correlated, balance measures may be useful to evaluate the validity of the assumption of no unobserved confounding. If observed confounders are well balanced between treatment groups, one could argue that this may also be the case for unobserved confounders (note that this is still an assumption; well-balanced distributions of observed confounders do not prove balance of unobserved confounders) (Schneeweis, Solomon, Wang, Rassen, & Brookhart, 2006). In contrast, if observed confounders are imbalanced between treatment groups, unobserved confounders are likely also to be imbalanced. As such, balance measures can be used as a means of falsifying the assumption of no unobserved confounding.

## Discrepancy between Predicted and Actual Treatment Status

A discrepancy between predicted probability of treatment (i.e., the propensity score) and the actual treatment received has been assumed to suggest unobserved confounding (Brooks & Ohsfeldt, 2013; Stürmer, Rothman, Avorn, & Glynn, 2010). The idea behind this is that for those units that have, for example, a very high probability of being treated (e.g., propensity score = 0.99) yet are not treated, there must be a reason (which is apparently unobserved) why this unit was not treated. Likewise, for those units that have a very low propensity score (e.g., propensity score = 0.01) and yet are treated, it is assumed that there must be an unobserved reason why those units were nevertheless treated. To state it differently, a clear discrepancy between the predicted probability and the actual treatment received is considered suggestive of unobserved reasons (confounders) for treatment allocation.

However, based on propensity score theory, such a discrepancy can—and in fact should—be present. Those who have a propensity score of 0.99 have a very high probability of being treated, yet it is still a probability. Hence, among 1,000 units with such a propensity score, we expect that on average 10 would be untreated. Actually, those 10 units are essential for making inferences about the effects of treatment for those who have a propensity score of 0.99. In the unfortunate situation in which we would not have any untreated unit with a propensity score of 0.99, we would not be able to make a valid comparison between treated and untreated units with a propensity score of 0.99. This situation is called nonpositivity, and it potentially biases results (Westreich & Cole, 2010). Thus, any discrepancy (or consistency) between the propensity score and the actual treatment status cannot be turned into a diagnostic for unobserved confounding.

## Goodness of Fit of the Propensity Score Model

Since the propensity score model is a model predicting treatment status based on observed confounders, one could expect—at first glance—that the model that is best in predicting treatment status is also best in controlling for confounding. There are several statistical goodness-of-fit measures to quantify the predictive performance of the propensity score model, including the likelihood of the model and the $c$-statistic. In the following we focus on the $c$-statistic, but we note that our conclusions also apply to other goodness-of-fit measures of the propensity score model (Weitzen, Lapane, Toledano, Hume, & Mor, 2005).

The $c$-statistic is the probability that for a random couple of a treated and an untreated unit, the treated unit will have the highest propensity score of the two. A $c$-statistic of 0.5 reflects that the propensity score model is no better in predicting treatment status than the flip of a coin, whereas a $c$-statistic close to 1.0 indicates that the propensity score model can perfectly discriminate between treated and untreated units. A $c$-statistic that is close to 0.5, is sometimes considered to be a sign of unobserved confounding, whereas a $c$-statistic value that is close to 1.0 may indicate that there is little room for unobserved confounding (Stürmer et al., 2006; Westreich, Cole, Funk, Brookhart, & Stürmer, 2011).

There are, however, several reasons why the value of the $c$-statistic cannot provide information on (the potential for) unobserved confounding. First, including variables that are so-called instruments (i.e., predictors of treatment that are not related to the outcome) will increase the $c$-statistic value, but since these instruments are not confounders, this will not control for confounding. Including instruments in the propensity score model may actually increase the bias (Brookhart et al., 2006; Westreich et al., 2011). Second, it is unclear what the optimal value of the $c$-statistic should be. In a large randomized controlled trial, the $c$-statistic is approximately 0.5 (due to the random allocation of treatment by design), but obviously there is no (unobserved) confounding (Groenwold et al., 2011). On the other hand, if the $c$-statistic value would be close to 1, the propensity score distributions of treated and untreated would be completely nonoverlapping. This is an example of extreme nonpositivity, in which case treatment effects cannot be estimated properly (Westreich et al., 2011).

To illustrate that the $c$-statistic is uninformative about bias due to unobserved confounding, we simulated different scenarios of observational studies (for detail, see Endnote 2). Results of these simulations are presented in Figure 13.2. If the variables that are included in the propensity score are actual confounders, the $c$-statistic indeed increases with the number of included confounders, while the bias reduces (Scenario A). The $c$-statistic also increases with inclusion of so-called instruments (variable related only to treatment but not to the outcome). However, in the presence of unobserved confounding (Scenario B), this may actually increase bias (Brookhart et al., 2006; Myers et al., 2011; Pearl, 2011). Adding instruments to the propensity score model, in the absence of unobserved confounding, increases the $c$-statistic value as well, yet does not induce bias (Scenario C). Finally, inclusion of risk factors for the outcome that are not related to treatment affects neither the $c$-statistic nor bias (Scenario D). In conclusion, although the $c$-statistic of the propensity score model increases when adding confounders to the propensity score model, an

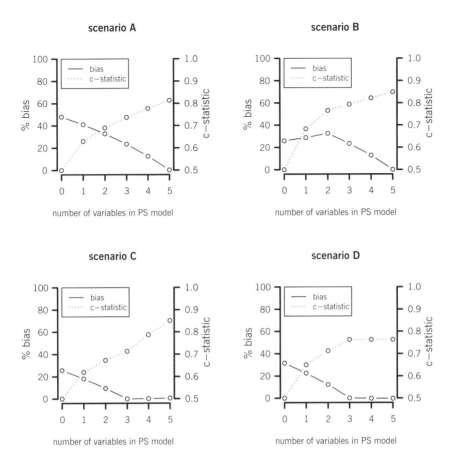

**FIGURE 13.2.** Relation between the number of confounders included in the propensity score (PS) model and the bias of treatment effect estimates from PS analysis and c-statistic of the PS model. *Note*: Figures are based on simulated datasets of 100,000 units that included five standard normally distributed covariates that were mutually independent. Covariates were either confounders (affecting treatment as well as outcome), instruments (affecting treatment only), or risk factor (affecting outcome only). The log(odds) of binary treatment increased by 0.2 per standard deviation (*SD*) increase of the confounders. The value of the continuous outcome increased by 0.2 per *SD* increase for each confounder and by 1.0 if the treatment was present. Instruments increased the log(odds) of treatment by 0.3 per *SD* increase but did not affect the outcome. Risk factors did not affect treatment but increased the outcome by 0.3 per *SD* increase. In Scenario A all covariates were confounders. In Scenario B the first two variables included in the PS model were instruments, whereas the last three were confounders. In Scenario C the first three variables included in the PS model were confounders, whereas the last two were instruments. In Scenario D, the first three variables included in the PS model were confounders, whereas the last two were risk factors for the outcome. Propensity scores were estimated using logistic regression, and treatment effect estimates were adjusted for confounding by including the PS as a covariate in the linear outcome model, in which the outcome was regressed on the treatment and the continuous PS.

increase in the $c$-statistic does not indicate better control for confounding. Furthermore, the absolute value of the $c$-statistic does not provide any information on the potential for unobserved confounding.

The $c$-statistic is just one of many measures of the statistical performance of the propensity score model in predicting treatment status. Just as no information on unobserved confounding can be derived from the $c$-statistic value, similarly other goodness-of-fit measures of propensity score model (e.g., the likelihood) do not yield information on the potential for unobserved confounding. We note that the $c$-statistic can provide information on the balance of observed confounders once propensity score matching has been applied (Franklin et al., 2014). In that case, the postmatching $c$-statistic is a metric of (multivariable) imbalance of observed confounders and highly predictive of bias due to any imbalance in observed confounders between treatment groups.

## Unexpected Findings in the Propensity Score Model

In general, characteristics of the propensity score model provide information solely on the association between the covariates included in the model and the treatment status. When evaluated in solitude, these characteristics do not provide information on unobserved confounders, which by definition involves the relation between covariates and the treatment as well as the outcome. However, when assessing characteristics of the propensity score model in combination with prior knowledge (external from the current study), these characteristics may tell something about unobserved confounding. For example, if the direction (i.e., sign) of the relation between a variable included in the propensity score model and treatment is opposite to what is expected, this could indicate the presence of unobserved confounding (Schuit et al., 2013). If researchers expect, for example, a positive association, yet a negative association is observed in the propensity score model, one possible reason for this discrepancy is unobserved confounding. A clear downside to this approach is that it may not be clear what to expect, and therefore misleading with regard to the assessment of unobserved confounding. The amount of unobserved confounding probably needs to be quite large in order to completely switch the sign of the association (more likely the magnitude of the association will be affected by the unobserved confounding, but the sign will be according to expectation). Importantly, there are more possible reasons from unexpected signs of the confounder–treatment relation, including misclassification, selection, and multicollinearity (Schuit et al., 2013).

Researchers may particularly have prior knowledge on the direction (or even magnitude) of the confounder–outcome relation. Since confounders are risk factors for the outcome (or proxies of those risk factors), the direction of their relation with outcome is typically known. However, this is not necessarily the case for the confounder–treatment relation, of which the direction and magnitude can be obtained by the propensity score model. For example, in an observational study of the effect of lipid-lowering drugs (i.e., statins) on the primary prevention of cardiovascular disease, statins were mainly prescribed to high-risk patients (Maitland-van der Zee et al., 2004). However, in an observational study on the secondary prevention of cardiovascular disease (i.e., effects of statins among patients who already experienced a first myocardial infarction), statins were predominantly prescribed to those units that had the lowest risk of the outcome (Klungel et al., 2002). Hence, in these two empirical examples, the direction of the confounder–treatment relation was opposite, which in fact did not suggest unobserved confounding in either of the two studies, but rather reflects the variation in treatment decisions that differs between settings of primary and secondary prevention.

It is important to understand that the data that are observed and used for analysis (i.e., the observed confounders) do not necessarily contain information on the data that were not observed (unobserved confounders). Hence, it is not straightforward (if possible at all) to make inferences on unobserved variables using the observed ones only.

## SENSITIVITY ANALYSIS OF UNOBSERVED CONFOUNDING IN PROPENSITY SCORE ANALYSIS

In the previous section, we indicated that considering the data at hand by themselves does not provide information on the likelihood, let alone the magnitude, of unobserved confounding. In this section, we will discuss methods to quantify the impact of unobserved confounding by means of sensitivity analysis. Sensitivity analyses are often conducted in addition to the main analysis of a study, in order to assess how sensitive results are to certain assumptions made in the main analysis (Greenland, 1996, 2005). One of the assumptions underlying propensity score analysis is that all confounders are observed and appropriately included in the propensity score model (i.e., no model misspecification). Sensitivity analysis can be applied to evaluate how robust results from propensity score analysis are to violations of this assumption.

There are two typical ways by which sensitivity analysis of unobserved confounding is used (Phillips, 2003). In one approach, the impact of a known, yet unobserved, confounder is evaluated (often through simulations). Smoking status is an example of a known, yet unobserved, confounder in studies of influenza vaccine effectiveness: we know smoking is a risk factor for various health outcomes and related to vaccination status, yet it is usually not routinely collected in health care registries (Groenwold, Nelson, Nichol, Hoes, & Hak, 2010). Another approach deals with unknown unobserved confounding; that is, the researchers do not have a clear picture of the kind of unobserved variable that could be a confounder. In that case, a wide range of scenarios of unobserved confounding is evaluated to quantify how much unobserved confounding is required in order to nullify the observed effect (Schneeweiss, 2006).

A distinct type of unobserved confounding is confounding by variables that are included in the propensity score model, yet without sufficient level of detail or measured with error. An example is smoking, which is often dichotomized (smoking yes/no), yet modeling it in a continuous way (e.g., number of pack years smoked) will probably better control for confounding by smoking. Sensitivity analysis can also be applied to quantify the impact of such simplifications of the confounder information. In the remainder of this chapter, however, we focus on unobserved confounding by confounders that are completely omitted from the propensity score model.

Sensitivity analysis of unobserved confounding can be conducted in two ways. One approach is to simulate the unobserved confounder(s), based on certain assumptions, which allows actually incorporating the unobserved confounder(s) in the propensity score model (Groenwold et al., 2010). Another approach is to apply analytical methods to adjust the treatment effect estimate obtained by propensity score analysis, again based on certain assumptions about the unobserved confounding. An analytical method for sensitivity analysis of unobserved confounding that is straightforward to apply is the one described by Lin, Psaty, and Kronmal (1998), which we will discuss here in more detail. Although we focus on the application of this method in a propensity score study, we note that it is applicable in any observational study, regardless of the methods used to control for confounding.

## A Method for Sensitivity Analysis of Unobserved Confounding

The method proposed by Lin, Psaty, and Kronmal (1998) makes the assumptions of a rare outcome it also assumes that observed and unobserved confounders are independent of each other. If these assumptions hold and the treatment–outcome relation is expressed as an odds ratio (OR), there is a simple relation between the observed treatment–outcome relation (OR*) and the true (unbiased) treatment–outcome relation (OR), had the unobserved confounders been observed:

$$OR = OR^*/Q \qquad (13.7)$$

The factor $Q$ is a simple correction factor of which the magnitude depends on assumptions made about unobserved confounders. When considering a single unobserved confounder, the factor $Q$ can be expressed as

$$Q = [\zeta_1 p_1 + (1 - p_1)]/[\zeta_0 p_0 + (1 - p_0)] \qquad (13.8)$$

where $\zeta_1$ represents the odds ratio of the outcome associated with the unobserved confounders among those treated, $\zeta_0$ represents the odds ratio of the outcome associated with the unobserved confounders among those untreated, $p_1$ is the prevalence of the unobserved confounder among the treated units, and $p_0$ is the prevalence of the unobserved confounder among the untreated units. If we assume no interaction between the treatment and the unobserved confounder, $\zeta_1$ and $\zeta_0$ are equal.

In the aforementioned example of an observational study on the effect of influenza vaccination on mortality risk among the elderly, smoking was an unobserved potential confounder. After adjustment for routinely collected confounders (demographic, comorbidity status, and medication use), the observed odds ratio of the relation between influenza vaccination and mortality was 0.56, with a 95% confidence interval 0.45–0.69 (Groenwold, Hoes, et al., 2009). No information was available on the potential confounder smoking status. For simplicity, we assume smoking status to be a dichotomous confounder, which is independent of the observed confounders. To evaluate the potential impact of this unobserved confounder, assume that the odds for mortality is twofold increased in those who smoke, compared to those who do not smoke, regardless of influenza vaccination status: $\zeta_1 = \zeta_0 = 2$. Furthermore, let's assume that smoking is twice as prevalent among vaccinated subjects, compared to unvaccinated subjects, e.g., $p_1 = 0.4$ and $p_0 = 0.2$. With these assumptions, the correction factor $Q$ can be calculated to be 1.17, and the "true" association between influenza vaccination and mortality risk would be 0.48 (= 0.56 / 1.17). The correction factor $Q$ equally applies to the confidence interval, resulting in a 95% confidence interval around the OR of 0.48: 95% confidence interval 0.38–0.59. Note that in reality the assumption that the unobserved confounders smoking is independent of the observed confounders (e.g., comorbidity status, such as COPD) seems unlikely to hold.

## Multiple Unobserved Confounders

It seems unlikely that in observational research only one potential confounder is unobserved. Instead, one could easily think of multiple unobserved potential confounders. One could apply methods for sensitivity analysis of unobserved confounding (as the one mentioned above) consecutively for multiple times. However, the joint effect of multiple confounders can be summarized by the effect of a single confounder for which the associations with treatment and outcome are stronger than for the individual confounders (Greenland, 2005). Hence, instead of applying the method of Lin, Psaty, and Kronmal (1998) multiple times, one could summarize the characteristics of multiple confounders (e.g., their joint effect on treatment, their joint effect on the outcome) before conducting sensitivity analysis of unobserved confounding.

As a final remark, we note that sensitivity analysis of unobserved confounding is not the ultimate solution for unobserved confounding, regardless of the method used to control for confounding (i.e., propensity score methods or, e.g., covariate adjustment using regression analysis). Sensitivity analysis of unobserved confounding does not actually control for unobserved confounding, but merely quantifies the impact of assumptions about unobserved confounding made by the researcher. As such, they can be informative to guide the discussion about the potential for and the impact of unobserved confounding in observational studies.

## CONCLUSION

In this chapter we discussed the impact and handling of unobserved confounding in observational studies that use the propensity score to control for confounding. Using information on confounders from a subset of the population, propensity score calibration can potentially control for unobserved confounding in the overall population. Furthermore, indirect adjustment (e.g., through hd-PS), meaning controlling for observed confounders by including them in the propensity score model, may indirectly control for part of the confounding by unobserved confounders that are not included in the propensity score model. This phenomenon will only be present if the unobserved confounders are correlated to the observed confounders. In contrast, particularly unobserved confounders that are (close to) independent of the observed confounders will have a large impact on the bias of treatment effect estimates. Propensity scores are not suitable as a diagnostic tool for detecting unobserved confounding and may be misleading. We stress that characteristics of the propensity score model (e.g., goodness-of-fit statistics such as the $c$-statistic) typically hold little information about the potential for unobserved confounding. However, balance measures may be useful as a means of falsifying the assumption of unobserved confounding. Evaluating the impact of unobserved confounding relies on assumptions that are grounded in knowledge from earlier studies. Sensitivity analysis to assess the impact of these assumptions on unobserved confounding can always be conducted and should become a routine extension to propensity score analysis in observational studies.

## NOTES

1. To illustrate the impact of correlation between observed and unobserved confounders, data were simulated and analyzed as follows. Datasets of 100,000 units were created by sampling five confounders from a multivariate normal distribution. All confounders were standard, normally distributed variables, that is, $\sim N(0,1)$. Their mutual correlation was varied in different simulations between 0 and 0.5. Binary treatment status was generated using the model $PT = \alpha_1 C_1 + \alpha_2 C_2 + \alpha_3 C_3 + \alpha_4 C_4 + \alpha_5 C_5 + \varepsilon_1$, where $C_1, \ldots, C_5$ indicate the five confounders; $\alpha_1, \ldots, \alpha_5$ indicate the effect of confounders on the probability of treatment, and $\varepsilon_1 \sim N(0, 0.5^2)$. The values of $\alpha_1, \ldots, \alpha_5$ were either 0.1 or 0.2, but within a simulation $\alpha_1, \ldots, \alpha_5$ were equal. If $PT > 0$ treatment was 1, otherwise 0. Next, outcomes were generated using the model $Y = T + \beta_1 C_1 + \beta_2 C_2 + \beta_3 C_3 + \beta_4 C_4 + \beta_5 C_5 + \varepsilon_2$, where $T$ indicates binary treatment; $C_1, \ldots, C_5$ indicate the five confounders, $\beta_1, \ldots, \beta_5$ indicate the effect of confounders on the outcome; and $\varepsilon_2 \sim N(0, .5^2)$. The values of $\beta_1, \ldots, \beta_5$ were either 0.1 or 0.2, but within a simulation, $\beta_1, \ldots, \beta_5$ were equal.

Propensity scores were estimated by means of logistic regression, including one, two, three, four, or five confounders. Adjustment for confounding using the propensity score was done by including the propensity score as a continuous covariate in a linear model regressing the outcome on the treatment and propensity score. All simulations and analyses were performed in R for Windows, version 2.13.1 (R Development Core Team, 2008).

2. To illustrate the relation between the $c$-statistic of the propensity score model and bias due to unobserved confounding, data were simulated and analyzed as follows. Datasets of 100,000 units were created by independently sampling five variable confounders from a standard normal distribution, that is, $\varepsilon_1 \sim N(0, 1)$. Binary treatment status was generated using the model $PT = \alpha_1 Z_1 + \alpha_2 Z_2 + \alpha_3 Z_3 + \alpha_4 Z_4 + \alpha_5 Z_5 + \varepsilon_1$, where $Z_1, \ldots, Z_5$ indicate the five variables; $\alpha_1, \ldots, \alpha_5$ indicate the effect of these variables on the probability of treatment; and $\varepsilon_1 \sim N(0, .5^2)$. The values of $\alpha_1, \ldots, \alpha_5$ were varied across scenarios: in Scenario A, $\alpha_1, \ldots, \alpha_5$ were 0.2; in Scenario B, $\alpha_1$ and

$\alpha_2$ were 0.3, while $\alpha_3$, $\alpha_4$, and $\alpha_5$ were 0.2; in Scenario C, $\alpha_1$, $\alpha_2$, and $\alpha_3$ were 0.2, while $\alpha_4$ and $\alpha_5$ were 0.3; in Scenario D, $\alpha_1$, $\alpha_2$, and $\alpha_3$ were 0.2, while $\alpha_4$ and $\alpha_5$ were 0. If PT > 0 treatment was 1, otherwise 0. Next, outcomes were generated using the model: $Y = \beta_1 Z_1 + \beta_2 Z_2 + \beta_3 Z_3 + \beta_4 Z_4 + \beta_5 Z_5 + \varepsilon_1$, where $Z_1, \ldots, Z_5$ indicate the five variables; $\beta_1, \ldots, \beta_5$ indicate the effect of these variables on the outcome; and $\varepsilon_2 \sim N(0, .5^2)$. The values of $\beta_1, \ldots, \beta_5$ were varied across scenarios: in Scenario A, $\beta_1, \ldots, \beta_5$ were 0.2; in Scenario B, $\beta_1$ and $\beta_2$ were 0, while $\beta_3$, $\beta_4$, and $\beta_5$ were 0.2; in Scenario C, $\beta_1$, $\beta_2$, and $\beta_3$ were 0.2, while $\beta_4$ and $\beta_5$ were 0; in Scenario C, $\beta_1$, $\beta_2$, $\beta_3$ were 0.2, while $\beta_4$ and $\beta_5$ were 0.3.

Propensity scores were estimated by means of logistic regression, including one, two, three, four, or five confounders. For each propensity score model, the $c$-statistic was estimated. Adjustment for confounding using the propensity score was done by including the propensity score as a continuous covariate in a linear regression model regressing the outcome on the treatment and propensity score. All simulations and analyses were performed in R for Windows, version 2.13.1 (R Development Core Team, 2008).

# REFERENCES

Austin, P. C. (2009). Balance diagnostics for comparing the distribution of baseline covariates between treatment groups in propensity-score matched samples. *Statistics in Medicine*, 28(25), 3083–3107.

Belitser, S. V., Martens, E. P., Pestman, W. R., Groenwold, R. H., de Boer, A., & Klungel, O. H. (2011). Measuring balance and model selection in propensity score methods. *Pharmacoepidemiology and Drug Safety*, 20(11), 1115–1129.

Brookhart, M. A., Schneeweiss, S., Rothman, K. J., Glynn, R. J., Avorn, J., & Stürmer, T. (2006). Variable selection for propensity score models. *American Journal of Epidemiology*, 163(12), 1149–1156.

Brooks, J. M., & Ohsfeldt, R. L. (2013). Squeezing the balloon: Propensity scores and unmeasured covariate balance. *Health Services Research*, 48(4), 1487–1507.

Fewell, Z., Davey Smith, G., & Sterne, J. A. (2007). The impact of residual and unmeasured confounding in epidemiologic studies: A simulation study. *American Journal of Epidemiology*, 166(6), 645–655.

Franklin, J. M., Rassen, J. A., Ackermann, D., Bartels, D. B., & Schneeweiss, S. (2014). Metrics for covariate balance in cohort studies of causal effects. *Statistics in Medicine*, 33(10), 1685–1699.

Greenland, S. (1996). Basic methods for sensitivity analysis of bias. *International Journal of Epidemiology*, 25(6), 1107–1116.

Greenland, S. (2005). Multiple bias modelling for analysis of observational data. *Journal of the Royal Statistical Society A*, 168(2), 267–306.

Grobbee, D. E., & Hoes, A. W. (2008). *Clinical epidemiology: Principles, methods, and applications for clinical research*. Sudbury, MA: Jones and Bartlett.

Groenwold, R. H., Hak, E., & Hoes, A. W. (2009). Quantitative assessment of unobserved confounding is mandatory in nonrandomized intervention studies. *Journal of Clinical Epidemiology, 62*(1), 22–28.

Groenwold, R. H., Hoes, A. W., & Hak, E. (2009). Impact of influenza vaccination on mortality risk among the elderly. *European Respiratory Journal, 34*(1), 56–62.

Groenwold, R. H., Hoes, A. W., Nichol, K. L., & Hak, E. (2008). Quantifying the potential role of unmeasured confounders: The example of influenza vaccination. *International Journal of Epidemiology, 37*(6), 1422–1429.

Groenwold, R. H., Nelson, D. B., Nichol, K. L., Hoes, A. W., & Hak, E. (2010). Sensitivity analyses to estimate the potential impact of unmeasured confounding in causal research. *International Journal of Epidemiology, 39*(1), 107–117.

Groenwold, R. H., de Vries, F., de Boer, A., Pestman, W. R., Rutten, F. H., Hoes, A. W., & Klungel, O. H. (2011). Balance measures for propensity score methods: A clinical example on beta-agonist use and the risk of myocardial infarction. *Pharmacoepidemiology and Drug Safety, 20*(11), 1130–1137.

Jones, A. S., D'Agostino Jr., R. B., Gondolf, E. W., & Heckert, A. (2004). Assessing the effect of batterer program completion on reassault using propensity scores. *Journal of Interpersonal Violence, 19*(9), 1002–1020.

Klungel, O. H., Heckbert, S. R., de Boer, A., Leufkens, H. G., Sullivan, S. D., Fishman, P. A., et al. (2002). Lipid-lowering drug use and cardiovascular events after myocardial infarction. *Annals of Pharmacotherapy, 36*(5), 751–757.

Klungel, O. H., Martens, E. P., Psaty, B. M., Grobbee, D. E., Sullivan, S. D., Stricker, B. H., et al. (2004). Methods to assess intended effects of drug treatment in observational studies are reviewed. *Journal of Clinical Epidemiology, 57*(12), 1223–1231.

Lin, D. Y., Psaty, B. M., & Kronmal, R. A. (1998). Assessing the sensitivity of regression results to unmeasured confounders in observational studies. *Biometrics, 54*(3), 948–963.

Lockheed, M., Harris, A., & Jayasundera, T. (2010). School improvement plans and student learning in Jamaica. *International Journal of Educational Development, 30*, 54–66.

Lunt, M., Glynn, R. J., Rothman, K. J., Avorn, J., & Stürmer, T. (2012). Propensity score calibration in the absence of surrogacy. *American Journal of Epidemiology, 175*(12), 1294–1302.

Maitland-van der Zee, A. H., Klungel, O. H., Stricker, B. H., Verschuren, W. M., Witteman, J. C., Stijnen, T., et al. (2004). Comparison of two methodologies to analyze exposure to statins in an observational study on effectiveness. *Journal of Clinical Epidemiology, 57*(3), 237–242.

Miettinen, O. S. (1983). The need for randomization in the study of intended effects. *Statistics in Medicine, 2*(2), 267–271.

Myers, J. A., Rassen, J. A., Gagne, J. J., Huybrechts, K. F., Schneeweiss, S., Rothman, K. J., et al. (2011). Effects of adjusting for instrumental variables on bias and precision of effect estimates. *American Journal of Epidemiology, 174*(11), 1213–1222.

Pearl, J. (2011). Invited commentary: Understanding bias amplification. *American Journal of Epidemiology, 174*(11), 1223–1227.

Phillips, C. V. (2003). Quantifying and reporting uncertainty from systematic errors. *Epidemiology, 14*(4), 459–466.

R Development Core Team. (2008). *R: A language and environment for statistical computing.* Vienna, Austria: R Foundation for Statistical Computing.

Rosenbaum, P. R., & Rubin, D. B. (1983). The central role of the propensity score in observational studies for causal effects. *Biometrika, 70*(1), 41–55.

Rosenbaum, P. R., & Rubin, D. B. (1984). Reducing bias in observational studies using subclassification on the propensity score. *Journal of the American Statistical Association, 79*(387), 516–524.

Schneeweiss, S. (2006). Sensitivity analysis and external adjustment for unmeasured confounders in epidemiologic database studies of therapeutics. *Pharmacoepidemiology and Drug Safety, 15*(5), 291–303.

Schneeweiss, S., Rassen, J. A., Glynn, R. J., Avorn, J., Mogun, H., & Brookhart, M. A. (2009). High-dimensional propensity score adjustment in studies of treatment effects using health care claims data. *Epidemiology, 20*(4), 512–522.

Schneeweiss, S., Solomon, D. H., Wang, P. S., Rassen, J., & Brookhart, M. A. (2006). Simultaneous assessment of short-term gastrointestinal benefits and cardiovascular risks of selective cyclooxygenase 2 inhibitors and nonselective nonsteroidal antiinflammatory drugs: An instrumental variable analysis. *Arthritis Rheumatism, 54*(11), 3390–3398.

Schuit, E., Groenwold, R. H., Harrell, F. E. Jr., de Kort, W. L., Kwee, A., Mol, B. W., et al. (2013). Unexpected predictor-outcome associations in clinical prediction research: Causes and solutions. *CMAJ, 185*(10), E499–E505.

Smith, G. D., Lawlor, D. A., Harbord, R., Timpson, N., Day, I., & Ebrahim, S. (2007). Clustered environments and randomized genes: A fundamental distinction between conventional and genetic epidemiology. *PLoS Medicine, 4,* e352.

Stürmer, T., Joshi, M., Glynn, R. J., Avorn, J., Rothman, K. J., & Schneeweiss, S. (2006). A review of the application of propensity score methods yielded increasing use, advantages in specific settings, but not substantially different estimates compared with conventional multivariable methods. *Journal of Clinical Epidemiology, 59*(5), 437–447.

Stürmer, T., Rothman, K. J., Avorn, J., & Glynn, R. J. (2010). Treatment effects in the presence of unmeasured confounding: Dealing with observations in the tails of the propensity score distribution—a simulation study. *American Journal of Epidemiology, 172*(7), 843–854.

Stürmer, T., Schneeweiss, S., Avorn, J., & Glynn, R. J. (2005). Adjusting effect estimates for unmeasured confounding with validation data using propensity score calibration. *American Journal of Epidemiology, 162*(3), 279–289.

Stürmer, T., Schneeweiss, S., Rothman, K. J., Avorn, J., & Glynn, R. J. (2007). Performance of propensity score calibration—a simulation study. *American Journal of Epidemiology, 165*(10), 1110–1118.

Swanson, S. A., & Hernán, M. A. (2013). Commentary: How to report instrumental variable analyses (suggestions welcome). *Epidemiology, 24*(3), 370–374.

Toh, S., García Rodríguez, L. A., & Hernán, M. A. (2011). Confounding adjustment via a semi-automated high-dimensional propensity score algorithm: An application to electronic medical records. *Pharmacoepidemiology and Drug Safety, 20*(8), 849–857.

Toh, S., García Rodríguez, L. A., & Hernán, M. A. (2012). Analyzing partially missing confounder information in comparative effectiveness and safety research of therapeutics. *Pharmacoepidemiology and Drug Safety, 21*(Suppl. 2), 13–20.

Vandenbroucke, J. P. (2004). When are observational studies as credible as randomised trials? *Lancet, 363*(9422), 1728–1731.

Weitzen, S., Lapane, K. L., Toledano, A. Y., Hume, A. L., & Mor, V. (2005). Weaknesses of goodness-of-fit tests for evaluating propensity score models: The case of the omitted confounder. *Pharmacoepidemiology and Drug Safety, 14*(4), 227–238.

Westreich, D., & Cole, S. R. (2010). Invited commentary: Positivity in practice. *American Journal of Epidemiology, 171*(6), 674–677.

Westreich, D., Cole, S. R., Funk, M. J., Brookhart, M. A., & Stürmer, T. (2011). The role of the $c$-statistic in variable selection for propensity score models. *Pharmacoepidemiology and Drug Safety, 20*(3), 317–320.

## CHAPTER 14

# Propensity-Score-Based Sensitivity Analysis

**Lingling Li
Changyu Shen
Xiaochun Li**

Propensity-score-based methods are popular in analysis of observational data to reduce bias and increase efficiency. The propensity score is the conditional probability of assignment to a certain treatment condition on given measured (or observed) covariates (Rosenbaum & Rubin, 1983b). Unlike in a randomized clinical trial in which treatment is randomly assigned with the propensity score fixed regardless of individual covariates, measured or unmeasured, treatment assignment in observational data is often influenced by covariates and possibly some unmeasured confounders as well. Consequently, a simple treatment effect estimate such as the difference in group means may be biased and can be to a large extent due to the differences in units' (e.g., subjects') characteristics between the two groups. The propensity score can be used to balance the covariates between the groups. Analogous to the use of randomization in a randomized clinical trial to balance covariates between groups, the distribution of covariates conditioning on the propensity score is the same across groups under *certain* assumptions (Rosenbaum & Rubin, 1983b).

One key assumption for valid propensity-score-based analysis is that there is no uncontrolled confounding. This assumption is not verifiable using observed data, and may be merely well-wishing in actual data analyses. Since the validity of study results hinges on this assumption, it is of great interest to examine the extent to which the study conclusion is sensitive to the violation of this assumption. Uncontrolled confounding remains a major concern for the validity of results from observational studies. Thus, evaluation of the impact of potential uncontrolled confounding is an important component of causal inference in observational studies. The initial idea of sensitivity analysis was proposed by Cornfield et al. (1959) in the context of the relation between smoking and lung cancer. Similar concepts were later discussed by Bross (Bross, 1966, 1967).

The general strategy in sensitivity analysis involves postulation of various assumptions on the nature of the associations of the unmeasured confounders with treatment assignment and outcomes, followed by examination of the bias induced (Lash, Fox, & Fink, 2009). Usually, these assumptions are in the format of plausible values of parameters not identifiable from the observed data that characterize those associations. Rosenbaum (2002) developed a logistic model in the randomization-based framework, where a single parameter measuring the strength of association between the unmeasured confounders and treatment assignment conditional on covariates already included is linked to a minimum and a maximum $p$-values of the inference. The $p$-values under different values of this parameter allow one to assess the sensitivity to uncontrolled confounding. Rosenbaum and Rubin (1983a) proposed an approach for binary outcome with one categorical covariate, where the sensitivity of the estimate to different values of nonestimable parameters (due to unmeasured confounders) in the full likelihood function was examined. The same authors also examined the bias due to incomplete matching (Rosenbaum & Rubin, 1985). Brumback, Hernan, Haneuse, and Robins (2004) developed an approach where the mean difference between treatment groups within each covariate stratum is used to examine the impact of residual confounding, which uses a similar type of strategy reported previously (Cole, Hernan, Margolick, Cohen, & Robins, 2005; Ko, Hogan, & Mayer, 2003; Robins, 1999a). Lin, Psaty, and Kronmal (1998) studied bias induced by uncontrolled confounding in the parametric regression setting. It was shown that under certain conditions there exists a simple algebraic relationship between the true effect and the "apparent" effect when there is uncontrolled confounding; see Hernan and Robins (1999) for more discussions. MacLehose, Kaufman, Kaufman, and Poole (2005) and Kuroki and Cai (2008) proposed linear programming methods to derive the upper and lower bounds for the causal effect on a binary outcome. Greenland (2005) developed a general Bayes framework to correct bias due to confounding, missing data, and classification error by including a bias model with relevant bias parameters. Other methods include Arah, Chiba, and Greenland (2008), Copas and Li (1997), Flanders and Khoury (1990),

Greenland and Neutra (1981), Imbens (2003), McCandless, Gustafson, and Levy (2008), Schlesselman (1978), and Sturmer, Schneeweiss, Rothman, Avorn, and Glynn (2007a, 2007b). Also, see Chapters 12 and 13 in this book for related discussions of missing data and unobserved confounding in propensity score analysis.

In this chapter, we introduce two sensitivity analysis approaches that were published before (Li, Shen, Wu, & Li, 2009; Shen, Li, Li, & Were, 2011). Some text, tables, and figures in this chapter were extracted from the published papers. Both methods are based on the inverse probability weighting estimator (Hernan, Brumback, & Robins, 2000; Robins, Hernan, & Brumback, 2000), but extend it to account for uncontrolled confounding from different perspectives. As a sensitivity analysis is about postulating various assumptions on the nature of the associations of the unmeasured confounders with treatment assignment and outcomes and such assumptions are not verifiable using observed data, these two approaches offer users greater flexibility in choosing the framework that suits their study best. Users can also use these two approaches to complement each other and conduct a more comprehensive sensitivity analysis.

In the next section, we first introduce the Lindner Center study, which is used as a real-life example to demonstrate the two sensitivity analysis approaches. Then, we introduce the inverse probability weighting approach, whose validity requires the absence of unmeasured confounders and is the base of the two sensitivity analysis approaches in this chapter, followed by two sections to explain (1) the sensitivity analysis Approach 1, which provides a general framework for sensitivity analysis of inference that supports both parametric and nonparametric modeling of the propensity score and (2) the sensitivity analysis Approach 2 which quantifies the hidden bias due to uncontrolled confounding using a one-dimensional sensitivity function that depends on the propensity score only. Although in answering a specific scientific question, there are issues of study design and analytical options, data sources, and model misspecifications where sensitivity analyses should also be addressed, they are beyond the length and scope of this chapter.

## THE LINDNER CENTER STUDY

Multiple placebo-controlled randomized trials had been conducted to demonstrate the unequivocal efficacy of platelet glycoprotein (GP) IIb/IIIa blockade administered during percutaneous coronary intervention (PCI) for reducing the risk of periprocedural ischemic events. However, results from clinical trials usually cannot be directly extrapolated to real-world settings due to the selected study populations and "protocol-driven" practice patterns.

To validate the clinical efficacy and cost effectiveness of these agents in real-world clinical practice settings, an observational study was conducted at The Christ Hospital, Cincinnati, Ohio, in 1997 to evaluate the impact of adjunctive pharmacotherapy with abciximab platelet GP IIb/IIIa blockade during PCI on costs and clinical outcomes in a high-book interventional practice (Kereiakes et al., 2000). We refer to this study as the Lindner Center study as it was primarily led by investigators and staff at the Carl and Edyth Lindner Center for Research and Education at The Christ Hospital. The Lindner Center dataset consists of observations on 996 patients who received an initial PCI at Ohio Heart Health Center of The Christ Hospital, in 1997 and were followed for at least 6 months. Among them, 698 of them were assigned to treatment with the abciximab platelet GP IIb/IIIa blockade, and the remaining 298 patients received usual-care-alone while undergoing their initial PCI.

In the Lindner Center study, confounding bias exists as the treatment was not assigned by a random mechanism. Alternatively, patients with worse baseline health status were more likely to be assigned to receive abciximab. In the original publication, the propensity score stratification method was used to adjust for confounding bias. The average reduction in mortality rate at 6 months after abciximab therapy increases from the crude 3.4 to 4.9% after the propensity score stratification adjustment.

Due to issues of data privacy and confidentiality, only a subset of the study data is included in the R package *twang* (Ridgeway, McCaffrey, & Morral, 2009) for public use. This dataset will be used in this chapter to illustrate two sensitivity analysis approaches.

In Table 14.1, we list the 10 variables that exist in the *twang* package and a standardized cost variable (std.cardbill), which we use as our outcome variable in the applications. Mean baseline characteristics, 6-month mortality after the patient's initial PCI, and medical cost during the 6 months after PCI are summarized by treatment, abciximab ($z=1$) or not ($z=0$), in Table 14.2.

From this simple summary, the two cohorts of patients do not appear to be readily comparable. The abciximab-treated patients seem to be in worse pretreatment cardiac-related conditions than the usual-care patients. For example, the proportion of patients who had acute myocardial infarction prior to PCI in the abciximab-treated cohort is three times that in the usual-care cohort. If we look at the outcomes numerically, the abciximab-treated cohort has a 6-month mortality rate 3% lower than the

**TABLE 14.1. List of Variables in the Lindner Center Data**

| Variable name | Definition |
|---|---|
| lifepres | Mean life years preserved due to survival for at least 6 months following PCI, 0 if died within 6 months, or 11.6 years otherwise |
| cardbill | Cardiac-related costs incurred within 6 months of patient's initial PCI |
| abcix | Treatment indicator: 1 for abciximab and 0 for usual-care-alone |
| stent | Coronary stent deployment: 1 for yes and 0 for no |
| height | Height in centimeters |
| female | 1 for female and 0 for male |
| diabetic | Diagnosis of diabetes mellitus: 1 for yes and 0 for no |
| acutemi | Acute myocardial infarction within the 7 days prior to PCI: 1 for yes and 0 for no |
| ejecfrac | The left ventricular ejection fraction |
| ves1proc | Number of vessels involved in the patient's initial PCI |
| Std.cardbill | $\log_{10}(cardbill)/\max(\log_{10}(cardbill))$ |

**TABLE 14.2. Summary of Lindner Data, Mean Values within Each Exposure Group**

| Variable name | Usual care | Abciximab | Variable name | Usual care | Abciximab |
|---|---|---|---|---|---|
| Height | 171.45 | 171.44 | Stent | 0.58 | 0.70 |
| Diabetic | 0.27 | 0.20 | Female | 0.39 | 0.33 |
| Ejecfrac | 52.29 | 50.40 | Acutemi | 0.06 | 0.18 |
| 6-month mortality[a] | 0.05 | 0.02 | Ves1proc | 1.20 | 1.46 |
| Cardbill | 14514.22 | 16126.68 | Std.cardbill | 0.78 | 0.79 |

[a]Six-month mortality is a recoded version of lifepres, that is, $I(\text{lifepres} = 0)$.

usual-care cohort, but with about $1,500 more cost. An obvious question is the cost and effectiveness of the treatment, after adjusting for the confounding factors.

## METHODS AND APPLICATIONS

In this section, we first introduce the inverse probability weighting estimator whose consistency requires the absence of uncontrolled confounding and is the base of the two sensitivity analysis approaches in this chapter. Then we introduce the two sensitivity analysis approaches and their applications to the Lindner Center study.

### The Inverse Probability Weighting Estimator in the Absence of Uncontrolled Confounding

Suppose we have $n$ i.i.d. copies of data, $\{(r_i, z_i, \mathbf{x}_i), i = 1, \ldots, n\}$, where $r_i$ denotes unit $i$'s observed outcome; $z_i$ the dichotomous treatment variable, with 1 for treatment and 0 for control; and $\mathbf{x}_i$, a vector of measured confounders, either continuous or discrete. We also define $r_{1i}$ and $r_{0i}$ as the potential outcome for treatment and control, respectively. We define the propensity score to be $e(\mathbf{x}_i) \equiv \text{PR}(z_i = 1|\mathbf{x}_i)$. The parameter of interest is the average treatment effect, $\psi = E[r_{1i}] - E[r_{0i}]$. Our results can be easily extended to other causal measures such as risk ratios and odds ratios for binary outcomes.

The inverse probability weighting approach has been well established to derive causal inference of $\psi$ in observational studies in the absence of uncontrolled confounding (Hernan et al., 2000; Robins et al., 2000). Its heuristic idea is to construct a pseudo-population consisting of $w_i = \left[ e(\mathbf{x}_i)^{z_i} \left(1 - e(\mathbf{x}_i)\right)^{1-z_i} \right]^{-1}$ copies of unit $i$'s data $(r_i, z_i, \mathbf{x}_i)$ to remove confounding. The weight equals the inverse of the propensity score for a treated unit and equals the inverse of (1 − propensity score) for a control unit. Propensity score is typically unknown and estimated via a logistic regression model. Let $\hat{e}(\mathbf{x}_i)$ and $\hat{w}_i \equiv \left[ \hat{e}(\mathbf{x}_i)^{z_i} \left(1 - \hat{e}(\mathbf{x}_i)\right)^{1-z_i} \right]^{-1}$ denote the estimated propensity score and the estimated weight for unit $i$, respectively; then the inverse probability weighting estimator of $\psi$ is defined as $\hat{\psi} \equiv \hat{\mu}_1 - \hat{\mu}_0$, where

$$\hat{\mu}_1 \equiv \left( \sum_{i=1}^{n} I(z_i = 1) \hat{w}_i \right)^{-1} \sum_{i=1}^{n} I(z_i = 1) \hat{w}_i r_i \qquad (14.1)$$

$$\hat{\mu}_0 \equiv \left(\sum_{i=1}^{n} I(z_i = 0)\hat{w}_i\right)^{-1} \sum_{i=1}^{n} I(z_i = 0)\hat{w}_i r_i \qquad (14.2)$$

An alternative definition is to replace the denominators in $\hat{\mu}_1$ and $\hat{\mu}_0$ with the sample size $n$. The two definitions are asymptotically equivalent. The idea of inverse probability weighting originates from survey sampling (Horvitz & Thompson, 1952), and has been further generalized to address many issues such as confounding bias in observational studies and missing data (Hernan et al., 2000; Robins et al., 2000; Robins, Rotnitzky, & Zhao, 1994, 1995). When there is no uncontrolled confounding, the potential outcomes are independent of the treatment variable given the measured covariates, that is, $(r_{1i}, r_{0i}) \coprod z_i | \mathbf{x}_i$, where $\coprod$ indicates independence in probability. As a direct consequence, the potential outcomes are also independent of $z_i$ given the propensity score, that is, $(r_{1i}, r_{0i}) \coprod z_i | e(\mathbf{x}_i)$ (Rosenbaum & Rubin, 1983b). Therefore,

$$E\left[\frac{rI(z=t)}{e(\mathbf{x})^t(1-e(\mathbf{x}))^{1-t}}\right] = E[r_t], \; t = 0, 1 \qquad (14.3)$$

Weighting removes the confounding bias introduced by a nonrandom treatment selection process. Under regularity conditions, it can be shown that $\hat{\psi}$ is a consistent estimator of $\psi$ as long as there is no uncontrolled confounding and $\hat{e}(\mathbf{x}_i)$ consistently estimates the true propensity score. But $\hat{\psi}$ is likely to be biased if there exist unmeasured confounders in addition to $\mathbf{x}_i$.

## Approach 1: A Feasible Region-Based Approach

### General Framework

To describe Approach 1 (Shen et al., 2011), we drop the subscript $i$ in all notations for simplicity. Equation 14.3 is the basis for unbiased estimation of the marginal mean of the outcome under each treatment and the causal effect using inverse probability weighting. When there is uncontrolled confounding, $r_t$ ($t = 0,1$) and $z$ are not independent conditional on $\mathbf{x}$. We assume that $r_t \perp z | \mathbf{x}, \mathbf{x}^*$ ($t = 0,1$), where $\mathbf{x}^*$ is a vector of covariates that are either not observed or not included in the analysis. Although $e(\mathbf{x})$ is still a conditional probability, it will not be equal to the true propensity score $e^*(\mathbf{x}, \mathbf{x}^*) = E(z | \mathbf{x}, \mathbf{x}^*)$ with probability 1. From now on, we call $e(\mathbf{x})$ the *pseudo-propensity score* to distinguish it from $e^*(\mathbf{x}, \mathbf{x}^*)$. The basic idea of our method is to develop bounds of the causal effect (or marginal means if those are of interest) by accounting for the error in using $e(\mathbf{x})$ to approximate $e^*(\mathbf{x}, \mathbf{x}^*)$. The bounds will allow us to assess the sensitivity of the result to uncontrolled confounding.

By $\varepsilon_1 = e^*/e (0 < \varepsilon_1 < \infty)$, we denote the multiplicative error of $e$ with respect to $e^*$. Here $\varepsilon_1$ is a measure of the quality of the pseudo-propensity score in approximating the true propensity score. The variance of $\varepsilon_1$ is a measure of the overall deviation of $e$ from $e^*$, with larger variance indicating more deviation. The relationship between $e$ and $e^*$ can be characterized by

$$e = E(e^* \mid e) \tag{14.4}$$

where the expectation is with respect to the distribution of $(\mathbf{x}, \mathbf{x}^*)$ within a pseudo-propensity score stratum with value $e$. To see this, note that

$$e = E(z \mid \mathbf{x}) = E[E(z \mid \mathbf{x}, \mathbf{x}^*) \mid \mathbf{x}] = E(e^* \mid \mathbf{x}) \Rightarrow E(e^* \mid e) = e \tag{14.5}$$

Equation 14.5 says that $e^*$ will center at $e$ within each stratum of $e$. It also implies, by the law of iterated expectation and decomposition of variance, that

$$\begin{aligned} E(\varepsilon_1) &= E\left(\frac{E(e^* \mid e)}{e}\right) = 1, \ \mathrm{Var}(\varepsilon_1) = \mathrm{Var}\left(\frac{E(e^* \mid e)}{e}\right) + E\left(\frac{\mathrm{Var}(e^* \mid e)}{e^2}\right) \\ &= E\left(\frac{\mathrm{Var}(e^* \mid e)}{e^2}\right) \end{aligned} \tag{14.6}$$

Since $e$ is not the true propensity score when there is uncontrolled confounding, the inverse probability weighting based on $e$ may be biased. As an example, consider the assessment of the magnitude of bias in estimating the mean of $r_1$. First, we observe that

$$\begin{aligned} E\left(\frac{rz}{e}\right) &= E\left(\frac{r_1 z}{e}\right) = E\left(E\left(\frac{r_1 z}{e} \mid (\mathbf{x}, \mathbf{x}^*, r_1)\right)\right) = E\left(\frac{r_1 E(z \mid \mathbf{x}, \mathbf{x}^*, r_1)}{e}\right) \\ &= E\left(\frac{r_1 e^*}{e}\right) = E(r_1 \varepsilon_1) \end{aligned} \tag{14.7}$$

where the fourth equality is due to the independence of $z$ and $r_1$ conditional on $(\mathbf{x}, \mathbf{x}^*)$. Then we have

$$E\left(\frac{rz}{e}\right) - E(r_1) = E(r_1 \varepsilon_1) - E(\varepsilon_1) E(r_1) = \rho_1 [\mathrm{Var}(r_1) \mathrm{Var}(\varepsilon_1)]^{1/2} \tag{14.8}$$

Here $\rho_1$ is the correlation coefficient between $r_1$ and $\varepsilon_1$. Equation 14.8 represents the key idea of our method. It says that the bias of $rz/e$ in estimating $E(r_1)$ is governed by two nonestimable quantities in addition to the variance of $r_1$ (also nonestimable), the correlation between the multiplicative error $\varepsilon_1$ in propensity score due to unmeasured confounders and the potential outcome $r_1$, and the variance of $\varepsilon_1$. The first quantity, in some sense, characterizes the strength of the association between the unmeasured confounders and the potential outcome. It can be interpreted as a measure that captures the concordance between the outcome value and the amount of extra weight assigned to the outcome value due to unmeasured confounders. The second quantity, as seen later in the parametric model, characterizes the strength of the association between the unmeasured confounders and the treatment assignment. Stronger correlation and higher variation in $\varepsilon_1$ will lead to higher bias. Intuitively, since higher $\varepsilon_1$ means that $e$ severely underestimates $e^*$, a positive correlation implies that higher $r_1$ values are overduplicated, whereas lower $r_1$ values are underduplicated in the pseudo-population. Therefore, the inverse probability weighting estimator based on $e$ overestimates $E(r_1)$. Similarly, a negative correlation implies an underestimate of $E(r_1)$. On the other hand, the variance of $\varepsilon_1$ characterizes the quality of $e$, and higher value of the variance indicates more severe deviation from $e^*$ and therefore more bias in estimating $E(r_1)$.

## Continuous Outcome

To derive the bounds for marginal means and the causal effect, we will assume that $r_1, r_0 \in [0,1]$. As in most practical problems, continuous outcomes can be monotonically transformed to the unit interval based on conservative estimates of the range of the outcomes, this assumption has quite general applicability. It can be shown that

$$\rho_1^2 v_1 \psi [E(r_1)(E(r_1) - 2\mu_1) + d] \leq (E(rz/e) - E(r_1))^2$$
$$\leq \rho_1^2 v_1 [E(r_1)(1 - E(r_1)) - b] \quad (14.9)$$

where $\mu_1 = E(r_1|z=1)$, $v_1 = \text{Var}(\varepsilon_1)$, $\psi = E(z)/(1-E(z))$, $b = E(z)(E(r_1|z=1) - E(r_1^2|z=1))$, and $d = E(z)[E(r_1|z=1)]^2 + (1-E(z))E(r_1^2|z=1)$. Equation 14.9 defines two intervals for $E(r_1)$, one for positive $\rho_1$ and one for negative $\rho_1$. We will call the interval that corresponds to the intended sign of $\rho_1$ the *feasible region* of $E(r_1)$. Note that the only parameters involved in defining the limits of the intervals that are not directly estimable are $\rho_1$ and $v_1$. In Figure 14.1, we illustrate the idea through a geometric demonstration.

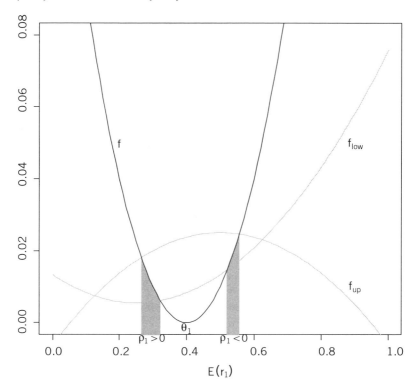

**FIGURE 14.1.** Illustration of the feasible regions of $E(r_1)$ defined by Equation 14.9. $f_{low}$, $f$, and $f_{up}$ can be viewed as three functions of $E(r_1)$ that correspond to the three terms in Equation 14.9: $\rho_1^2 v_1 \psi [E(r_1)(E(r_1) - 2\mu_1) + d]$, $f = (\theta_1 - E(r_1))^2$, and $f_{up} = \rho_1^2 v_1 [E(r_1)(1 - E(r_1)) - b]$. The two intervals on X-axis under the gray regions correspond to the feasible regions under $\rho_1 > 0$ and $\rho_1 < 0$, respectively. Here, $\theta_1 = E(rz/e) = 0.4$, $|\rho_1| = 0.5$, $v_1 = 0.5$, $\mu_1 = 0.25$, $\psi = 1$, $b = 0.05$, and $d = 0.10625$. From Shen, Li, Li, and Were (2011). Reprinted with permission from the authors.

Essentially, Figure 14.1 shows that the *feasible region* for $E(r_1)$ is determined by the positions and shapes of three second-order polynomials. The distances between $E(rz|e)$ and the two shaded regions on the X-axis represent possible magnitude of bias depending on the sign of $\rho_1$. The width of the interval originates from uncertainty on the relationship between $E(r_1)$ and $\text{Var}(r_1)$. For any given $(\rho_1, v_1)$, one can solve equations in Equation 14.9 to obtain the lower $(l_1)$ and upper $(L_1)$ limits of the interval. These limits set the boundaries for $E(r_1)$ after adjusting for the error in estimating the propensity score $(v_1)$ and its correlation with the potential outcome $(\rho_1, v_1)$. By examining $l_1$ and $L_1$ under different values of $(\rho_1, v_1)$, one can gain insight into the robustness of the estimate of $E(r_1)$. The same type of bounds $l_0$ and $L_0$ can also be derived for $E(r_0)$ for a fixed pair of $(\rho_0, v_0)$, where $v_0$ is the variance of $\varepsilon_0 = (1 - e^*)/(1 - e)$ and $\rho_0$ is the correlation coefficient of $r_0$ and $\varepsilon_0$.

## Binary Outcome

It can be shown that

$$(E(rz/e) - E(r_1))^2 = \rho_1^2 v_1 E(r_1)(1 - E(r_1)) \tag{14.10}$$

For any fixed $(\rho_1, v_1)$ the region defined by Equation 14.10, if it exists, is a point. Therefore, $l_1 = L_1$. Similarly, $l_0 = L_0$.

## Bounds for Average Treatment Effect

It is obvious that $l_1 - L_0$ and $L_1 - l_0$ are a set of lower and upper bounds for the causal effect. To assess the sensitivity of the pseudo-propensity score to uncontrolled confounding, one needs to specify $(\rho_1, v_1)$ and $(\rho_0, v_0)$. As the correlation coefficient is a popular and sensible measure to most users, the variance of the error term might not be sensible enough to be specified easily. Since a random variable taking values in the unit interval with mean $\mu$ has the maximum variance of $\mu(1 - \mu)$, we have

$$v_1 = \mathrm{Var}(\varepsilon_1) = E\left(\frac{\mathrm{Var}(e^* \mid e)}{e^2}\right) \leq E\left(\frac{e(1-e)}{e^2}\right) = E\left(\frac{1-e}{e}\right) = V_1 \tag{14.11}$$

Therefore, instead of proposing a value of $v_1$, we can postulate the percentage of the maximum possible variance $\lambda_1 = v_1/V_1$. Similarly, we can propose $\lambda_0 = v_0/V_0$, where $V_0 = E[e/(1 - e)]$.

In practice, a propensity score model is first fitted to the data and the estimated propensity score will play the role of pseudo propensity score. The lower and upper limits are then derived using parameters from the empirical distributions. It often provides sufficient insight into the robustness of the result by setting $|\rho_1| = |\rho_0| = \rho$ and $\lambda_1 = \lambda_0 = \lambda$ (as long as $\lambda_1$ and $\lambda_0$ are compatible, see next session) so that one needs only to assess the sensitivity of the estimates by examining various values of $(\rho, \lambda)$. Nevertheless, one will still need to decide on the signs of $\rho_1$ and $\rho_0$, which can often be chosen to work against the finding of the original analysis to examine the robustness. Inference can also be made on the limits. For instance, if a positive treatment effect is found (i.e., treatment has higher outcome value), one would be interested in testing $H_0: l_1 - L_0 \leq 0$ versus $H_1: l_1 - L_0 > 0$ under certain values of $(\rho, \lambda)$. Rejection of the null will increase the confidence of the finding.

## Compatibility of $\lambda_1$ and $\lambda_0$

Certain values of $\lambda_1$ and $\lambda_0$ may not be compatible due to their connection through the distribution of $e$ and $\text{Var}(e^*|e)$. The following result establishes the range of compatible $\lambda_0$ for a fixed $\lambda_1$.

## Results

For a fixed $\lambda_1$, $E[I(e \leq q_1)e/(1-e)]/V_0 \leq \lambda_0 \leq E[I(e \leq q_2)e/(1-e)]/V_0$, where $q_1$ and $q_2$ satisfy $E[I(e \leq q_1)(1-e)/e] = E[I(e \geq q_2)(1-e)/e] = v_1 = \lambda_1 V_1$. Note that both bounds of $\lambda_0$ are estimable from the observed data given $\lambda_1$.

## A Parametric Model

In this section, we introduce a parametric model that provides a more mechanistic view on how the uncontrolled confounding introduces bias in the inference and therefore provides some guidance on the scale of $\lambda$.

Considering the following probit model as the true propensity score model:

$$e = \Pr(z = 1 | \mathbf{x}, \mathbf{x}^*) = \Phi(w(\mathbf{x}) + \tau u(\mathbf{x}^*)) \tag{14.12}$$

Here $\Phi$ is the cumulative distribution function of a standard normal variable. Equation 14.12 states that the contribution of $\mathbf{x}$ and $\mathbf{x}^*$ to $\Phi^{-1}(e^*)$ is additive. We will assume that $u$ is a standard normal variable and independent of $\mathbf{x}$, and $\tau$ is a measure of the strength of association between the unmeasured confounders and treatment assignment after adjustment of $w(\mathbf{x})$. In Table 14.3, we show the odds ratios of being treated associated with one interquartile range (IQR) increase in $u$ for different values of $\tau$. Note that because the odds ratio depends on the value of $w$ (and therefore $e^*$), we list the range of the odds ratios for $e^*$ between 0.1 and 0.9.

It is well known that integrating out $u$ leads to

$$e = \Pr(z = 1 | \mathbf{x}) = \Phi\left(\frac{w(\mathbf{x})}{\sqrt{1+\tau^2}}\right) \tag{14.13}$$

TABLE 14.3. Odds Ratio Ranges Associated with One Interquartile Range Increase in u for e* Ranging from 0.1 to 0.9

| $\tau$ | OR Range[a] |
|---|---|
| 0.1 | 1.24–1.31 |
| 0.2 | 1.54–1.73 |
| 0.3 | 1.91–2.31 |
| 0.4 | 2.37–3.13 |
| 0.5 | 2.95–4.29 |
| 0.6 | 3.68–5.97 |
| 0.7 | 4.58–8.43 |

[a]The first number corresponds to the OR at $e^* = 0.1$, and the second number corresponds to the OR at $e^* = 0.1$.

Thus, the pseudo-propensity score is still a probit model. This means although we miss $u$, the probit model remains the correct model for $E[z|\mathbf{x}]$. In addition, it can be shown that

$$\mathrm{Var}_\tau(e^*|e) = F_\tau\left(\sqrt{1+\tau^2}\Phi^{-1}(e), \sqrt{1+\tau^2}\Phi^{-1}(e)\right) - e^2 \qquad (14.14)$$

where $F_\tau(\cdot,\cdot)$ is the cumulative distribution function of a bivariate normal vector, with both variables having mean 0 and variance $1 + \tau^2$, and a covariance of $\tau^2$. $\mathrm{Var}_\tau(e^*|e)$ is a monotonically increasing function of $\tau$ for fixed $e$. It has the limit of $e(1 - e)$ as $\tau$ goes to infinity. Thus, the stronger is the association between the unmeasured confounders with the treatment assignment, the higher is the conditional variance of the true propensity score within each pseudo-propensity score stratum. Since $\lambda_1 = E(\mathrm{Var}(e^*|e)/e^2)/V_1$ and $\lambda_0 = E(\mathrm{Var}(e^*|e)/(1-e)^2/V_0$, both parameters are functions of $\tau$. Thus, instead of specifying the lambda values, we only need to specify $\tau$ in the sensitivity analysis, provided we are willing to accept the parametric model 14.12. If we do not want to impose a parametric model, then the properties of the model 14.12 can still guide us on the choice of $\lambda$. For example, starting from a fixed $\tau$, we can consider the following value of $\lambda$ and the conditional variance of $e^*$ given $e$:

$$\lambda(\tau) = \mathrm{Max}_e\left(\frac{\mathrm{Var}_\tau(e^*|e)}{e(1-e)}\right) = \left(\frac{\mathrm{Var}_\tau(e^*|e)}{e(1-e)}\right)_{e=0.5} = 4F_\tau(0,0) - 1 \qquad (14.15)$$
$$\mathrm{Var}_\lambda(e^*|e) = \lambda e(1-e)$$

Therefore, $\lambda$ is the maximum proportion of $\text{Var}_r(e^*|e)$ relative to the maximum conditional variance of $e^*$ across all $e$. $\lambda$ is more conservative than $\tau$ in the sense that $\text{Var}_\lambda(e^*|e)$ is always higher than $\text{Var}_r(e^*|e)$ for all $e$, suggesting a more severe impact of the unmeasured confounders on the probability of treatment assignment.

## Application to the Lindner Center Study

We focus on the standardized cost as our outcome of interest to illustrate how our method can be used to analyze a continuous outcome. We first did a logarithm transformation of the original cost variable, and then we divided the transformed variable by its maximum to keep it bounded below 1. There are a total of 996 patients, among whom 698 received abciximab and 298 did not. A two-sample $t$-test shows that the intervention group had significantly higher cost than the control group (0.792 vs. 0.777, $t$-test $p < .0001$, two sided). To account for potential confounders, we fit a probit propensity score model that includes coronary stent deployment (Yes/No), acute myocardial infarction within seven days prior to PCI (Yes/No), diagnosis of diabetes mellitus (Yes/No), and the left ventricular ejection fraction (continuous). These factors univariately correlate with at least one of the two measures: cost or abciximab usage. The inverse propensity score weighting leads to an estimate of the treatment effect of 0.024 (Z-test, $p < .0001$, two sided), suggesting again an increase in cost in the intervention group after adjustment.

To investigate potential uncontrolled confounding, we conducted a similar sensitivity analysis. Since the outcome is continuous, the sensitivity analysis will generate estimates of the lower and upper bounds. For this example, it was the lower bound of the causal effect that is of our interest as a positive treatment effect was found. The result is shown in Figure 14.2. Clearly, the positive intervention effect is sensitive to uncontrolled confounding. For the estimate of the lower bound of the intervention effect to go below 0, $\rho$ only needs to be a bit over 0.1 when $\tau = 0.4$ for both $\text{Var}_r(e^*|e)$ and $\text{Var}_\lambda(e^*|e)$ based analyses. Similarly, for $\tau = 0.2$, the estimate of the lower bound of the intervention effect goes below 0 when $\rho > .25$ regardless of the method used. The lower limit of the 90% confidence interval (one sided) of the lower bound for $\tau = 0.3$ shows that as $\rho > .11$ the confidence intervals will contain 0. Hence, the sensitivity analysis suggests that the significant intervention effect could have been induced by mild confounding. If we fix $\lambda_1$ at 0.0063, 0.0245, 0.0526, and 0.0881, the compatible regions of $\lambda_0$ are (0.0001, 0.32), (0.0009, 0.48), (0.003, 0.57), and (0.005, 0.64). Therefore, the common values are legitimate.

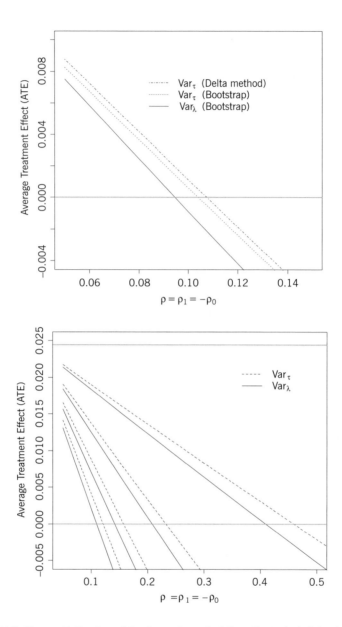

**FIGURE 14.2.** Upper: Estimates of the lower bound of the effect of abciximab on cost under different combinations of $\rho = \rho_1 = -\rho_0$ and $\tau$. Dashed lines are the estimates of the ATE based on $\text{Var}_\tau(e^* \mid e)$ (Equation 14.9), and solid lines are the ATE based on $\text{Var}_\lambda(e^* \mid e)$ (Equation 14.10). The four dashed lines correspond to (from top to bottom) $\tau = 0.1, 0.2, 0.3$, and $0.4$. The four solid lines correspond to (from top to bottom), $\lambda(0.1) = 0.0063$, $\lambda(0.2) = 0.0245$, $\lambda(0.3) = 0.0526$, and $\lambda(0.4) = 0.0881$. The horizontal gray line on the top is the estimated ATE assuming no uncontrolled confounding. Lower: The lower limit of the one-sided 90% confidence interval of the lower bound of the intervention effect for $\tau = 0.3$ for different values of $\rho = \rho_1 = -\rho_0$. From Shen, Li, Li, and Were (2011). Reprinted with permission from the authors.

In fact, we intentionally ignored a covariate in our probit model for the pseudo-propensity score: the number of vessels involved in the patient's initial PCI. Univariate analysis shows that this variable is correlated with both treatment assignment and the cost. When included in the probit model after normalization, $\hat{\tau} = 0.29$ (Wald test, $p < .0001$, two-sided). Therefore, this variable may be a potential confounder that induces the "treatment effect." The sensitivity analysis shows that when $\hat{\tau} = 0.3$, a weak correlation $\rho_1 = -\rho_0 > 0.11$ could be responsible for the "significant" increase in cost. In fact, when we use the propensity score obtained from the revised probit model with the number of vessels added, the intervention effect is not significant ($-0.0019$, Z-test, $p = 0.91$, two-sided).

## Approach 2: A Sensitivity-Function-Based Sensitivity Analysis Approach

In this section, we introduce an alternative sensitivity analysis approach (Li et al., 2009) that uses a propensity-score-based sensitivity function (SF) to quantify the hidden bias due to unmeasured confounders.

### Sensitivity Function

In the presence of uncontrolled confounding, $(r_{1i}, r_{0i})$ is likely to be correlated with the treatment variable $z$ conditional on $e(\mathbf{x}_i)$. Thus, we cannot obtain a valid estimate of the causal effect by directly comparing the outcome means between the two treatment groups in the weighted pseudo-population. To address this issue, we propose a SF defined below to quantify the hidden bias:

$$c(t, e) = E[r_t | z = 1, e(\mathbf{x}) = e] - E[r_t | z = 0, e(\mathbf{x}) = e] \qquad (14.16)$$

For $t \in \{0, 1\}$ and $0 < e < 1$. That is, for the subpopulation with the same $e(\mathbf{x}) = e$, $c(t, e)$ is the mean difference for the potential outcome $r_t$ between the treated ($z = 1$) and untreated ($z = 0$) groups. In other words, $c(t, e)$ quantitatively measures the impact of unmeasured confounders on the difference in potential outcomes between the treated and untreated units conditional on $e(\mathbf{x})$, the propensity score of measured covariates. The range of the SF $c(t, e)$ reflects the magnitude of uncontrolled confounding bias. Under the assumption of no uncontrolled confounding, $c(t, e) = 0$ for any value of $(t, e)$.

Our sensitivity analysis method was developed along the lines of the work by Robins (1999a, 1999b) and Brumback et al. (2004), in which the uncontrolled confounding is quantified using the between-group difference conditional on the values of all measured confounders, that is, $c^*(t, \mathbf{x}) = E[r_t|z = 1, \mathbf{x}] - E[r_t|z = 0, \mathbf{x}]$. On the web, in the appendix of our paper (Li et al., 2009), we proved that $c(t, e) = E[c^*(t, \mathbf{x})|e(\mathbf{x}) = e]$. Therefore, if $c^*(t, \mathbf{x})$ is constant, $c(t, e) = c^*(t, \mathbf{x})$, and both methods are the same. Nonetheless, when $\mathbf{x}$ is a high-dimensional vector, our approach is much easier to implement because our SF depends only on a single random variable $e(\mathbf{x})$, a one-dimensional summary of $\mathbf{x}$, instead of a high-dimensional vector. Note that in performing a sensitivity analysis, an analyst needs to specify not only the functional form of the SF but also the values of the coefficients. For instance, $c^*(t, \mathbf{x})$ equals $\beta_1 \times$ age $+ \beta_1 \times$ race where $\beta_1 = 0.2$ and $\beta_2 = 0.1$. When $c^*(t, \mathbf{x})$ depends on multiple confounders, such specifications will be difficult, and the imposed working functional form is unlikely to accurately reflect the complex relationships between the measured and unmeasured confounders and the potential outcomes. Furthermore, since we cannot empirically verify the imposed assumptions using the observed data, it is a common practice to vary these assumptions in sensitivity analysis to evaluate the corresponding causal estimates. When $c^*(t, \mathbf{x})$ depends on multiple coefficients, it will be technically difficult to do so as we would need to vary many coefficients in $c^*(t, \mathbf{x})$ simultaneously.

Our approach nicely reduces the dimension of the SF and makes it much easier to vary sensitivity assumptions to explore plausible scenarios. In practice, the specified SF is likely to be incorrect. Nonetheless, since the new SF is one-dimensional, low-order polynomials (e.g., linear, quadratic) should be able to provide reasonable approximations as long as the true SF $c(t, e)$ is continuous with respect to $e$ in interval $[0, 1]$ (Rudin, 1973, 1976). We suggest conducting a sensitivity analysis with constant, linear, or quadratic SFs with the coefficients varying over a set of plausible values, which should be selected based on the observed data, literature, and subject matter knowledge specific to the application setting. For instance, suppose the outcome of interest is death and the treated units are relatively sicker than the untreated, then before conducting sensitivity analysis, we need to understand how different the treated and untreated groups are after controlling for measured confounders. Suppose we expect an average 5 ~ 10% excess risk for the treated units compared to the untreated units even if, contrary to fact, they were given the same treatment. We would vary $c(t, e)$ between 0.05 and 0.1 when considering a constant SF. If we expect the amount of hidden bias to vary approximately linearly across levels of $e(\mathbf{x})$, we would use a linear SF. Since $e \in (0, 1)$, we would select the intercept and slope of the linear SF based on likely values of excess risks for those with very large or very small propensity scores. For instance, $c(t, e) = 0.05$

+ 0.05$e$ if we expect $c(t, e)$ to increase with $e$ or $c(t, e) = 0.1 - 0.05e$ if we expect $c(t, e)$ to decrease with $e$. Later, we provide more specific illustrations and instructions in the context of the Lindner Center study example.

## SF-Corrected Inverse Probability Weighting Estimators

Given a SF $c(t, e)$, we construct the SF-corrected inverse probability weighting estimators by replacing the observed outcome $r$ in the original estimator $\hat{\psi}$ with the SF-corrected outcomes

$$r^{SF} \equiv r - (E[r_z|z, e(\mathbf{x})] - E[r_z|e(\mathbf{x})]) \\ = \begin{cases} r - (1 - e(\mathbf{x}))c(1, e) & \text{if } z = 1 \\ r + e(\mathbf{x})c(0, e) & \text{if } z = 0 \end{cases} \quad (14.17)$$

Then, $\hat{\psi}^{SF} \equiv \hat{\mu}_1^{SF} - \hat{\mu}_0^{SF}$, where, for $t = 0, 1$,

$$\hat{\mu}_t^{SF} \equiv \left( \sum_{i=1}^n I(z_i = t)\hat{w}_i \right)^{-1} \sum_{i=1}^n I(z_i = t)\hat{w}_i r_i^{SF} \quad (14.18)$$

We proved the consistency of $\hat{\psi}^{SF}$, on the web, in the appendix of our paper (Li et al., 2009). The intuitive idea is straightforward that we simply remove the hidden bias in the pseudo-population by applying the SF to the observed outcome. Then the causal effect can be consistently estimated by the between-group difference of the means of the SF-corrected outcomes.

Note that for noncontinuous outcomes (e.g., binary outcomes), instead of using an additive SF defined above, we may use a multiplicative SF $c(t, e) \equiv \log[E[r_z|z = 1, e(\mathbf{x})]/E[r_z|z = 0, e(\mathbf{x})]]$ and remove residual bias by defining $r^{SF} \equiv r E[r_z|e(\mathbf{x})]/E[r_z|z,e(\mathbf{x})]$, which equals $r \times [e(\mathbf{x}) + \exp(-c(1, e(\mathbf{x}))) \times (1 - e(\mathbf{x}))]$ if $z = 1$ and $r[1 - e(\mathbf{x}) + \exp(c(0, e(\mathbf{x}))e(\mathbf{x})]$ if $z = 0$. Then it can be easily shown that $E[r^{SF}|z = t, \mathbf{x}] = E[r_t|e(\mathbf{x})]$. In addition, $r^{SF}$ is guaranteed to be positive. Nonetheless, with binary outcomes, the estimates of the marginal means $\hat{\mu}_1^{SF}$ and $\hat{\mu}_0^{SF}$ may still be outside the plausible range [0, 1]. This in turn guides analysts in the selection of sensible parameters in the SF. Otherwise, multiplicative SFs can be implemented in exactly the same manner.

To appropriately account for the variation in the estimated propensity scores and the IPW estimator, we estimate the variance of $\hat{\psi}^{SF}$ via a nonparametric bootstrap method (Cole & Hernan, 2008; Efron & Tibshirani, 1997) and construct the 95% CI using the 2.5% and 97.5% percentiles from the bootstrap samples.

## Application to the Lindner Center Study

We implemented the SF-based sensitivity analysis approach (Approach 2) on the Lindner Center study data to illustrate its use. In this application, we address a different question from the question we addressed in the application of Approach 1. Specifically, we adjust for all measured covariates, including the number of vessels involved in the patient's initial PCI procedure (ves1proc), and assess how the results vary with any possible residual confounding bias.

We estimated the propensity scores via a logistic regression model including all measured covariates. After adjusting for the estimated propensity scores via propensity score quintile stratification, the marginal distributions for the measured baseline covariates are balanced between the two treatment groups without significant difference. Even though we used the logistic link here instead of the probit link for Approach 1, the estimated propensity scores are almost identical. We use the parametric regression models in this application because the number of covariates is relatively small and the imposed regression model appears to be reasonable as covariate balance is greatly improved with propensity score adjustment. A parametric propensity score model has the advantage of providing an analytic form for the relationship between the treatment variable and the covariates. However, if the number of covariates is large and the propensity score functional form appears to be complex, we recommend using the generalized boosted models, a nonparametric, data-adaptive approach, to estimate propensity scores (McCaffrey, Ridgeway, & Morral, 2004; Ridgeway & McCaffrey, 2007).

The patients thought to have more severe disease status were assigned to the intervention group. The crude mean difference for the standardized cost equals 0.015 (95% CI [0.010, 0.020]) and the inverse probability weighting-adjusted mean difference equals 0.009 (95% CI [0.001, 0.016]), adjusting for all measured covariates. We conducted 2000 bootstrap replications to calculate the 95% CIs.

In the sensitivity analysis, we consider constant, linear, and quadratic SFs. Our sensitivity assumptions in this application are made based on observed data, literature, and subject matter knowledge for this specific application, and may not apply to other settings.

## Constant SF

We first consider $c(t, e) = c_t$ for $t \in \{0, 1\}$. Since we expect the intervention group to have more severe disease status even after controlling for measured covariates, we expect $c_0$ and $c_1$ to be non-negative constants as the sicker patients in the intervention group ($z = 1$) are expected to have a higher cost than the less sick control group ($z = 0$) even if, contrary to fact, they received the same treatment. We do not expect the difference in the mean potential cost with the abciximab-augmented care ($r_1$) between the two groups to be greater than the observed crude difference when the two groups did receive different care, therefore we vary the value of $c_1$ in the range of [0, 0.015]. We allow the possibility that $c_0$ is greater than $c_1$, that is, the uncontrolled confounding has a bigger impact on the potential outcome for usual care alone ($r_0$) than on the potential outcome for abciximab ($r_1$).

Let $d = c_0/c_1$ indicate the ratio between the two constant SFs. In Figure 14.3, we present four plots for $d$ that equal 1.0, 1.2, 1.5, and 2, respectively. The solid lines indicate the point estimates of the mean difference, while the dotted lines indicate the lower and upper limits for the 95% CIs. The horizontal line represents the null value of 0.

As expected, the mean difference estimates decrease when either $c_1$ or $d$ increases. This is intuitively plausible because the more the uncontrolled

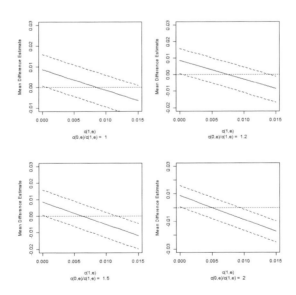

**FIGURE 14.3.** Point (solid line) and Interval Estimates (dotted lines) of mean difference on standardized cost between abciximab and usual care among patients who received an initial percutaneous coronary intervention. We assume constant SFs that $c(1,e) = c_1$ and $c(0,e) = d \times c_1$. We vary the value of $c_1$ between 0.000 and 0.015 and the value of $d = c(0,e)/c(1,e)$ in (1.0, 1.2, 1.5, 2.0). The CIs were obtained using the 2.5% and 97.5% percentiles among the 2,000 bootstrap replications.

confounding is assumed to exist, the further the SF-corrected estimator decreases as we attribute an increasing proportion of the observed difference to the effect of uncontrolled confounding. Under the assumption of no unmeasured confounder, inverse probability weighting-adjusted mean difference equals 0.009 (95% CI [0.001, 0.016]). Let's first examine the plot on the upper left corner with $d = 1$ (i.e., $c(t = 1, e) = c(t = 0, e) = c_1$). The 95% CI became insignificant with a very small amount of residual confounding bias, as the 95% CI with $c_1 = 0.002$ includes the null value of zero. The 95% CI remained statistically insignificant within the considered range of $c_0 = c_1 \leq 0.015$. In other plots with higher $d$ values, the 95% CI may become significant with fairly large $c_1$ and $c_0$ values (e.g., $c_1 = 0.015$ and $c_0 = 0.0225$). We cannot rule out the possibility that $c_0$ is greater than the observed crude difference as the intervention group may incur a much higher cost if they, contrary to fact, received the usual care which is suboptimal for them and caused them to suffer a much slower and prolonged recovery process. But such values are likely to occur only under extreme scenarios.

### Linear and Quadratic Sensitivity Functions

We also consider a linear SF $c(t, e) = c_t + s_t e$, that is, the effect of uncontrolled confounding changes linearly with the propensity score. In this example we expect the magnitude of residual confounding to increase with the propensity score (i.e., $s_t$ is positive) since patients with higher propensity scores are expected to be sicker at baseline. In this application, propensity score is in the range of [0.2, 1.0]; thus, $c_t + 0.2s_t$ and $c_t + s_t$ indicate the lower and upper bounds of $c(t, e)$, respectively.

In Table 14.4, we present the results for a set of scenarios in which the lower bound $(c_1 + 0.2s_1)$ varies between 0 and 0.02 and the upper bound $(c_1 + s_1)$ varies between 0 and $0.02 - (c_1 + 0.2s_1)$. We consider three possible values (i.e., 1.0, 1.5, 2.0) for the ratio $d = c(0, e)/c(1, e)$. The numbers presented in Table 14.4 suggest that the results are similar to those in Figure 14.3. The point and interval estimates of the mean difference keep decreasing when $c_1$, $s_1$, or $d$ increases. The more the uncontrolled confounding is assumed to exist, the smaller the mean difference estimates are. The 95% CI became insignificant with a small amount of residual bias, and the CI became significant, again indicating a negative mean difference only under extreme scenarios.

To evaluate the effect of violations of linear structures, we further consider the quadratic SF $c(t, e) = a_t + b_t e + q_t e^2$. For each linear structure $c^l(t, e) = c_t + s_t e$, we consider two quadratic SF functions $c_1^q(t, e)$ and $c_2^q(t, e)$ such that $c_1^q(t, e = 0.2) = c_2^q(t, e = 0.2) = c^l(t, e = 0.2)$, $c_1^q(t, e = 1) = c_2^q(t, e = 1) =$

**TABLE 14.4. Point and Interval Estimates of Mean Difference on Standardized Cost between Abciximab and Usual Care among Patients Who Received an Initial Percutaneous Coronary Intervention, with Linear SFs**

| | | $d = 1.0$ | | $d = 1.5$ | | $d = 2.0$ | |
|---|---|---|---|---|---|---|---|
| $c_1 + 0.2s_1$ | $c_1 + s_1$ | $\hat{\psi}^{SF}$ | 95% CI | $\hat{\psi}^{SF}$ | 95% CI | $\hat{\psi}^{SF}$ | 95% CI |
| 0.00 | 0.000 | .009 | (.001, .016) | .009 | (.001, .016) | .009 | (.001, .016) |
| | 0.005 | .005 | (−.003, .013) | .004 | (−.004, .012) | .003 | (−.005, .011) |
| | 0.010 | .002 | (−.006, .010) | .000 | (−.009, .007) | −.003 | (−.011, .005) |
| | 0.015 | −.001 | (−.009, .006) | −.005 | (−.013, .003) | −.009 | (−.017, .001) |
| | 0.020 | −.005 | (−.013, .003) | −.010 | (−.018, −.002) | −.014 | (−.023, −.006) |
| 0.005 | 0.000 | .007 | (−.000, .015) | .007 | (−.001, .015) | .007 | (−.001, .014) |
| | 0.005 | .004 | (−.004, .012) | .003 | (−.005, .010) | .001 | (−.007, .009) |
| | 0.010 | .001 | (−.007, .008) | −.002 | (−.010, .006) | −.005 | (−.013, .003) |
| | 0.015 | −.003 | (−.011, .005) | −.007 | (−.015, .001) | −.011 | (−.019, −.003) |
| 0.010 | 0.000 | .006 | (−.001, .014) | .006 | (−.002, .013) | .005 | (−.003, .012) |
| | 0.005 | .003 | (−.005, .011) | .001 | (−.007, .009) | −.001 | (−.009, .007) |
| | 0.010 | .000 | (−.008, .007) | −.004 | (−.011, .004) | −.007 | (−.015, .001) |
| 0.015 | 0.000 | .005 | (−.003, .013) | .004 | (−.004, .012) | .003 | (−.005, .011) |
| | 0.005 | .002 | (−.006, .009) | .000 | (−.008, .007) | −.003 | (−.010, .005) |
| 0.020 | 0.000 | .004 | (−.004, .012) | .003 | (−.005, .010) | .001 | (−.006, .009) |

*Note.* We assume the SF follows a linear structure such that $c(t = 1, e) = c_1 + s_1 e$ and $c(t = 0, e) = c_1 \times c(t = 0, e)$. The CIs were obtained using the 2.5% and 97.5% percentiles from 2,000 bootstrap samples.

$c^l(t, e = 1)$, $c_1^q(t, e = 0.6) = c^l\, t, e = 0.2) + 1/4(c^l(t, e = 1) - c^l\, t, e = 0.2))$, $c_2^q(t, e = 0.6) = c^l\, t, e = 0.2) + 3/4(c^l(t, e = 1) - c^l(t, e = 0.2))$. Note that $c^l(t, e = 0.6) = c^l\, t, e = 0.2) + 1/2(c^l(t, e = 1) - c^l(t, e = 0.2))$. The difference between $c_1^q(t, e = 0.6)$ and $c^l(t, e = 0.6)$ and the difference between $c_2^q(t, e = 0.6)$ and $c^l(t, e = 0.6)$ indicate the deviation of the SF from the linear structure. A sample of the results are presented in Table 14.5 for $d = 1.0$, where $d = c(0, e)/c(1, e)$. The results for $d = 1.5$ and 2.0 are similar to those for $d = 1.0$. The point and interval estimate do differ from the estimates from the corresponding linear SF, but the results reflect the same messages.

In summary, we conducted a comprehensive sensitivity analysis for the Lindner Center study considering constant, linear, and quadratic SFs and various sets of coefficients. The inverse probability weighting

**TABLE 14.5. Point and Interval Estimates of Mean Difference on Standardized Cost between Abciximab and Usual Care among Patients Who Received an Initial Percutaneous Coronary Intervention, with Linear and Quadratic SFs**

| Minimum of $c(1,e)$ | Maximum of $c(1,e)$ | Linear SF $\hat{\psi}^{SF}$ | 95% CI | Quadratic SF 1 $\hat{\psi}^{SF}$ | 95% CI | Quadratic SF 2 $\hat{\psi}^{SF}$ | 95% CI |
|---|---|---|---|---|---|---|---|
| 0.00 | 0.000 | .009 | (.001, .016) | .009 | (.001, .016) | .009 | (.001, .016) |
|  | 0.005 | .005 | (−.003, .013) | .006 | (−.002, .014) | .004 | (−.004, .012) |
|  | 0.010 | .002 | (−.006, .010) | .004 | (−.004, .012) | .000 | (−.008, .008) |
|  | 0.015 | −.001 | (−.009, .006) | .002 | (−.007, .009) | −.004 | (−.012, .003) |
|  | 0.020 | −.005 | (−.013, .003) | −.001 | (−.009, .007) | −.009 | (−.017, .001) |
| 0.005 | 0.000 | .007 | (−.000, .015) | .006 | (−.001, .014) | .008 | (.001, .016) |
|  | 0.005 | .004 | (−.004, .012) | .004 | (−.004, .012) | .004 | (−.004, .012) |
|  | 0.010 | .001 | (−.007, .008) | .002 | (−.006, .010) | .000 | (−.008, .007) |
|  | 0.015 | −.003 | (−.011, .005) | .000 | (−.009, .007) | −.005 | (−.012, .003) |
| 0.010 | 0.000 | .006 | (−.001, .014) | .004 | (−.004, .012) | .008 | (.000, .016) |
|  | 0.005 | .003 | (−.005, .011) | .002 | (−.006, .010) | .004 | (−.004, .012) |
|  | 0.010 | .000 | (−.008, .007) | .000 | (−.008, .007) | .000 | (−.008, .007) |
| 0.015 | 0.000 | .005 | (−.003, .013) | .002 | (−.006, .010) | .008 | (.000, .016) |
|  | 0.005 | .002 | (−.006, .009) | .000 | (−.008, .007) | .004 | (−.004, .011) |
| 0.020 | 0.000 | .004 | (−.004, .012) | .000 | (−.008, .007) | .008 | (.000, .016) |

*Note.* We assume the SF follows a linear structure $c^l(t,e = 0.2) = c_t + s_t e$ and two quadratic structures $c_1^q(t,e)$ and $c_2^q(t,e)$ such that (i) $c_1^q(t,e = 0.2) = c_2^q(t,e = 0.2) = c^l(t,e = 0.2)$, (ii) $c_1^q(t,e = 1) = c_2^q(t,e = 1) = c^l(t,e = 1)$, (iii) $c_1^q(t,e = 0.6) = c^l(t,e = 0.2) + ¼(c^l(t,e = 1) − c^l(t,e = 0.e))$, and (iv) $c_2^q(t,e = 0.6) = c^l(t,e = 0.2) + ¾(c^l(t,e = 1) − c^l(t,e = 0.2))$. The CIs were obtained using the 2.5% and 97.5% percentiles from 2,000 bootstrap samples. In this table, $d = c(0,e)/c(1,e) = 1.0$.

estimator for the average treatment effect on the standardized cost is very sensitive to residual bias due to uncontrolled confounding. The 95% CI includes the null value of 0 with a small amount of potential residual bias.

## DISCUSSION AND CONCLUSION

We introduced two recently developed sensitivity analysis approaches. Both approaches are based on inverse probability weighting, but extend it from different perspectives. Approach 1 proposes a general framework and a parametric model for sensitivity. The essential idea is that the data allow us to estimate the bounds of the treatment effects under different postulations about parameters not directly estimable by observed data. The reason that we can only estimate the bounds of the treatment effect for continuous outcome (instead of the treatment effect itself) is the lack of knowledge on the variance–mean relationship for the potential outcomes, which cannot be identified even with infinite data points. For practical purposes, a key to construct a sensitivity analysis is simple and sensible parameters, the scales of which are familiar to investigators. We choose to base our sensitivity analysis on $(\rho, \tau)$ as these two measures are of broad familiarity with clear and sensible scales. From the analytical standpoint, in many cases sensitivity analysis will generate some bounds. These bounds add another level of uncertainty in addition to sampling variation. Therefore, for a sensitivity analysis to be useful and informative, these bounds should be as sharp as possible to accurately characterize the robustness. Although we consider compatibility of $\lambda_1$ and $\lambda_0$ in our analysis, the compatibility between $\lambda_1$ and $\rho_1$ (or between $\lambda_0$ and $\rho_0$) is more complicated and is not studied here. Therefore, our bounds are unlikely to be sharp. Nevertheless, the approach proposed is a balance of simplicity/sensibility and sharpness to be useful and accessible to medical researchers and scientists.

The motivation to restrict a continuous variable to the [0, 1] interval is to bound the variance of the potential outcomes (from both up and below) by estimable parameters and the non-estimable target (e.g., $E(r_1)$) to avoid the need to specify the variance and issue of the compatibility of the mean and variance. Practically, it is often feasible to scale a continuous variable to [0, 1] using reasonable lower and upper bounds. Even without assumptions of the upper and lower bounds, one can still use monotone nonlinear transformations (i.e., probit and inverse logit functions) to rescale the original variable to [0, 1]. The bounds of the mean of the potential outcome in the original scale can be obtained by Taylor expansion, followed by plugging in the bounds of the mean and the variance of the transformed scale (Kereiakes et al., 2000).

Approach 2 uses an SF to quantify residual bias due to unmeasured confounders and uses the SF-corrected inverse probability weighting estimator to assess the effect of possible uncontrolled confounding on causal effect estimates. As we have shown through its application to the Lindner Center study, the new method can be easily implemented to provide valuable insight on the impact of uncontrolled confounding. The SF is a one-dimensional function of the propensity score. If strong prior information is available, appropriate functional forms and coefficients can be directly imposed. Otherwise, low-order (e.g., linear, quadratic) polynomials are expected to provide reasonably well approximations of the continuous SF.

We suggest varying the coefficients over a set of plausible values, which should be determined on the basis of observed data, literature, and subject matter knowledge. The sensitivity assumptions we made in the application of the Lindner Center study were appropriate for this specific study and need to be examined and potentially modified before the approach is applied to other studies.

The proposed approach is a direct extension of another sensitivity analysis approach in which the SF depends on the entire covariate vector **x**. The motivation of our approach is to reduce the dimension of the SF to facilitate the implementation of a comprehensive sensitivity analysis. Nonetheless, a good understanding of the relation between the propensity score and the outcome is still required in order to impose reasonable parametric assumptions on the one-dimensional SF. In some settings, patients who have similar propensity scores may have totally different disease risks and thus are subject to different amounts of hidden bias (e.g., relatively healthy patients and very severely impaired patients may both have low propensities of receiving the intervention). Then it would be less straightforward to impose assumptions on the one-dimensional SF, since we collapse units that have similar propensity scores but different disease risks together. In such settings, we suggest taking an intermediate step to balance the trade-off between reducing the dimension of the SF and keeping subjects with different disease risks separate. Specifically, we could define the SF as the conditional mean difference in the potential outcomes between the treated and untreated subgroups, conditional on not only the propensity score but also one or several elements in **x** that were strong predictors of the outcome (e.g., a dummy variable indicating whether the patient was severely impaired). The subsequent application of the approach is exactly the same as we showed above.

The two approaches assess the impact of the assumption of absence of unmeasured confounders on the causal effect estimates from two different angles. There is no one-size-fit-all advice for all situations. Since this situation is shrouded in complete unknowns, a set of assumptions is necessary to explore the impact of unmeasured confounders on causal effect estimates. Researchers should examine the whole set of assumptions of an approach and choose one that is more plausible and appropriate to the observed data at hand, literature, and the subject domain knowledge.

Sensitivity analysis is a critical component for causal inference using observational data due to the potential impact of unmeasured confounders. Nevertheless, it has not been widely incorporated into observational studies due in part to the lack of user-friendly and intuitive software to facilitate the sensitivity analysis. An important future direction is to develop such software to improve how observational data are analyzed and interpreted. R code to facilitate the implementation of the two sensitivity analysis approaches can be downloaded from *www.populationmedicine.org/research/biostatistics/software.*

## REFERENCES

Arah, O. A., Chiba, Y., & Greenland, S. (2008). Bias formulas for external adjustment and sensitivity analysis of unmeasured confounders. *Annals of Epidemiology, 18*(8), 637–646.

Bross, I. D. (1966). Spurious effects from an extraneous variable. *Journal of Chronic Diseases, 19*(6), 637–647.

Bross, I. D. (1967). Pertinency of an extraneous variable. *Journal of Chronic Diseases, 20*(7), 487–495.

Brumback, B. A., Hernan, M. A., Haneuse, S. J., & Robins, J. M. (2004). Sensitivity analyses for unmeasured confounding assuming a marginal structural model for repeated measures. *Statistics in Medicine, 23*(5), 749–767.

Cole, S. R., & Hernan, M. A. (2008). Constructing inverse probability weights for marginal structural models. *American Journal of Epidemiology, 168*(6), 656–664.

Cole, S. R., Hernan, M. A., Margolick, J. B., Cohen, M. H., & Robins, J. M. (2005). Marginal structural models for estimating the effect of highly active antiretroviral therapy initiation on CD4 cell count. *American Journal of Epidemiology, 162*(5), 471–478.

Copas, J. B., & Li, H. G. (1997). Inference for non-random samples. *Journal of the Royal Statistical Society, Series B, 59*, 55–95.

Cornfield, J., Haenszel, W., Hammond, E. C., Lilienfeld, A. M., Shimkin, M. B., & Wynder, E. L. (1959). Smoking and lung cancer—Recent evidence and a discussion of some questions. *Journal of the National Cancer Institute, 22*(1), 173–203.

Efron, B., & Tibshirani, R. (1997). *An introduction to the bootstrap.* London: Chapman & Hall/CRC.

Flanders, W. D., & Khoury, M. J. (1990). Indirect assessment of confounding: Graphic description and limits on effect of adjusting for covariates. *Epidemiology, 1*(3), 239–246.

Greenland, S. (2005). Multiple-bias modelling for analysis of observational data. *Journal of the Royal Statistical Society Series A, Statistics in Society, 168*, 267–291.

Greenland, S., & Neutra, R. (1981). An analysis of detection bias and proposed corrections in the study of estrogens and endometrial cancer. *Journal of Chronic Diseases, 34*(9–10), 433–438.

Hernan, M. A., Brumback, B., & Robins, J. M. (2000). Marginal structural models to estimate the causal effect of Zidovudine on the survival of HIV-positive men. *Epidemiology, 11*(5), 561–570.

Hernan, M. A., & Robins, J. M. (1999). Method for conducting sensitivity analysis. *Biometrics, 55*(4), 1316–1317.

Horvitz, D. G., & Thompson, D. J. (1952). A generalization of sampling without replacement from a finite universe. *Journal of the American Statistical Association, 47*(260), 663–685.

Imbens, G. W. (2003). Sensitivity to exogeneity assumptions in program evaluation. *American Economic Review, 93*, 126–132.

Kereiakes, D. J., Obenchain, R. L., Barber, B. L., Smith, A., McDonald, M., Broderick, T. M., et al. (2000). Abciximab provides cost-effective survival advantage in high-book interventional practice. *American Heart Journal, 140*(4), 603–610.

Ko, H., Hogan, J. W., & Mayer, K. H. (2003). Estimating causal treatment effects from longitudinal HIV natural history studies using marginal structural models. *Biometrics, 59*(1), 152–162.

Kuroki, M., & Cai, Z. (2008). Formulating tightest bounds on causal effects in studies with unmeasured confounders. *Statistics in Medicine, 27*(30), 6597–6611.

Lash, T. L., Fox, M. P., & Fink, A. K. (2009). *Applying quantitative bias analysis to epidemiologic data*. New York: Springer.

Li, L., Shen, C. Y., Wu, A. C., & Li, X. (2009). Propensity score-based sensitivity analysis method for uncontrolled confounding. *American Journal of Epidemiology, 174*(3), 345–358.

Lin, D. Y., Psaty, B. M., & Kronmal, R. A. (1998). Assessing the sensitivity of regression results to unmeasured confounders in observational studies. *Biometrics, 54*(3), 948–963.

MacLehose, R. F., Kaufman, S., Kaufman, J. S., & Poole, C. (2005). Bounding causal effects under uncontrolled confounding using counterfactuals. *Epidemiology, 16*(4), 548–555.

McCaffrey, D. F., Ridgeway, G., & Morral, A. R. (2004). Propensity score estimation with boosted regression for evaluating causal effects in observational studies. *Psychological Methods, 9*(4), 403–425.

McCandless, L. C., Gustafson, P., & Levy, A. R. (2008). A sensitivity analysis using information about measured confounders yielded improved uncertainty assessments for unmeasured confounding. *Journal of Clinical Epidemiology, 61*(3), 247–255.

Ridgeway, G., & McCaffrey, D. F. (2007). Comment: Demystifying double robustness: A comparison of alternative strategies for estimating a population mean from incomplete data. *Statistical Science, 22*(4), 540–580.

Ridgeway, G., McCaffrey, D. F., & Morral, A. R. (2009). *twang R package manual*. Available at *http://cran.r-project.org/web/packages/twang/twang.pdf*.

Robins, J. M. (1999a). Association, causation, and marginal structural models. *Synthese, 121*(1–2), 151–179.
Robins, J. M. (1999b). Marginal structural models versus structural nested models as tools for causal inference. In E. Halloran & D. Barry (Eds.), *Statistical models in epidemiology: The environment and clinical trials* (pp. 95–134). New York: Springer-Verlag.
Robins, J. M., Hernan, M. A., & Brumback, B. (2000). Marginal structural models and causal inference in epidemiology. *Epidemiology, 11*(5), 550–560.
Robins, J. M., Rotnitzky, A., & Zhao, L. P. (1994). Estimation of regression coefficients when some regressors are not always observed. *Journal of the American Statistical Association, 89*, 846–866.
Robins, J. M., Rotnitzky, A., & Zhao, L. P. (1995). Analysis of semiparametric regression-models for repeated outcomes in the presence of missing data. *Journal of the American Statistical Association, 90*(429), 106–121.
Rosenbaum, P. R. (2002). *Observational studies* (2nd ed.). New York: Springer.
Rosenbaum, P. R., & Rubin, D. B. (1983a). Assessing sensitivity to an unobserved binary covariate in an observational study with binary outcome. *Journal of the Royal Statistical Society, Series B, 45*, 212–218.
Rosenbaum, P. R., & Rubin, D. B. (1983b). The central role of the propensity score in observational studies for causal effects. *Biometrika, 70*(1), 41–55.
Rosenbaum, P. R., & Rubin, D. B. (1985). The bias due to incomplete matching. *Biometrics, 41*(1), 103–116.
Rudin, W. (1973). *Functional analysis*. New York: McGraw-Hill.
Rudin, W. (1976). *Principles of mathematical analysis* (Vol. 3). New York: McGraw-Hill.
Schlesselman, J. J. (1978). Assessing effects of confounding variables. *American Journal of Epidemiology, 108*(1), 3–8.
Shen, C. Y., Li, X., Li, L., & Were, M. C. (2011). Sensitivity analysis for causal inference using inverse probability weighting. *Biometrical Journal, 53*(5), 822–837.
Sturmer, T., Schneeweiss, S., Rothman, K. J., Avorn, J., & Glynn, R. J. (2007a). Performance of propensity score calibration—A simulation study. *American Journal of Epidemiology, 165*(10), 1110–1118.
Sturmer, T., Schneeweiss, S., Rothman, K. J., Avorn, J., & Glynn, R. J. (2007b). Propensity score calibration and its alternatives. *American Journal of Epidemiology, 165*, 1122–1123.

# CHAPTER 15

# Prognostic Scores in Clustered Settings

**Ben Kelcey
Christopher M. Swoboda**

A central issue in nonexperimental research is identifying comparable units that received alternative treatments. When units from different treatment conditions are similar in their distribution of pretreatment covariates, observed differences in outcomes are plausibly due to differences among treatment conditions rather than preexisting differences. As we have seen throughout this book, one common way to identify comparable units in the presence of a high-dimensional covariate space is through propensity score methods (Rosenbaum & Rubin, 1983). These methods identify comparable units by constructing a model of the treatment assignment that balances pretreatment characteristics across treatment conditions.

In parallel to the propensity score, recent literature has developed the prognostic score to construct models of the potential outcomes (Hansen, 2008). Whereas the propensity score provides a unidimensional description of how pretreatment covariates relate to the probability of selecting into a treatment group, the prognostic score provides a summary of how pretreatment covariates relate to the expected response under the control condition. Prognostic scores are constructed by estimating the relationship between the response and observed covariates using only units in the control group (or a selected treatment group) and then applying those relationships to everyone in the sample to predict their expected response under the control condition.

In this chapter, we extend prognostic scores to incorporate data from multilevel or clustered settings. Similar to single-level prognostic scores, multilevel prognostic scores attempt to identify units that have comparable expected responses under the control condition (i.e., their prognoses) but do so by considering both the influence of individual covariates and the influence of cluster covariates and membership. We start with a brief review of prognostic scores and then describe their extension to clustered or multilevel settings. We then provide an illustration of multilevel prognostic scores to study the impact of participating in a prekindergarten program on students' mathematical achievement in kindergarten.

## PROGNOSTIC SCORES

Propensity scores summarize the associations between covariates and the treatment assignment mechanism using the conditional probability of receiving the treatment:

$$e(\mathbf{X}) = P(Z = 1 | \mathbf{X}) \qquad (15.1)$$

Let $e(\mathbf{X})$ be the propensity score, $\mathbf{X}$ be the observed covariates, and $Z$ the treatment indicator that takes a value of one with treatment and zero otherwise. If adjustment on the measured covariates, $\mathbf{X}$, is sufficient for unbiased estimation of the treatment effect, then so is adjustment on propensity scores, $e(\mathbf{X})$ (Rosenbaum & Rubin, 1983). Propensity scores are sufficient statistics that act as unidimensional balancing scores in which all the information relevant to balancing the covariates, $\mathbf{X}$, across the treatment assignment, $Z$, is extracted in the propensity score, $e(\mathbf{X})$. As a result, units with similar propensity score values but different treatment assignments can help to construct estimates of the counterfactual or the unobserved potential outcome. See Chapter 1 for an overview of propensity score analysis.

Similar to propensity scores, prognostic scores reduce the dimensionality of the observed covariate space. In contrast to propensity scores, however, prognostic scores summarize the associations between the potential responses in the control condition and the observed covariates. More specifically, a prognostic score is a summary that induces conditional independence between the potential responses and the observed covariates. That is, the prognostic score, $\Psi(\mathbf{X})$, is sufficient (in the prognostic sense) for the potential responses under the control condition, $r^{(0)}$, if it renders conditional independence between the potential responses under the control condition and covariates, $X$, $r^{(0)} \perp X | \Psi(X)$ (Hansen, 2006).

For instance, analogous to canonical propensity scores with binary treatment conditions (Equation 15.1 above), a prognostic score for a binary outcome can be defined as the conditional probability of success under the control condition (also known as a disease risk score):

$$\Psi(X) = p(r^{(0)} = 1 | X) \qquad (15.2)$$

Here, we use $r^{(0)}$ to denote the potential responses under the control condition (as opposed to the potential response under the treatment condition, $r^{(1)}$) and $X$ to denote the observed covariates. Prognostic scores, $\Psi(X)$, are thus summaries that capture the information relevant to balancing the covariates, $X$, across the potential responses under the control condition, $r^{(0)}$. As a result, prognostic scores induce independence between the potential responses under the control condition, $r^{(0)}$, and observed covariates, $X$, such that $r^{(0)} \perp X | \Psi(X)$.

In a simple case where there are no effect moderators, prognostic scores are simply the predicted response under the control condition. If the potential outcome of interest follows a generalized linear model, then a prognostic score is the linear predictor of the potential response under the control condition. Thus, within a generalized linear model framework, prognostic scores might be obtained by estimating an outcome model using only the units that experienced the control condition and then applying this model to all units in the sample to predict their responses under the control condition.

The principal benefit of prognostic scores is that they constrain variation in the outcome due to sources other than the treatment, thereby favorably reducing both bias and variance of treatment effect estimators (Hansen, 2006). Because prognostic scores are estimated as a function of the covariates using only the control observations, prognostic scores postpone commitment to a functional form for both potential outcomes without risk of inducing subjective bias associated with the use of outcomes in the design stage (Iacus, King, & Porro, 2011). This separation of control and treatment groups is, in part, what differentiates prognostic scores and helps them outperform other approaches (Hansen, 2006).

Many of the useful properties of prognostic scores parallel those of the propensity score. For instance, a key property of propensity scores is that if adjustment for observed covariates is sufficient for an unbiased estimate of the treatment effect, adjustment for the propensity score is also sufficient for an unbiased estimate of the effect (Rosenbaum & Rubin, 1983). The prognostic score also shares a form of this property. Given that there is no bias from unobserved covariates (e.g., unobserved covariates confounding the treatment–outcome relationship), if adjustment for the observed covariates is sufficient to support conditional independence between the potential responses under the control condition and the treatment assignment, then adjustment on prognostic scores is also sufficient:

$$r^{(0)} \perp Z|X \Rightarrow r^{(0)} \perp Z|\Psi(X) \tag{15.3}$$

This property also extends to the potential responses under the treatment condition:

$$r^{(1)} \perp Z|X \Rightarrow r^{(1)} \perp Z|\Psi(X) \tag{15.4}$$

However, as discussed below, this extension is dependent on the assumption that there are no effect modifications (e.g., interactions between covariates and the treatment).

Similarly, a useful diagnostic feature of the propensity score is its balancing property; units with the same propensity score, regardless of treatment condition, should have the same distribution of observed covariates (Rosenbaum & Rubin, 1983):

$$X \perp Z|e(X) \tag{15.5}$$

Prognostic scores also bring about a form of balance termed *prognostic balance* (Hansen, 2008). Prognostic balance suggests that when comparing units with similar prognostic scores (predicted response under the control condition), the distributions of covariates across units with different potential responses under the control condition should be comparable:

$$r^{(0)} \perp X|\Psi(X) \tag{15.6}$$

This balancing property also extends to stratifications that demonstrate prognostic balance. Hansen (2006) showed that if $b(X)$ is some stratification that provides prognostic balance such that $r^{(0)} \perp X|b(X)$, then with probability 1,

$$E[\Psi(X)|b(X)] = \Psi(X) \tag{15.7}$$

Absent hidden bias, stratifications that produce prognostic balance are also unconfounded such that

$$r^{(0)} \perp Z \mid b(X) \tag{15.8}$$

Despite reducing the dimensionality of X and constraining variation in the outcome, prognostic scores have several important limitations. Perhaps first and foremost is that use of prognostic scores requires the (partial) use of outcome data in the design and formation of matches. Although prognostic scores rely on only the outcomes for the control condition, such an approach potentially deviates from the clear separation of the design and analysis phases that many have advocated for (Rubin, 2007; Stuart, 2010). In particular, literature has suggested that nonexperimental studies should be purposefully designed by constructing subgroups of similar treated and control units using only pretreatment information (i.e., without access to any outcome information). Only after these subgroups have been constructed should outcome data be introduced into the analysis (Rubin, 2007).

Other inherent limitations of the prognostic score result largely from their asymmetric estimation (i.e., they are constructed using only the control units). For instance, an invaluable method to probe the quality of a set of propensity scores is to assess the balance of pretreatment covariates across treatment conditions for subgroups with similar propensity scores. Because propensity scores are estimated using treatment and control units, propensity score balance can be assessed across the entire sample. In contrast, prognostic scores intentionally exclude the treated sample, and, as a result, balance can only be appraised in the control sample. Consequently, prognostic score balance assessments may be less informative and provide weaker evidence concerning their quality in practice than propensity score balance assessments.

Asymmetric estimation of prognostic models may also make them particularly susceptible to multiple types of model misspecification (Hansen, 2008). Take, for example, overfitting. Overfitting can occur when the estimated prognostic model describes random error as part of the underlying relationships among the outcome and covariates in ways that do not replicate to the out of sample treatment group.

Similarly, when control and treatment groups differ substantially on pretreatment covariates, applying the outcome model constructed with the control group to the treatment group may rely heavily on the extrapolation of the relationship between pretreatment covariates and the outcome. Misspecification may arise when prognostic models that fail to capture the presence of nonlinear relationships or interactions between the treatment and a covariate may miss important differences in response formation. Prognostic scores that do not appropriately adjust for such nonlinearities or interactions may not be sufficient for deconfounding the treatment assignment and potential responses under both the control and treatment condition. In order to safeguard the full benefits of prognostic score adjustment, prognostic score models thus need to capture such complexities despite no access to observed outcomes for the treatment group.

Related limitations also concern the extent to which prognostic scores are fully transferable from the control to the treatment condition. Because prognostic score models will often need to accommodate a range of outcomes (e.g., continuous, categorical, and ordinal), prognostic scores are not necessarily scalars. For outcomes described by a linear regression model such that the error variance also depends on the observed covariates, a score defined by the regression function alone would not be sufficient. Rather, a prognostic score would be two-dimensional—the regression and variance function together. As a result, misspecification may arise when unidimensional prognostic models do not fully capture the multidimensional nature of the response.

For these reasons, prognostic scores are more likely to be seen as a complement to propensity scores rather than an alternative (Hansen, 2006). Instances of prognostic scores in the literature have focused on their use alongside propensity scores and have largely come through the use of Mahalanobis distances. Specifically, propensity and prognostic scores are combined into a single index using

$$D_M = \sqrt{(\mathbf{P} - \boldsymbol{\mu})^T \mathbf{S}^{-1} (\mathbf{P} - \boldsymbol{\mu})} \qquad (15.9)$$

where $\mathbf{P}$ are the prognostic scores and propensity scores with means $\boldsymbol{\mu}$ and sample covariance matrix $\mathbf{S}$. A key feature of this metric is that it intentionally adjusts for the variance and covariance of the scores so that resulting distances are scale-invariant. When the covariance matrix is diagonal (i.e., covariance between scores is zero) the distances reduce to normalized Euclidean distances. Mahalanobis metric matching has been shown to be effective in controlling for selection bias (Rubin, 1976, 1979). In addition, Mahalanobis metric matching has been shown to be equal percent bias reducing under commonly assumed distributional conditions (Rubin, 1976). For each matching covariate or linear combination of matching covariates, equal percent bias reducing methods produce the same percent reduction in expected bias.

More practically, Mahalanobis distance provides an equal percent bias reducing measure of the similarity between any two units so that the comparability of all control and treatment units (e.g., subjects) is defined by a single index, $D_M$. Matching along this combined index has shown to be effective at both reducing bias and variance above and beyond, for example, covariance adjustment or propensity score matching (Hansen, 2006). Use of prognostic scores in combination with propensity scores through Mahalanobis metric matching tends to be particularly favorable in the presence of nonlinear relationships because it, to some extent, alleviates assumptions of functional form (Rubin, 1979).

## PROGNOSTIC SCORES IN CLUSTERED SETTINGS

In many studies, individuals are nested or clustered within hierarchical groups, and the composition or context they cultivate can contribute to potential responses. Take, for example, the increasing literature base concerning teacher effects and effectiveness. Students are often considered to be nested or clustered within classrooms and schools such that which classroom and school a student attends has important implications for his or her cognitive development (Nye, Konstantopoulous, & Hedges, 2004). The importance of addressing the influence of hierarchical units (e.g., classrooms and schools) in estimating treatment effects has been demonstrated in multiple studies (e.g., Hong & Raudenbush, 2006; Kelcey, 2011a; Kim & Seltzer, 2007; Rosenbaum, 1986). These studies have, however, largely focused on extending the propensity score to multilevel settings. Below, we describe how the influence of cluster membership can be incorporated to extend prognostic scores to multilevel settings.

As described above in the unclustered case, $\Psi(X)$ is a prognostic score if the potential responses under the control condition are independent from the observed covariates given a statistic $\Psi(X)$. In this way, it is implicitly assumed that the potential responses under the control condition are unclustered and are solely influenced by individual-level covariates ($X$). In multilevel settings, however, the potential responses under the control condition are likely influenced by a much broader range of effects. For instance, responses are potentially shaped by individual-level covariates, $X$, cluster-level covariates and their cross-level interactions, $W$, and unobserved cluster-level effects and their cross-level interactions, $U$. As a result, prognostic scores constructed on the basis of individual-level covariates will generally not be sufficient to render potential responses under the control condition independent from systematic cluster differences.

To accommodate the impact of clusters, we expand the prognostic score to incorporate effects originating from individual and cluster levels and their interactions. If the potential responses under the control condition are independent from the observed effects given a statistic $\Psi(X, W, U)$, then $\Psi(X, W, U)$ is a prognostic score. That is,

$$r^{(0)} \perp X, W, U \mid \Psi(X, W, U) \tag{15.10}$$

We use X to represent observed individual-level covariates, W to represent observed cluster-level covariates (and their cross-level interactions), and U to represent unobserved cluster-specific effects that potentially include both simple shifts, $U_s$ (i.e., random intercept), and interactions between individual-level covariates and cluster-specific effects (i.e., random slopes).

The conditional independence between the potential responses under the control condition and the systematic roots of those responses can be achieved in a number of ways that depend on the setting. Let us first consider a situation where the potential responses follow a linear model that depends on individual covariates, X, cluster covariates, W, and cluster membership only up to shifts in the cluster mean ($U_{0k}$) (e.g., a hierarchical linear model with random intercepts). Under this scenario, clusters are associated with shifts in the responses, but the predictive nature of individual covariates is constant across clusters and each cluster has a constant and uniform influence on all of its individuals.

Under this scenario, several simple approaches suggest prognostic scores. First, one could construct a common (across all clusters) linear model for the potential responses under the control condition using only individual-level covariates, X, and restrict matches to within clusters (Rosenbaum, 1986):

$$r_{jk}^{(0)} = \beta_0 + \sum_{p=1}^{P} \beta_p X_{pjk} + \varepsilon_{jk} \tag{15.11}$$

We use $r_{jk}^{(0)}$ as the potential response of individual $j$ in cluster $k$ under the control condition, $\beta_0$ as the intercept, $X^{pjk}$ as the value of covariate $p$ for individual $j$ in cluster $k$ with corresponding coefficient $\beta_p$, and $\varepsilon_{jk}$ as the normally distributed error with mean zero and variance $\sigma_\varepsilon^2$.

Using the expected value from Equation 15.8, $E(r^0|X)$, as the prognostic score and matching within clusters will be sufficient because cluster-level covariates, W, and cluster-specific shifts, $U_{0k}$, are constant for individuals within the same cluster. This approach affords estimation of cluster-specific treatment effects as well as an overall estimate of the treatment effect and its variability across clusters. Practically, however, this approach is limited by within-cluster sample sizes and the availability of (high-quality) matches within clusters.

A second type of prognostic model under this scenario would be to use fixed effects to adjust for differences among cluster means:

$$r_{jk}^{(0)} = \beta_{0k} + \sum_{p=1}^{P}\beta_p X_{pjk} + \sum_{k=1}^{K}\gamma_k I_k + \varepsilon_{jk} \qquad (15.12)$$

Here, Equation 15.12 introduces as indicators of cluster membership with $\gamma_k$ as the cluster-specific adjustments in the mean response. In contrast to Equation 15.11, this approach incorporates cluster membership, $C$, directly into the model so that the prognostic score accommodates any shift differences among clusters in terms of observed effects, $W$, and unobserved effects, $U_{0k}$. As a result, prognostic scores could be constructed using $\Psi(X, C) = E[r^{(0)}|X, C]$. Absent bias from unobserved covariates, prognostic scores are now comparable across clusters so that matches can be had within clusters and/or across clusters. As a result, the approach potentially alleviates the aforementioned within-cluster sample size problems concerning the availability of suitable matches within a given cluster. However, the approach may also introduce unstable estimation when there are many clusters (Neyman & Scott, 1948).

A third approach is to construct a prognostic model using the potential responses under the control condition using a multilevel model:

$$r_{jk}^{(0)} = \beta_{0k} + \sum_{p=1}^{P}\beta_p X_{pjk} + \sum_{m=1}^{M}\gamma_m W_{mk} + u_{0k} + \varepsilon_{jk} \qquad (15.13)$$

Here we introduce $u_{0k}$ as the cluster-specific random effects that take on a normal distribution centered at zero with variance $\tau_0^2$. Similar to the fixed-effect approach, the prognostic model accommodates unobserved cluster-specific shifts in the average response through $U_{0k}$ and systematic shifts resulting from cluster differences in observed effects, $W$. As a result, prognostic scores could be constructed using $\Psi(X, W, U_{0k}) = E[r^{(0)}|X, W, U_{0k}]$ (best linear unbiased predictors). Absent bias from unobserved covariates, it also allows for within- and/or across-cluster matching. As a result, the approach potentially lessens the aforementioned within-cluster sample size problems and potentially alleviates the incidental parameter problem of fixed effects.

Let us now consider the more realistic and complex case where the impacts of the individual covariates ($X$) also vary with cluster membership ($X_{qjk} u_{qk}$) (e.g., a hierarchical linear model with random intercepts and slopes). Such coefficient variation across clusters indicates that the potential responses ought to be represented by different prognostic models for each cluster. As a result, the aforementioned approaches will generally no longer be sufficient because the rank ordering of prognostic scores within and across clusters will depend on the ways in which individual-level covariates interact with cluster membership.

Use of a common prognostic model across all clusters and within-cluster matching, for instance, may fail to provide a sufficient prognostic score because the prognostic model differs by cluster (i.e., β differ by cluster). In theory, one could modify this approach by constructing a separate prognostic model for each cluster and then restrict matches to other units within a cluster. However, practically this would require large within-cluster sample sizes to estimate parameters and match individuals. Similarly, the fixed-effect approach (15.12) could also be modified to include interactions among the indicators and individual-level covariates such that

$$r_{jk}^{(0)} = \beta_{0k} + \sum_{p=1}^{P} \beta_p X_{pjk} + \sum_{k=1}^{K} \gamma_k I_k + \sum_{n=1}^{N} \pi_n X_{njk} I_k + \varepsilon_{jk} \quad (15.14)$$

where $\pi_n$ describes interactions between cluster- and individual-level covariates. Such an approach would sufficiently accommodate the complex differences among clusters; however, within-cluster sample size for both parameter estimation and matching are likely to be issues.

When the predictive capacities of the individual-level covariates vary across clusters, a more practical option is to extend the aforementioned multilevel (random intercept) approach (Equation 15.13) to include random slopes:

$$r_{jk}^{(0)} = \beta_{0k} + \sum_{p=1}^{P} \beta_p X_{pjk} + \sum_{m=1}^{M} \gamma_m W_{mk} + \sum_{q=1}^{Q} X_{qjk} u_{qk} + u_{0k} + \varepsilon_{jk} \quad (15.15)$$

We introduce random slopes, $u_{qk}$, to capture the cluster-specific deviations of the effect of individual covariates (assumed to have a multivariate normal distribution with $u_{0k}$). Prognostic scores could then be constructed using $\Psi(X, W, U) = E[r^{(0)}|X, W, U]$. Such an approach accommodates the potential for different outcome processes to occur in each cluster and, lacking bias from unobserved covariates, allows both within- and across-cluster matching.

Prognostic scores in clustered settings share the same important limitations as their unclustered counterparts, but also have additional limitations. Limitations, in part, stem from the introduction of new covariates. For instance, in unclustered settings a sufficient statistic for $r^{(0)}$ may not be sufficient for $r^{(1)}$ because of effect modification by a covariate or function of the covariate. In clustered settings, this effect modification can additionally arise from, for example, cross-level interactions between the treatment and cluster-level covariates.

Other limitations stem more from cluster membership. In clustered settings, the inference space associated with a research question can introduce complexities in estimating the potential responses under the control condition for individuals who received the treatment condition. The complexity has to do with the difference between unit-specific or population-average inquiries (Raudenbush & Bryk, 2002). If we are trying to capture relationships that are occurring within each cluster and how these cluster-specific relationships differ over a population of clusters (i.e., holding constant cluster membership), then our inference space is unit-specific. However, if we are trying to describe the average relationships across all clusters in a population (i.e., ignoring cluster membership), then we are trying to address a population average inquiry.

To see the difference between these two spaces, let us consider the case where the potential responses under the control condition follow a linear model in which the intercept and individual-level slopes vary across clusters (e.g., Equation 15.15). Let us further consider a research question that examines the impact of being retained or held back in kindergarten on students' achievement in schools that freely allow retention. If we are trying to describe the potential responses under the control condition (not being retained) of students who were retained holding constant students' school membership, then our inference space is unit-specific. Thus, the counterfactual might be defined as the student's predicted achievement level when not being retained in the same kindergarten school of record. As a result, prognostic scores for retained students might be constructed using both the fixed and random effects as described in Equation 15.15.

In contrast, if we are trying to describe the conditional average potential responses under the control condition (not being retained) of students who were retained regardless of students' current school membership, then we need a population-average approach. We could define the counterfactual here as the student's predicted achievement level in a typical school when not retained. Thus, the potential response can be viewed as the average of the school-specific prognostic scores for the student. In this case, predictions for the achievement levels of retained students had they not been retained might be constructed using only the fixed effects in Equation 15.15.

The within-school sample size and the type or level of treatment can also dictate the inference space. Consider a research question that concerns the impact of a cluster-level treatment on an individual-level outcome that follows a random intercept and slope linear model. Cluster-level treatments may preclude estimation of cluster-specific random effects under the control condition for individuals who actually received the treatment because parameter estimation in the prognostic model is based only on those who actually experienced the control condition. Thus, absent a separate sample, cluster-level random effects under the control condition are not available for treatment clusters and cannot be incorporated in the construction of the prognostic scores.

In many instances with cluster-level treatment, a particular inference space may also be insensible. For instance, consider the impact of attending a private (treatment condition) versus a public school (control condition) in kindergarten. The population-average approach reasonably asks, for students who attended private schools, what their achievement would be if they attended a typical or average public school. In contrast, the unit-specific approach asks, for students who attended private schools, what their achievement would be if they had attended that same school and it had been a public school. Although theoretically possible, such an estimand may be of little interest. In this way, the data, the research question, and the type of treatment help determine the appropriate inference space.

## DEMONSTRATION

Prior investigations have indicated that the proportion of children in the United States participating in prekindergarten programs has increased markedly in the past five decades (U.S. Department of Education, 2003). Although there is a strong literature describing the positive impacts of high-quality early education interventions on student cognitive development (e.g., Brooks-Gunn, 2003; Waldfogel, 2002), studies describing the impacts of participation in a prekindergarten program at scale are sparse (Magnuson, Ruhm, & Waldfogel, 2007). For the few studies that have examined the impact of participation in prekindergarten programs, they have largely drawn on observational designs and unconditional comparisons between students who had participated in prekindergarten programs with those who had not. However, the validity of such unconditional comparisons has been called into question because, for example, research has demonstrated that children who belong to less educated and lower income families are less likely to attend prekindergarten programs (Bainbridge, Meyers, Tanaka, & Waldfogel, 2005). As a result, observed differences between those children who did and did not participate in prekindergarten programs may owe to preexisting differences rather than causal effects of participation in the prekindergarten program. In this section, we briefly illustrate the use of prognostic scores within clustered settings by examining the extent to which participation in a prekindergarten program impacts students' kindergarten mathematics achievement. Our application is presented only as a simple illustration of the methods and is not meant to inform the value of participation in a prekindergarten program.

## Method

To investigate the effects of participation in a typical prekindergarten program, we drew on data from the Early Childhood Longitudinal Study—Kindergarten Cohort (ECLS-K). ECLS-K was a nationally representative observational study that measured students and their schools along a wide array of dimensions. In our analyses, we took participation in a center-based prekindergarten program to be the treatment condition, whereas the control condition was a lack of participation in a prekindergarten program. We structured our analyses so that students were nested within schools such that students were considered as level one and schools were considered as level two. Additional nesting structures could be considered (e.g., students could also be considered to be nested within classrooms) but are omitted in these analyses for ease of presentation.

Our analyses focused on a subsample of the original data—we removed all units with incomplete data and, for simplicity, removed schools with only a few students. Furthermore, although many factors may influence both the likelihood a child participates in a prekindergarten program and his or her mathematics achievement, our analyses considered only four pretreatment (child-level) covariates: mother's education, family socioeconomic status, free/reduced lunch status, and child's gender. Descriptive statistics for the included variables are shown in Table 15.1.

**TABLE 15.1. Descriptive Information for Sample ECLS-K Data**

| Variable | Not in prekindergarten (49%) | | In prekindergarten (51%) | |
|---|---|---|---|---|
| | Mean | SD | Mean | SD |
| Mathematics achievement[a] | 18.80 | 7.23 | 20.61 | 8.37 |
| Mother's education[a] | 3.90 | 1.77 | 4.48 | 1.80 |
| Student gender | 0.49 | 0.50 | 0.50 | 0.50 |
| Free and reduced lunch eligibility | 0.40 | 0.49 | 0.46 | 0.50 |
| Family socioeconomic status[a] | −0.34 | 0.68 | −0.14 | 0.78 |

Note. [a]Difference between prekindergarten groups significant, $p < .05$.

## Prognostic and Propensity Score Models

*Prognostic Score Model.* To develop a prognostic model, we used students who did not participate in a prekindergarten program. We constructed several simple unidimensional prognostic models, each progressively more complex, using the four aforementioned covariates. We note that we considered only a small subset of student covariates and did not consider school-level covariates. A more complete analysis would consider, for example, richer sets of student and school covariates, the interactions among these covariates, and probe for evidence of multidimensionality in the prognostic scores.

The first model we estimated was a single-level prognostic model that incorporated only the predictive capacity of the student covariates

$$r_{jk}^{(0)} = \beta_{0k} + \sum_{p=1}^{4} \beta_p X_{pjk} + \varepsilon_{jk} \tag{15.16}$$

Here we used $r_{jk}^{(0)}$ to denote the potential mathematics achievement under the control condition for student $j$ in school $k$, $\beta_{0k}$ as the intercept, $X_{pjk}$ as covariate $p$ (where $p = 4$ and the covariates are mother's education, socioeconomic status, free/reduced lunch status, or gender) for student $j$ in school $k$ with corresponding coefficient $\beta_p$, and $\varepsilon_{jk}$ as normally distributed error terms with mean zero and variance $\sigma_\varepsilon^2$.

The second model we considered was a random intercept multilevel model. Whereas the single-level model implicitly assumes that incorporating school membership does not improve the model's prognostic value, the random intercept model supposes that prediction is improved by including school membership. The random intercept model was

$$r_{jk}^{(0)} = \beta_{0k} + \sum_{p=1}^{4} \beta_p X_{pjk} + \varepsilon_{jk}$$
$$\beta_{0k} = \gamma_{00} + u_{0k} \tag{15.17}$$

Continuing with the aforementioned notation, the multilevel random intercept model introduces a random intercept term $u_{0k}$, which has a normal distribution centered at zero and variance $\tau_0^2$. In this model, the prediction of students' mathematics achievement is amended by allowing school membership to be associated with achievement such that each school has a constant and uniform effect on all of its students (i.e., through $u_{0k}$). As a result, it is assumed that the predictive nature of student covariates is constant across schools (i.e., the relationship between each predictor and the outcome do not vary across schools so that $\beta_p$ are constant across schools).

The third model we considered further expanded the multilevel approach by incorporating random slopes. We can write this model as

$$r_{jk}^{(0)} = \beta_{0k} + \sum_{p=1}^{4} \beta_{pk} X_{pjk} + \varepsilon_{jk}$$
$$\beta_{0k} = \gamma_{00} + u_{0k}$$
$$\beta_{pk} = \gamma_{p0} + u_{pk}$$

(15.18)

Here we introduce $u_{pk}$ as a random slope term for student-level covariate $p$ and along with $u_{0k}$, $u_{pk}$ is assumed to have multivariate normal distribution with mean 0 and unstructured covariance matrix $\Sigma$. The introduction of random slopes is intended to capture the degree to which the coefficients associated with student-level covariates vary by school. As a result, it is no longer assumed that the predictive nature of student covariates is constant across schools. Rather, the random intercept and slopes model suggests that although schools have effects on all their students' mathematics achievement, these effects vary depending on students' background (e.g., their mother's education, their gender, etc.).

To assess the relative fit of these models, we compared the models' likelihood and corresponding information criteria. The proposed prognostic models represent a set of nested or restricted models, and, as a result, the distribution of the difference in deviances between a larger model and a more restrictive model should have an approximate $\chi^2$ distribution with degrees of freedom equal to the difference in the number of parameters (Raudenbush & Bryk, 2002). Such comparisons help suggest which prognostic model best describes the potential responses under the control condition.

Evaluations of relative fit can provide guidance as to the general structure of the model (e.g., whether random intercepts/slopes are needed). However, such evaluations are fundamentally concerned with relative fit rather than balance. As a result, such comparisons are insufficient to ensure prognostic balance. Rather, a sufficient prognostic model requires an iterative process that respecifies the prognostic model until balance can be achieved. For this reason, we iteratively (re)specified the prognostic score models using higher-order terms and interactions until we achieved balance on each of the four covariates.

Although we investigated the fit of several different models, it is important to note the illustrative nature of our analysis and inherent limitations of the small set of covariates and models considered. As noted above, prognostic score models are particularly sensitive to many types of model misspecification because of their asymmetric estimation. Similar to adjustments on the propensity score, estimates of treatment effects can be sensitive to prognostic score model specification. We caution readers to carefully consider and investigate the specification of prognostic score models and their transferability to the treatment group.

Propensity Score Model. To estimate the propensity scores, we used logistic regression with the full sample of (treatment and control) students and considered models using each of the four aforementioned covariates. Based on approaches outlined in this book, we iteratively (re)specified the propensity score using higher-order terms and interactions until we achieved balance on each of the four covariates. Although we constructed the prognostic score model using a multilevel approach, our propensity score model was constructed using a single-level model. This difference reflects the fact that treatment decisions (participation in a prekindergarten program) occurred well before enrollment in a school and thus school membership could not have influenced the likelihood that a student would attend a prekindergarten program.

## Covariate Balance

A critical diagnostic benchmark of propensity-score-based analyses is demonstrating balance in covariate distributions across treatment groups in, for example, propensity-score-based strata or matches. Likewise, demonstrating prognostic balance is a key diagnostic. Given the prognostic strata, covariates (or function of covariates) should not demonstrate any association with the potential responses under the control condition. The lack of such associations provides evidence that by conditioning on the prognostic strata one has effectively conditioned on the prognostic score.

To provide an assessment of prognostic balance, we considered one such approach. We partitioned the control group into quintile-based strata using the estimated prognostic scores and assessed the residual association between each covariate (and several transformations of each covariate) and the response using a series of linear models within each prognostic stratum for each covariate. Similarly, we further assessed balance by examining the residual association between several transformations of each covariate (e.g., log transformation) and the response and by examining the intraclass correlation coefficient within each stratum. We followed a similar path for propensity score balance and assessed it using absolute standardized mean differences with and without propensity score adjustment (e.g., Rubin, 2001; Stuart, 2010; Stuart & Rubin, 2007). See Chapter 5 in this book for detailed discussion on how to evaluate covariate balance.

## Combining Scores

As described earlier, alone prognostic scores have several important limitations. When paired with propensity scores, however, prognostic scores have been shown to reduce both bias and variance of estimated treatment effects (Hansen, 2006). Prior literature has largely considered the concurrent adjustment for propensity scores and prognostic scores through Mahalanobis metric matching. Matching treated and control units along a single score defined by Mahalanobis distance attempts to equally weight the scores because net distances between units are formed by adding up the variance normalized squared distances of the scores. When estimated scores reflect similar levels of precision and importance, Mahalanobis distances are an effective way of measuring similarities among treated and control units (Rubin, 1979).

Combining prognostic and propensity scores into a single index, however, may not always be well suited for investigating treatment effects because the squaring of distances potentially allows one score to dominate information provided from another. Although Mahalanobis distances are designed to take into account differences in the distributions of the scores, it is possible for it to favor close matches on the prognostic scores and more coarse matches on propensity scores. For instance, poor performance of Mahalanobis metric matching has been noted in the presence of rare events because Mahalanobis metric matching tends to place undue emphasis on variables with low prevalence rates as a result of their small variance (Rubin & Thomas, 2000). Similarly, when scores contain outliers or contain excessive noise, the estimated variance can diminish its contributions to Mahalanobis distance. If, for example, the outcome represents low prevalence binary responses or contains outliers, Mahalanobis distance may privilege close matches on the prognostic score over the propensity score.

These drawbacks may be worsened by the fact that propensity scores and prognostic scores are constructed using different samples; propensity scores with the full data and prognostic scores with the control only. As a result, the variance in prognostic scores may often reflect a larger portion of error than do propensity scores. In part, the poor performance of Mahalanobis metric matching, especially in high-covariate space, is what in part led to the development of the propensity score (e.g., Rubin & Thomas, 2000).

Combining prognostic and propensity scores into a single index may not be optimal on theoretical grounds because there are critical differences between the scores. For instance, the balancing property of propensity scores can be explicitly appraised for the full sample, whereas prognostic balance can only be examined for the control sample. Although balance is a necessary but not sufficient condition for bias reduction, the authentication of prognostic balance using only control units inherently produces balance and results that are more sensitive to misspecifications. Similarly, our review of the literature suggests that bias reduction should be fundamentally more important than variance reduction in observational studies. Although prognostic scores help to address bias, propensity scores would seem to be more appropriately positioned to objectively address bias because they model treatment selection.

Rather than define discrepancies between potential matches by combining prognostic scores and propensity scores into a single index using Mahalanobis distance, we considered stratifying on prognostic scores and subsequently matching on propensity scores within prognostic strata (Kelcey, 2013). Propensity score matching within prognostic strata attempts to privilege propensity scores by using coarser matching on prognostic scores and finer matching on propensity scores. Limited evidence suggests that this alternative approach potentially improves the performance of the treatment effect estimator (Kelcey, 2013). However, the sequential use of prognostic scores and propensity scores may have the undesirable effect of reducing the availability of propensity score matches within strata, and the trade-off needs to be further investigated.

For the purposes of this demonstration, our adjustments for students' prognoses were implemented by stratifying on quintiles of the prognostic scores. To make use of the propensity scores, we used nearest neighbor matching within each of the five prognostic strata with a caliper of 0.10. As a result, we first subclassified the entire sample into five groups on the basis of students' prognostic scores and subsequently matched students with replacement on the basis of their propensity scores.

## Treatment Effects

To estimate the treatment effect, we further combined our propensity and prognostic score adjustments with regression adjustment. We estimated the effect of participating in a prekindergarten program using a multilevel model with indicators for matches. The model paralleled that of the prognostic scored, specifying mathematics achievement as a function of student predictors and school membership:

$$r_{jk} = \beta_{0k} + \sum_{p=1}^{4} \beta_{pk} X_{pjk} + \sum_{q=1}^{Q} \pi_q I_{jk} + \varepsilon_{jk}$$
$$\beta_{0k} = \gamma_{00} + u_{0k}$$
$$\beta_{pk} = \gamma_{p0} + u_{pk}$$

(15.19)

The notation remains unchanged from Equation 15.15 except that now we used $r_{jk}$ to denote observed mathematics achievement level and $I_{jk}$ as the match indicators with coefficients $\pi_q$.

## Results

### Prognostic and Propensity Score Models

Using the control group, we developed a prognostic model by iteratively constructing and comparing each of the three increasingly complex models described above. Our analyses were conducted in the statistical software package R and made use of the packages lme4 and *MatchIt* (Bates, Maechler, & Bolker, 2013; Ho, Imai, King, & Stuart, 2011; R Core Team, 2013). The results indicated that our measures of relative fit preferred a random intercepts and slopes model (Table 15.2). In particular, our analysis suggested that the contribution of schools to the outcome varied significantly, as did the predictive capacity of socioeconomic status only. Our final model was of the form

$$r_{jk}^{(0)} = \beta_{0k} + \beta_{1k}X_{1jk} + \sum_{p=2}^{4}\beta_{pk}X_{pjk} + \varepsilon_{jk}$$
$$\beta_{0k} = \gamma_{00} + u_{0k}$$
$$\beta_{1k} = \gamma_{10} + u_{1k}$$
(15.20)

where we use $\beta_{1k}$ to denote the coefficient associated student socioeconomic status, $X_{1jk}$, and $\beta_{pk}$ to denote the coefficients associated with parental education, gender, and free/reduced lunch eligibility.

To estimate prognostic scores, we drew on this multilevel random intercept and slope model using a unit-specific focus. Using the expected

**TABLE 15.2. Comparison of Prognostic Score Models**

| | Deviance | AIC | BIC | *p*-value[a] |
|---|---|---|---|---|
| Single level | 10430 | 10445 | 10482 | — |
| Multilevel—random intercepts | 10404 | 10420 | 10463 | $p < .001$[b] |
| Multilevel—random intercepts and slopes | 10390 | 10409 | 10463 | $p < .001$[c] |

[a]*p*-value is based on the likelihood ratio test.
[b]Comparing the single-level model to the multilevel model with random intercepts only.
[c]Comparing the multilevel model with random intercepts only to the multilevel model with random intercepts and slopes.

response given measured student covariates, school random intercepts and the interactions between student covariates and random school effects (i.e., random slopes) we estimated the prognostic scores as

$$\Psi(X, W, U_{0k}) = E[r^{(0)}|X, W, U_{0k}] \qquad (15.21)$$

After several iterative specifications of the propensity score model, our final propensity score model included several higher-order terms and interactions. The model was

$$\log\left(\frac{P(Z_j = 1)}{1 - P(Z_j = 1)}\right) = \beta_0 + \sum_{p=1}^{4} \beta_p X_{pj} + \varepsilon_j \qquad (15.22)$$

$Z_j$ is the treatment assignment for student $j$, and $\beta_p$ is used to denote the coefficients associated with family socioeconomic status, mother's education, the student's gender, free/reduced lunch status, each interaction between these variables, family socioeconomic status squared, and mother's education squared.

### Covariate Balance

Figure 15.1 and Table 15.3 describe the improvement in balance for each of the covariates considered (and the log of those variables) brought about by stratifying along quintiles of the prognostic scores using standardized regression coefficients and their $t$-values. Unconditional values (i.e., coefficients and $t$-values) express the magnitude of the relationship between

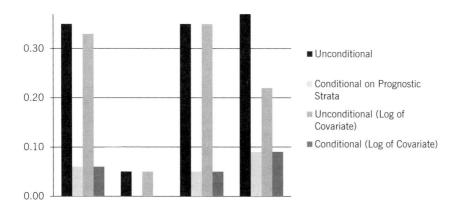

**FIGURE 15.1.** Prognostic balance.

**TABLE 15.3. Prognostic Score Balance Using Standardized Regression Coefficients**

|  | Mother's education | Student gender | Free and reduced lunch eligibility | Family socioeconomic status |
|---|---|---|---|---|
| Unconditional | 0.35 | 0.05 | 0.35 | 0.37 |
| Conditional | 0.06 | −0.01 | 0.05 | 0.09 |
| Unconditional (log of covariate) | 0.33 | 0.05 | 0.35 | 0.22 |
| Conditional (log of covariate) | 0.06 | −0.01 | 0.05 | 0.09 |
| Unconditional $t$-value | 14.70 | 1.83 | 14.90 | 15.60 |
| Conditional $t$-value | 0.93 | −0.18 | 0.83 | 1.51 |
| Unconditional $t$-value (log of covariate) | 13.90 | 1.83 | 14.90 | 8.84 |
| Conditional $t$-value (log of covariate) | 0.96 | −0.18 | 0.83 | 1.52 |

a covariate and the outcome and the associated significance. Conditional assessments describe similar quantities but are based on the average absolute value across each of the prognostic strata.

As is evident from these tables, stratifying along prognostic strata substantively improved prognostic balance on each covariate. Before prognostic stratification, other than gender each of the covariates and their log transformations was significantly related to mathematics achievement in the control group (Table 15.3). After stratifying on quintiles of the prognostic score, the relationship between the covariate and outcome was substantially reduced and was no longer statistically significant (Table 15.3). Similarly, whereas the unconditional intraclass correlation among all students in the control group was 0.21 and significant, the average intraclass correlation coefficient across the prognostic strata was reduced to less than 0.05 and its confidence interval included zero. Collectively, the minimal relationships between covariates and the outcome and lack of school-level variation within each of the prognostic strata suggested that students within a prognostic stratum were relatively homogeneous and balanced on observed characteristics as they related to their potential responses under the control condition.

Table 15.4 illustrates similar balance assessments capturing the differences in covariate distributions across treatment groups (i.e., propensity score balance) instead of covariate distributions across the potential responses under the control condition. Before incorporating adjustments for propensity score matches and/or prognostic strata, the absolute standardized mean difference across treatment conditions was moderate to large and significant for each of the observed covariates save gender. After matching on the propensity score, differences among students who attended a prekindergarten program and those who did not were reduced to nearly zero (Table 15.4). When we combined propensity score matching with stratification on prognostic scores, the average absolute standardized mean difference of covariates between treatment conditions (i.e., propensity score balance) and across prognostic strata decreased markedly from the unconditional differences, but these differences increased slightly from those found with using only the propensity score. Balance might be improved with alternative respecifications. However, the imbalances found were acceptable by most standards and suitable for the purposes of this example (Rubin, 2001; Stuart, 2010; Stuart & Rubin, 2007).

The small reductions in propensity score balance found when integrating adjustments for propensity and prognostic scores (see Table 15.4) demonstrated important trade-offs. The small reductions in propensity score balance are associated with the relative importance we place on covariates in constructing matches and strata and the relationships each covariate has with treatment assignment and the outcome (Brookhart et al., 2006; Stuart, Lee, & Leacy, 2013). In constructing matches and strata, giving more weight to covariates that are predictive of the treatment assignment tends to provide precise propensity score balance on predictors (i.e., balance across treatment conditions). Such precise balance on covariates

**TABLE 15.4. Propensity Score Balance Using Absolute Standardized Mean Difference**

|  | Mother's education | Student gender | Free and reduced lunch | Socioeconomic status |
|---|---|---|---|---|
| No adjustment | 0.33* | 0.01 | 0.12* | 0.25* |
| Propensity score only | 0.00 | 0.01 | 0.03 | 0.02 |
| Propensity score within prognostic strata | 0.00 | 0.07 | 0.04 | 0.03 |

*Differences are significant at the $p < .05$ level.

predictive of the treatment assignment tends to address overt bias (e.g., bias introduced by observed covariates), but tends to be less efficient and miss more obscure bias (e.g., bias emerging from covariates weakly predictive of the treatment but strongly predictive of the potential outcomes; Brookhart et al., 2006; Westreich, Cole, Funk, Brookhart, & Sturmer, 2011). In contrast, constructing matches and strata using covariates predictive of the potential outcomes (i.e., the prognostic score), regardless of the degree to which they predict treatment assignment, tends to trade precise propensity score balance on covariates that are highly predictive of the treatment assignment for a coarser propensity score balance on all covariates and better prognostic balance on covariates (Kelcey, 2011b, 2013). In turn, research has demonstrated that such balance (on propensity and prognostic balance) tends to be an effective strategy for reducing bias and variance because it produces more precise balance on covariates that are most predictive of the potential responses, as such covariates could introduce the most bias if left unbalanced (Brookhart et al., 2006; Hansen, 2006; Stuart, Lee, & Leacy, 2013).

## Treatment Effects

Under the artificial assumption that there is no bias from unobserved covariates, we estimated the treatment effects using (1) no adjustments, (2) adjustments for only the propensity score, and (3) adjustments for the propensity and prognostic score. The results are presented in Table 15.5. Unconditional comparisons among students who participated in a prekindergarten program and those who did not suggested that attending a prekindergarten program significantly improved students' mathematics achievement by about 0.71 standard deviations (Table 15.5). However, comparisons that took into account the differences between the treatment and control groups through propensity score matching suggested that at least some of the unadjusted effect could be explained by selection bias (see Table 15.5, rows 1 and 2). Although the propensity-score-based estimator suggested that the treatment effect was still statistically significant, it indicated that the effect was about 20% less than the unadjusted differences. When taking into account both propensity and prognostic scores, the estimate of the effect considerably reduced further. Adjusting for both scores suggested that the effect size was less than half of that based on the propensity score only and that the estimate was not statistically different from zero (Table 15.5).

Collectively, the results of our application suggested that subclassification based on a combination of the propensity and prognostic scores

**TABLE 15.5. Treatment Effect Estimates by Propensity Score Method**

|  | Estimated effect | Standard error | $t$-value |
|---|---|---|---|
| No propensity score adjustment | 0.71* | 0.25 | 2.87 |
| Propensity score only | 0.55* | 0.27 | 2.03 |
| Propensity score within prognostic strata | 0.24 | 0.27 | 0.88 |

*Treatment effect estimate is significant at the $p < .05$ level.

produced substantively different effect sizes as compared to subclassification on the propensity score only. Because our application represents an (artificial) empirical study and the true treatment effect is unknown, the authority of the treatment effect estimate based on adjustment for both the propensity and prognostic scores over alternative estimators is unclear. However, very limited research into the comparative performance of propensity and/or prognostic-score-based treatment effect estimators would suggest that adjustment for both the propensity and prognostic scores yields a less biased and more efficient estimator (Hansen, 2006; Kelcey, 2013). However, much more work needs to be done to study the efficacy of such methods and the conditions under which use of prognostic scores in combination with the propensity scores outperform alternative approaches.

## CONCLUSION

In this chapter, we described how prognostic scores might be extended to accommodate clustered or multilevel data. The critical consideration is how to take into account both the effects of clusters and the extent to which the strength of individual-level predictors varied across these clusters. We considered several different approaches that paralleled more general approaches to clustered data and found the multilevel random intercepts and slopes approach to be the most flexible.

We provided an example investigating the effects of prekindergarten program participation on kindergarten mathematics achievement using a small set of covariates and several unidimensional prognostic score models. The results of the application suggested that the multilevel random intercepts and slopes model best captured students' potential responses under the control condition.

Although there is evidence that when combined with propensity scores, prognostic scores improve treatment effect estimates, the size and scope of studies examining the value of introducing the prognostic score alongside the propensity score is limited. For this reason, it is important that future research consider the limitations of prior research in several areas. We highlight six important areas.

First, literature has largely demonstrated use of prognostic scores with only a relatively small number of covariates. However, as with propensity score applications, most investigations potentially involve many covariates. The approaches outlined in this chapter can become complicated quickly by increasing the number of covariates considered. For instance, although it is reasonable to consider a multilevel model with only a few random slopes, estimating a multilevel model with many random slopes can be challenging because for many models the dimensions of integration increase with the number of random effects.

Second, there is little research that has investigated strategies for integrating propensity and prognostic scores. Hansen (2006) suggested combining them through Mahalanobis distance and we opted to combine them using matching and stratification. Although limited simulations suggested that propensity score matching within prognostic strata perform well, there are clearly situations in which this strategy will fail and there are clearly many viable alternative strategies (e.g., prognostic score matching within propensity score strata or combinations of weighting and stratifying) that have not been fully investigated.

Third, to date there has been little research considering the dimensionality of prognostic scores. More specifically, for continuous outcomes following a normal distribution, the prognostic score reduces to a scalar only if the error variance is constant. If instead the error variance depends on the observed covariates the prognostic score would be two-dimensional. Future work should investigate the extent to which the benefits of incorporating a scalar prognostic score are sensitive to the dimensionality of the prognostic score. Similarly, there has been little research examining the diagnosis and impact of model misspecification in prognostic score models. It would appear that the potential to develop diagnostic tools for detecting misspecification in prognostic score models would be high.

A fourth limitation not considered in this chapter was whether prognostic matches should be restricted to within a school or whether matches across schools should be permitted. Literature has noted that propensity-score-based methods tend to perform less well when matches are constructed using units from different social contexts. Extending this to prognostic scores challenges whether, for example, we should construct prognostic strata or matches solely within a school or whether we should allow the subclassifications to cross school boundaries. The choice offers a tradeoff. Restricting subclassifications to students within schools may shield against residual bias from unobserved school-level factors. However, such protection is often coupled with a lack of comparable matches within each school because restricting comparisons to within schools generally requires a large reservoir of treatment and control students in each school to ensure high-quality matches. In constrast, allowing subclassifications to contain students from different schools likely improves the reservoir of potential matches and often leads to higher quality matches. Because the multilevel random intercepts and slopes approach outlined above takes into account both school membership and how the predictive capacities of covariates vary across schools, the estimated responses under the control condition are more comparable across schools. As a result, multilevel prognostic score models technically make it reasonable to create subclassifications using students from different schools. The advantage of matching across schools, however, is paired with the assumption that there are no unobserved school-level covariates.

Fifth, as we discussed before there is a significant risk of overfitting in estimating a prognostic model because it is estimated using only the control portion of the sample. Although the seminal paper by Hansen (2008) noted this concern, there has been little research examining overfitting and its impact on treatment effect estimates. Future work needs to critically examine the conditions under which adjustment on prognostic scores are useful in the presence of overfitting.

A sixth area of research involves examining the extent to which the use of prognostic scores reduces study objectivity. As discussed earlier, many researchers advocate for a clear separation of the design and analysis phases of study so that, for example, matching is conducted without the use of observed outcomes. In theory, such separation supports the objectivity of a study because matches will not have been chosen to yield a particular result. Prognostic scores and the theory that supports them suggest that the conditions of such separation should be more flexible and allow the use of outcomes for the control units (but not the treated units). Future research needs to continue to examine the tradeoff between the value of objectivity and properties of estimators.

In conclusion, when used in conjunction with propensity scores, prognostic scores have shown significant potential to reduce the bias and variance of estimated treatment effects. This potential is largely built on the fact that prognostic score models complement propensity score models because they explicitly consider the relationships of covariates with the outcome. Because the bias reduction capacity of a covariate is proportional to the concurrent relationships it has with the outcome and treatment assignment, matching on both the propensity and the prognostic score privileges empirical confounders—those covariates that empirically demonstrate strong relationships with both the treatment assignment and the outcome. Despite the benefits of prognostic scores, their use blurs the clear separation of the design and analysis phases of a study. Prognostic scores and the theory that supports them, however, suggest that the conditions of such separation should be more flexible and allow for the use of outcomes for the control units (but not the treated units). Future research needs to continue to examine the trade-offs between the objectivity gained through complete separation and the bias and variance gains made by use of prognostic scores.

## REFERENCES

Bainbridge, J., Meyers, M., Tanaka, S., & Waldfogel, J. (2005). Who gets an early education?: Family income and the gaps in enrollment of 3–5 year olds from 1968 to 2000. *Social Science Quarterly, 86,* 724–745.

Bates, D., Maechler, M., & Bolker, B. (2013). lme4: Linear mixed-effects models using s4 classes [Computer software manual]. Retrieved from *http://cran.r--project.org/package=lme4* (R package version 0.999999–2)

Brookhart, M., Schneeweiss, S., Rothman, K., Glynn, R., Avorn, J., & Sturmer, T. (2006). Variable selection for propensity score models. *Practice of Epidemiology, 163,* 1149–1156.

Brooks-Gunn, J. (2003). Do you believe in magic? What we can expect from early childhood intervention programs? SRCD. *Social Policy Report, 17,* 3–14.

Hansen, B. (2008). The prognostic analogue of the propensity score. *Biometrika, 95,* 481–488.

Hansen, B. B. (2006). *Bias reduction in observational studies via prognostic scores.* (University of Michigan, Statistics Department, Technical Report 441). Retrieved March 2010 from *www.stat.lsa.umich.edu/~bbh/rspaper2006–06.pdf.*

Ho, D. E., Imai, K., King, G., & Stuart, E. A. (2011). MatchIt: Nonparametric preprocessing for parametric causal inference. *Journal of Statistical Software, 42*(8), 1–28.

Hong, G., & Raudenbush, S. (2006). Evaluating kindergarten retention policy: A case study of causal inference for multilevel observational data. *Journal of the American Statistical Association, 101,* 901–910.

Iacus, S. M., King, G., & Porro, G. (2011). *Causal inference without balance checking: Coarsened exact matching, political analysis.* Unpublished.

Kelcey, B. (2011a). Assessing the effects of teachers' reading knowledge on students' achievement using multilevel propensity score stratification. *Education Evaluation and Policy Analysis, 33,* 458–482.

Kelcey, B. (2011b). Covariate selection in propensity scores using outcome proxies. *Multivariate Behavioral Research, 46,* 453–476.

Kelcey, B. (2013). *Propensity score matching within prognostic strata.* Paper presented at the spring conference of the Society for Research on Educational Effectiveness.

Kim, J., & Seltzer, M. (2007). *Causal inference in multilevel settings in which selection processes vary across schools* (CSE Technical Report 708). Los Angeles: National Center for Research on Evaluation, Standards and Student Testing, University of California.

Magnuson, K., Ruhm, C., & Waldfogel, J. (2007). Does prekindergarten improve school preparation and performance? *Economics of Education Review, 26,* 33–51.

Neyman, J., & Scott, E. L. (1948). Consistent estimates based on partially consistent observations. *Econometrica: Journal of the Econometric Society,* 1–32.

Nye, B., Konstantopoulous, S., & Hedges, L. V. (2004). How large are teacher effects? *Education Evaluation and Policy Analysis, 26,* 327–357.

Raudenbush, S. W., & Bryk, A. S. (2002). *Hierarchical linear models: Applications and data analysis methods.* New York: Sage.

R Core Team. (2013). *R: A language and environment for statistical computing.* Vienna, Austria: R Foundation for Statistical Computing. Retrieved from www.R-project.org.

Rosenbaum, P., & Rubin, D. (1983). The central role of the propensity score in observational studies for causal effects. *Biometrika, 70,* 41–55.

Rosenbaum, P. (1986). Dropping out of high school in the United States: An observational study. *Journal of Educational Statistics, 11*(3), 207–224.

Rubin, D. (2007). The design *versus* the analysis of observational studies for causal effects: Parallels with the design of randomized trials. *Statistics in Medicine, 26,* 20–26.

Rubin, D. B. (1976). Multivariate matching methods that are equal percent bias reducing: I. Some examples. *Biometrics, 32,* 109–120.

Rubin, D. B. (1979). Using multivariate matched sampling and regression adjustment to control bias in observation studies. *Journal of the American Statistical Association, 74,* 318–328.

Rubin, D. B. (2001). Using propensity scores to help design observational studies: Application to the tobacco litigation. *Health Services and Outcomes Research Methodology, 2*(3–4), 169–188.

Rubin, D. B., & Thomas, N. (2000). Combining propensity score matching with additional adjustments for prognostic covariates. *Journal of the American Statistical Association, 95*(450), 573–585.

Stuart, E. A. (2010). Matching methods for causal inference: A review and a look forward. *Statistical Science, 25,* 1–21.

Stuart, E., Lee, B., & Leacy, F. (2013). Prognostic score-based balance measures can be a useful diagnostic for propensity score methods in comparative effectiveness research. *Journal of Clinical Epidemiology, 66*, 84–90.

Stuart, E., & Rubin, D. B. (2007). Best practices in quasi-experimental designs: Matching methods for causal inference. In J. Osborne (Ed.), *Best practices in quantitative social science* (pp. 155–176). Thousand Oaks, CA: Sage.

U.S. Department of Education. (2003). *The condition of education.* Washington, DC: National Center for Education Statistics.

Waldfogel, J. (2002). Child care, women's employment and child outcomes. *Journal of Population Economics, 15*, 527–548.

Westreich, D., Cole, S. R., Funk, M. J., Brookhart, M. A., & Sturmer, T. (2011). The role of the c-statistic in variable selection for propensity score models. *Pharmacoepidemiol Drug Safety, 20*, 317–320.

# Author Index

Abadie, A., 27, 75, 146, 152, 171
Ackermann, D., 306
Agresti, A., 6
Ahmed, A., 93, 102
Alexander, K. L., 79
Allison, P. D., 78
Alpert, A., 191
Anderson, G. M., 120, 249
Anthony, J. C., 54, 117, 118, 271
Arah, O. A., 321
Asparouhov, T., 199, 241
Austin, P. C., 7, 9, 12, 13, 15, 76, 115, 116, 117, 118, 120, 122, 123, 126, 133, 134, 137, 143, 146, 148, 154, 157, 165, 191, 193, 202, 249, 269, 306
Avorn, J., 299, 302, 307, 322

**B**

Bai, H., 3, 74, 75, 79, 116, 118, 124, 134
Bainbridge, J., 359
Ball, D. L., 79
Bang, H., 170
Bartels, D. B., 306
Barth, R. P., 7
Bates, D., 366
Bauer, K. W., 245
Belin, T., 275
Belitser, S. V., 306
Bentler, P. M., 203
Berger, V., 217
Berglund, P., 230
Bergstralh, E., 22
Berk, R. A., 117, 122
Biemer, P. P., 239, 240
Black, A. R., 231
Blackwell, M., 28, 29
Bloom, H. S., 217, 231
Bolker, B., 366
Bollen, K. A., 191, 195, 196, 207
Bosker, R. J., 192, 239
Bowers, J., 154
Bradshaw, C., 79

Breiman, L., 50, 51, 60
Brookhart, M. A., 13, 21, 56, 92, 192, 270, 306, 308, 369, 370
Brooks, J. M., 307
Brooks-Gunn, J., 359
Bross, I. D., 321
Brosseau-Liard, P. E., 202
Brumback, B. A., 11, 41, 98, 268, 321, 322, 335
Bryk, A. S., 192, 238, 358, 362
Bühlmann, P., 50
Burgette, L. F., 49, 54, 67, 202
Burstein, L., 223
Butcher, I., 217
Byar, D. P., 217

## C

Cai, Z., 321
Caliendo, M., 9, 74, 76, 81, 116, 133
Campbell, D. T., 74, 218, 253
Campbell, R. T., 231
Chambers, R. L., 237
Chen, F., 207
Chen, M.-H., 275
Cheong, J., 196
Chiba, Y., 321
Cho, Y. B., 269
Christ, S. L., 239, 240
Christenson, S. L., 79
Clark, M. H., 15, 74, 115, 116, 120, 133
Coca-Perraillon, M., 22, 25
Cochran, W. G., 7, 9, 58, 81, 116, 124, 217, 218, 219, 220, 252
Cohen, J., 58, 79
Cohen, M. H., 321
Cole, S. R., 307, 308, 321, 370
Cook, D., 8, 13, 14, 253, 254
Cook, E. F., 13, 21, 192, 270
Cook, T. D., 74, 120, 133, 253
Copas, J. B., 321
Cornfield, J., 321
Cox, D. R., 6
Crump, R. K., 171
Cundiff, N. L., 116, 123

Curran, P. J., 191, 192, 194, 195, 196, 207, 208
Czajka, J. C., 98

## D

da Veiga, P. V., 269
D'Agostino Jr., R. B., 108, 117, 270, 271, 272, 276, 279, 299
Davey Smith, G., 302
Davidian, M., 15, 150, 268, 292
Dehejia, R. H., 7, 29, 49, 75, 76, 77, 85, 86, 90, 173
Dempster, A. P., 271
Dendukuri, N., 270
Dennis, M. L., 62
Diamond, A., 7, 97, 201, 232
Diehr, P., 217
Donders, R. A. R. T., 272
Donner, A., 217
Drake, C., 55
Duell, O. K., 79
DuGoff, E. H., 237, 241
Duncan, S. C., 191
Duncan, T. E., 191

## E

Eisermann, J., 133
Enders, C. K., 200
Entwisle, D. R., 79

## F

Falconer, M. K., 116
Fan, X., 196
Faries, D. E., 24, 35, 41, 43
Ferguson, A. J., 238
Fewell, Z., 302
Fink, A. K., 321
Flanders, W. D., 321
Forbes, A., 292
Forthofer, R. N., 238

Fox, M. P., 321
Franklin, J. M., 306, 310
Fraser, M. W., 124, 250, 253
Freedman, D. A., 109, 117, 122
Freedman, L. S., 217
Freund, Y., 50
Friedman, J. H., 49, 50, 51, 70
Funk, M. J., 270, 308, 370

## G

Gao, X., 275
García Rodríguez, L. A., 304
Gentleman, J. F., 258
Gibbons, C., 7
Gilbert, S. A., 126
Glynn, R. J., 13, 21, 74, 192, 270, 299, 302, 307, 322
Goldstein, H., 192
Gondolf, E. W., 299
Gorney, D., 79
Graham, J. W., 268, 270
Graubard, B. I., 238
Green, S. B., 217
Greene, T., 141, 142, 143, 149, 151, 152, 153, 154, 158, 163
Greenland, S., 311, 314, 321, 322
Griffin, B. A., 49, 54, 67, 69, 202, 218
Grobbee, D. E., 297
Grobman, W. A., 126
Groenwold, R. H., 296, 297, 298, 299, 305, 308, 312, 313
Grootendorst, P., 120, 249
Gu, X. S., 7, 8, 74, 82, 86, 193, 201
Guo, S. Y., 7, 12, 124, 250, 253
Gustafson, P., 14, 322

## H

Hahs-Vaughn, D. L., 193, 217, 237, 240, 241, 242, 252, 260
Hak, E., 296, 297, 299, 312
Halloran, M. E., 6
Hancock, G. R., 194

Haneuse, S. J., 321
Hanley, J. A., 270
Hansen, B. B., 8, 30, 37, 98, 154, 348, 350, 351, 352, 353, 354, 364, 370, 371, 372, 373
Hanushek, E. A., 79
Harder, V. S., 54, 59, 117, 118, 121, 122, 124, 126, 134, 136, 271
Hardy, R. J., 217
Harrell Jr., F. E., 272
Harris, A., 299
Hasselblad, V., 124
Hastie, T., 49, 50, 52
Haviland, A. M., 230, 231, 273, 275
Heck, R. H., 239, 240, 245
Heckert, A., 299
Heckman, J. J., 4, 8, 76, 198, 200, 218
Hedges, L. V., 124, 217, 354
Heimberg, R. G., 230, 231
Hernan, M. A., 11, 41, 98, 170, 268, 304, 321, 322, 325
Herring, A. H., 275
Hettmansperger, T. J., 180, 184
Hill, H., 79
Hill, J. L., 116, 174, 175, 272, 273, 287
Hirabayashi, S. M., 98
Hirano, K., 12, 31, 98, 122, 126, 150
Ho, D. E., 7, 10, 14, 21, 23, 37, 43, 58, 78, 81, 82, 86, 103, 153, 227, 366
Hodgkins, D., 62
Hoes, A. W., 296, 297, 299, 305, 312, 313
Hoffman, N. G., 133
Hogan, J. W., 321
Holland, P. W., 4, 91, 219
Holt, D., 236
Hong, G., 6, 217, 218, 354
Hornik, R., 237
Horvitz, D. G., 12
Hotz, V. J., 171
Houang, T. R., 221
Hudgens, M. G., 6
Hudson, C. M., 231
Huitema, B. E., 168, 170, 171, 174, 180
Hullsiek, K. H., 268
Humphries, J. E., 198

Hunt, P., 131, 133, 135
Hutter, R., 79
Hux, J. E., 117

## I

Iacus, S., 28, 29
Iacus, S. M., 89, 98, 350
Ibrahim, J. G., 275
Ichimura, H., 4, 76
Imai, K., 7, 9, 21, 58, 74, 78, 80, 99, 103, 108, 153, 154, 227, 249, 366
Imbens, G. W., 4, 5, 12, 27, 31, 55, 75, 98, 122, 126, 143, 145, 146, 150, 152, 169, 171, 192, 322

## J

Jayasundera, T., 299
Jimenez, F., 201
Joffe, M. M., 246
Jones, A. S., 299
Judd, C. M., 238

## K

Kain, J. F., 79
Kalton, G., 238, 239, 241, 260
Kang, J. D. Y., 8, 15, 117, 118, 119, 120, 133, 134, 135, 137, 150
Kaplan, D., 238
Karr, A. F., 270
Karter, A., 270
Kaufman, J. S., 321
Kaufman, S., 321
Kaya, Y., 201
Kelcey, B., 348, 354, 365, 370, 371
Kenny, D. A., 238
Kereiakes, D. J., 323, 343
Kessler, R. C., 230
Khoo, S. T., 196
Khoury, M. J., 321
Kim, E. S., 134, 242, 252
Kim, J., 354
King, G., 7, 9, 21, 28, 29, 58, 78, 80, 89, 99, 103, 108, 153, 154, 227, 249, 350, 366
Kirby, J. B., 207
Kish, L., 238, 239, 240
Klar, N., 217
Kloke, J. D., 181, 185
Klopfer, S. O., 30, 37
Klungel, O. H., 296, 311
Ko, H., 321
Koepsell, T. D., 217
Konstantopoulous, S., 354
Kopeinig, S., 9, 74, 76, 81, 116, 133
Korn, E. L., 238
Kosanke, J., 22
Kosten, S. F., 168, 174, 175, 176
Koth, C., 79
Kronmal, R. A., 312, 313, 314
Kuroki, M., 321
Kurth, T., 12, 15, 117, 118, 122, 126

## L

Laird, N. M., 271
LaLonde, R. J., 90, 91, 93, 94, 95, 96, 99, 100, 101, 102, 104, 105, 106
Landon, M. B., 126
Landrum, M. B., 145, 149
Lanehart, R. E., 35
Lang, W., 270
Langenskiold, S., 107
Lapane, K. L., 307
Lash, T. L., 321
Laupacis, A., 117
Lawrence, F. R., 194
Le, T., 245
Leacy, F., 369, 370
Leaf, P., 79
Lee, B. K., 14, 20, 33, 54, 59, 121, 122, 137, 369, 370
Lee, E. S., 238
Lee, M., 275
Lee, W. S., 154
Leite, W. L., 191, 194, 196, 201, 208

Leon, A. C., 24
Leon, S., 292
Lepkowski, J. M., 275
Lessler, J., 14, 20, 54, 59, 121, 270
Leuven, E., 22
Levy, A. R., 14, 322
Li, F., 145, 149, 191
Li, H. G., 321
Li, L., 141, 142, 143, 149, 151, 152, 153, 154, 158, 163, 320, 322, 334, 335
Li, X., 320, 322, 334
Lin, D. Y., 312, 314
Lipkovich, I., 275
Lipsitz, S. R., 275
Little, R. J. A., 78, 98, 269, 272, 279
Lockheed, M., 299
Lohr, S., 239
Louis, T. A., 268
Lu, B., 237
Luellen, J. K., 74, 116, 121, 133
Lumley, T., 238
Lunceford, J. K., 15, 150, 268
Lunt, M., 302

## M

MacCallum, R. C., 222
Macinnes, J. W., 201
Mackinnon, D. P., 196
MacLehose, R. F., 321
Mader, N. S., 198
Madigan, D., 50
Maechler, M., 366
Magnuson, K., 359
Mahoe, R., 239
Maitland-van der Zee, A. H., 311
Mamdani, M. M., 15, 116, 117, 118, 122, 133, 137
Margolick, J. B., 321
Maria Haro, J., 24
Markman, J. M., 79
Martin, D. C., 217
Mayer, K. H., 321
McArdle, J. J., 209

McCaffrey, D. F., 14, 20, 33, 49, 54, 56, 59, 60, 62, 67, 71, 117, 135, 192, 202, 218, 270, 323, 338
McCall, W. A., 218
McCandless, L. C., 14, 322
McKean, J. W., 168, 174, 177, 180, 181, 184, 185
Meyer, J. A., 56
Meyers, M., 359
Miettinen, O. S., 299
Ming, K., 29
Miratrix, L. W., 109
Mitnik, O. A., 171
Mitra, R., 201, 267, 273, 274, 275, 276, 277, 279, 282, 284, 285, 286, 288, 289, 290, 291, 292
Moons, K. G. M., 272, 279
Morgan, K. L., 109
Morgan, S. L., 4, 12, 13, 219
Morgan, T., 270
Morral, A. R., 14, 20, 33, 54, 56, 71, 117, 192, 202, 270, 323, 338
Mun, E. Y., 209
Murray, D. M., 217, 238
Muthén, B. O., 192, 194, 202, 208, 223, 225, 241
Muthén, L. K., 202, 225
Myers, J. A., 308

## N

Nagin, D. S., 230, 231, 273
Necowitz, L. B., 222
Nelson, D. B., 312
Neutra, R., 322
Neyman, J., 218, 356
Nichol, K. L., 299, 312
Nord, C., 245
Nye, B., 354

## O

Obenchain, R. L., 24
Ohsfeldt, R. L., 307

Olkin, I., 271
Olshen, R. A., 51
Onwuegbuzie, A. J., 193, 237, 241, 260
Ou, S. R., 200
Oudshoorn, C. G. M., 200

**P**

Pan, W., 3
Pane, J. F., 218
Parris, D., 116
Pattanayak, C. W., 89, 107, 109
Paxton, P., 207
Pearl, J., 308
Peng, S. S., 240
Perrin, E. B., 217
Peugh, J. L., 200
Pfeffermann, D., 238
Phillips, C. V., 312
Pitts, S. C., 208
Pohl, S., 133
Poole, C., 321
Porro, G., 28, 29, 89, 350
Prindle, J. J., 209
Psaty, B. M., 312, 314
Pyke, S. D. M., 217

**Q**

Qu, Y., 275

**R**

Raab, G. M., 217
Radbill, L., 239
Raghunathan, T. E., 275
Rao, J. N. K., 241
Rassen, J., 306
Rassen, J. A., 306
Raudenbush, S. W., 6, 192, 217, 218, 238, 354, 358, 362

Reiter, J. P., 174, 175, 201, 270, 272, 273, 274, 275, 276, 277, 279, 282, 284, 285, 286, 287, 288, 289, 290, 291, 292
Rhemtulla, M., 202
Richburg-Hayes, L., 231
Ridder, G., 12, 98
Ridgeway, G., 14, 20, 33, 49, 50, 54, 56, 71, 117, 192, 202, 270, 323, 338
Rivkin, S. G., 79
Robb, R., Jr., 4
Robins, J. M., 11, 12, 41, 98, 170, 268, 321, 322, 325, 335
Rosenbaum, P. R., 3, 4, 5, 6, 7, 8, 9, 10, 12, 13, 14, 29, 30, 31, 34, 37, 49, 56, 74, 75, 76, 80, 81, 82, 86, 89, 92, 97, 98, 117, 123, 137, 142, 158, 193, 201, 217, 237, 245, 246, 249, 268, 270, 273, 296, 306, 320, 321, 326, 348, 349, 351, 354, 355
Rosenthal, R., 250
Rosnow, R. L., 250
Rotheram-Borus, M., 275
Rothman, K. J., 299, 302, 307, 322
Rotnitzky, A., 326
Rounds, T., 79
Rowan, R. B., 79
Roznowski, M., 222
Rubin, D. B., 3, 4, 5, 6, 7, 8, 9, 10, 13, 14, 22, 34, 49, 56, 74, 75, 76, 77, 78, 80, 81, 86, 89, 90, 91, 92, 97, 98, 104, 105, 107, 108, 109, 117, 123, 124, 133, 137, 142, 158, 175, 217, 218, 219, 228, 229, 237, 249, 250, 252, 268, 269, 270, 271, 272, 273, 276, 279, 296, 306, 320, 321, 326, 348, 349, 351, 352, 353, 354, 363, 364, 369
Ruhm, C., 359
Rust, K. F., 240

**S**

Sandbach, R., 201
Särndal, C. E., 218

Satorra, A., 203
Sauer, B. C., 141
Savalei, V., 202
Schafer, J. L., 8, 15, 117, 118, 119, 120, 133, 134, 135, 137, 150, 268, 270, 271, 275, 276, 291
Schapire, R., 50
Schenker, N., 258
Schlesselman, J. J., 322
Schmidt, W. H., 221, 223
Schneeweiss, S., 13, 20, 74, 192, 270, 299, 305, 306, 312, 322
Schommer-Aitkins, M., 79
Schonlau, M., 50
Schuit, E., 310
Schuler, M., 20, 62, 63, 66, 237
Schuster, T., 12
Scott, A., 217
Scott, E. L., 356
Sekhon, J. S., 7, 97, 109, 193, 199, 201, 227, 232
Seltzer, M., 354
Setoguchi, S., 13, 14, 20, 33, 192, 270
Shadish, W. R., 15, 74, 116, 118, 119, 120, 122, 135, 137, 253
Shah, B. R., 117, 118
Shaikh, A. M., 154
Sheather, S. J., 177
Shen, C. Y., 320, 322, 326, 334
Sianesi, B., 22
Simonsen, M., 154
Sivo, S. A., 196
Skinner, C. J., 236, 237
Smith, A. J., 75
Smith, T. M. F., 217, 236
Snijders, T. A. B., 192, 239
Sobel, M. E., 4, 6
Soellner, R., 133
Solenberger, P., 275
Solomon, D. H., 306
Song, J., 275
Sorongon, A., 245
Stanley, J. C., 218
Stapleton, L. M., 202, 241
Stein, M. B., 230

Steiner, P. M., 8, 13, 14, 15, 116, 120, 133, 253, 254
Sterne, J. A., 302
Stijnen, T., 272
Stone, C. A., 117, 121, 122, 137
Stone, C. J., 51
Strumpf, G., 131, 133, 135
Strycker, L. A., 191
Stuart, E. A., 6, 7, 8, 9, 13, 14, 21, 30, 54, 58, 59, 78, 80, 98, 99, 103, 104, 108, 115, 116, 117, 118, 121, 124, 146, 153, 154, 191, 192, 227, 228, 229, 237, 249, 352, 363, 366, 369, 370
Stürmer, T., 74, 118, 299, 301, 307, 308, 322, 370
Swensson, B., 218
Swoboda, C. M., 348

T

Tanaka, S., 359
Tang, Y., 117, 121, 122, 137
Tannen, R. L., 271
Tanner, M. A., 285
Tate, R. F., 271
Thoemmes, F. J., 134, 242, 252
Thomas, N., 7, 364
Thomas, S. L., 240, 245
Thompson, D. J., 12
Thompson, S. G., 217
Tibshirani, R., 49, 50
Titus, J. C., 62
Todd, J. J., 12, 13
Todd, P. E., 4, 75, 76
Toh, S., 304
Tomarken, A. J., 194
Tourangeau, K., 244, 245
Tsiatis, A. A., 292
Turpie, A. G., 90

U

Unsicker, J., 62

## V

Van Buuren, S., 200, 275
van Dyk, D. A., 74
van Hoewyk, J., 275
Vandenbroucke, J. P., 299
von Eye, A., 209
Vytlacil, E. J., 154

## W

Wahba, S., 7, 29, 49, 75, 76, 77, 85, 86, 90, 173
Waldfogel, J., 359
Walkup, M., 270
Waller, N. G., 194
Wang, P. S., 306
Wang, Q., 217, 227
Weiner, M. G., 271
Were, M. C., 322, 334
Westreich, D., 270, 307, 308, 370
White, H. R., 209
White, M., 62
Wilder, R. P., 269
Wiley, D. E., 223, 225
Williamson, E., 292
Winship, C., 4, 219, 239
Witta, E. L., 196
Wolfe, R. G., 223, 225, 292
Wolter, K. M., 240
Wong, W. H., 285
Woo, M.-J., 270
Wooldridge, J. M., 55, 143, 145, 169
Wretman, J., 218
Wu, A. C., 322

## X

Xie, D., 271

## Y

Yildiz, N., 154
Yu, B., 50, 109

## Z

Zanutto, E. L., 237, 241, 245, 252, 272
Zaslavsky, A. M., 145, 149
Zhao, L. P., 326
Zubizarreta, J. R., 89, 97

# Subject Index

The letter *f* following a page number indicates figure; the letter *t* indicates table

*a priori* adjustments, 245
Absolute differences, 102–103, 102*f*
Absolute standardized mean difference (ASMD), 369–370, 369*t*. *See also* Standardized bias (SB)
Across and within methods
  examples of, 289–292, 291*f*
  missing data, 279–284, 280*t*, 281*t*, 282*t*
Actual treatment received, 307
Ad hoc imputation methods, 275–277
Adjustment computations
  complex survey samples, 244–246
  prognostic scores, 350–351
  propensity score adjustment, 134–135
Aggregated approach. *See* Design-based approach
Analysis of covariance (ANCOVA)
  estimands, 170
  latent growth modeling, 192
  observational study design, 169
Analysis of outcome. *See* Outcome analysis

Analysis of variance (ANOVA)
  latent growth modeling, 192
  propensity score adjustment, 116, 118, 126, 135
Assumptions
  of propensity scores, 5–6
  sensitivity analysis, 320–322, 336–337
Asymmetric estimation, 352
Average treatment effect (ATE). *See also* Population average treatment effect (PATE); Treatment effects
  complex survey samples, 253–258, 255*t*–256*t*, 257*f*
  generalized boosted modeling, 59, 63, 65, 66–67
  latent growth modeling, 192
  matching weights, 142
  missing data, 279–284, 280*t*, 281*t*, 282*t*
  multiple treatments, 60–62
  multiple-group latent growth model with a treatment factor (MG-LGM-TF), 195–196

Average treatment effect (cont.)
  outcome analysis, 12
  overview, 4–5
  propensity score adjustment, 117, 118–119, 122, 135, 136
  propensity score weighting, 32–34
  sensitivity analysis, 330–331, 334f
Average treatment effect for the treated (ATT). See also Population average treatment effect for the treated (PATT); Treatment effects
  complex survey samples, 253–258, 255t–256t, 257f, 259
  generalized boosted modeling, 59–60
  latent growth modeling, 192, 202
  longitudinal studies, 193
  matching methods, 21–22
  multiple treatments, 60–62
  multiple-group latent growth model with a treatment factor (MG-LGM-TF), 195–196
  outcome analysis, 10–11
  overview, 4–5
  propensity score adjustment, 117, 118–119, 122, 135, 136
  propensity score weighting, 32–34
  subclassification, 34–35
  treatment effects estimands, 54–55

# B

Balance. See also Covariate balance
  complex survey samples, 249–250
  dual matching, 218
  latent growth modeling, 200–201
  matching weights, 153–155, 157–160, 159f, 165, 165f
  missing data, 287
  prognostic scores, 351–352, 363, 364–365, 369–370
  propensity score adjustment, 118, 122, 132–133, 135–136
  propensity score matching, 79–85, 83t
  unobserved confounding, 306
Balance diagnostics, 37–42, 39f, 40f, 42f

Balance metrics
  generalized boosted modeling, 66–67
  propensity score estimation, 56–57
Balanced repeated replication (BRR) procedures, 240, 241
Bayesian procedures
  missing data, 277
  sensitivity analysis, 321–322
Bias. See also Bias reduction
  dual matching, 218–221
  matched-pairs observational study, 173–178, 174t
  multilevel data, 220–221
  prognostic scores, 352, 356
  sensitivity analysis, 321
Bias, estimation
  multilevel data, 230
  propensity score matching, 76
Bias, selection. See also Estimation selection bias
  dual matching, 218–219, 220, 220–221
  multilevel data, 217, 220–221
  overview, 74
  propensity score adjustment, 122, 123–124, 125t, 131–132
Bias, standardized. See also Absolute standardized mean difference (ASMD)
  generalized boosted modeling, 64–65, 67, 68f
  overview, 8–9
  propensity score adjustment, 127, 128t, 132
  propensity score estimation, 56–57
  propensity score matching, 84–85, 86
Bias reduction. See also Bias
  multilevel data, 217, 227, 227t, 231
  prognostic scores, 350, 353–354, 364–365, 373–374
  propensity score adjustment, 117, 118, 119–121
  propensity score matching, 77–86, 78t, 83t, 84t
Binary covariates, 100–104, 101f, 102f, 104
Binary outcome, 330, 337

## Subject Index

Binary treatment conditions, 63–66, 64f, 65f, 66f. *See also* Treatment conditions
Blocking, 169. *See also* Subclassification
Boosted regression, 49–50. *See also* Generalized boosted modeling (GBM); Regression model
Bootstrapping, 241
Box plot of propensity scores
 balance diagnostics, 40f
 missing data, 283–284, 291–292, 291f

## C

Caliper matching. *See also* Matching methods; Propensity score matching
 latent growth modeling, 201–202
 longitudinal studies, 193
 multilevel data, 230
 nearest neighbor matching, 24–25, 25
 outcome analysis after, 10
 overview, 7
 pair matching, 148
 propensity score adjustment, 124
 propensity score matching, 81–85, 83t
Categorical covariates
 coarsened exact matching (CEM), 28
 covariate balance, 100, 102
Categorical outcomes
 outcome analysis, 12
 propensity score adjustment, 121–135, 125t, 127f, 128t, 129t, 130t
Cauchy errors, 180t
Causal inference, 3–5
Causality
 covariate balance, 108–109
 matching weights, 142
 multilevel data, 230–231
 sensitivity analysis, 321–322, 335, 344–345
*cem* package, 28–29
Chi-squares, 116
Clustered settings, 354–359
Cluster-randomized trials (CRTs), 217, 218

Coarsened exact matching (CEM), 28–29. *See also* Matching methods
Coding form, 242
Common support, 76–77
Complete cases, 290–291
Complex data, 15
Complex sample (CS) adjustment, 245
Complex survey samples
 examples of, 243–258, 248t, 249f, 251t, 255t–256t, 257f
 issues in analyzing, 237–238
 overview, 236–237, 258–261
 propensity score analysis, 242–243
Comprehensive R Archive Network (CRAN), 185
Computation, adjustment
 complex survey samples, 244–246
 prognostic scores, 350–351
 propensity score adjustment, 134–135
Computer software. *See* Software
Conditional distribution *p*, 269–270
Confounding. *See also* Unobserved confounding
 overview, 296
 sensitivity analysis, 323, 335–336
 treatment effects, 309f
Confounding, unobserved. *See also* Confounding
 indirect control for, 302–305, 303f
 in medical research, 297–299
 overview, 296–297, 314–315
 propensity score as a diagnostic for, 306–311, 309f
 propensity score calibration, 299–302
 sensitivity analysis of, 311–314
Constant sensitivity function, 338–340, 339f
Continuous covariates
 coarsened exact matching (CEM), 28
 covariate balance, 104–107, 105f, 106f
Continuous distributions, 105–107
Continuous outcomes
 outcome analysis, 12
 propensity score adjustment, 121–135, 125t, 127f, 128t, 129t, 130t
 sensitivity analysis, 328–330, 329f, 333

Control groups, 80
Correlated confounders, 304–305
Counterfactual model, 219, 221
Covariate adjustment
  complex survey samples, 245
  propensity score adjustment, 117–118, 119–121, 122, 126, 134–135
  propensity score matching, 118–121
Covariate balance. *See also* Balance
  additional considerations, 107–109
  evaluating, 8–9, 98–107, 101*f*, 102*f*, 105*f*, 106*f*
  generalizability versus causality, 108–109
  latent growth modeling, 200–201
  matching weights, 153–155
  missing data, 107–108
  observational study design, 90–98, 93*f*, 94*f*, 95*f*, 96*t*
  overview, 89–90, 109
  prognostic scores, 363, 367–370, 367*f*, 368*t*, 369*t*
  propensity score adjustment, 123–124, 125*t*, 126–127, 127*f*, 132
  propensity score matching, 79–81
  propensity score weighting, 31–32
Covariate overlap, 180*t*
Covariate selection, 134
Covariates
  identification and prioritization of, 92–96, 93*f*, 94*f*, 95*f*, 96*t*
  propensity score estimation, 13–14
  separation from outcomes, 91–92
*c*-statistic, 308, 309*f*, 310, 315*n*–316*n*

# D

Data collection, 231
Data source. *See also* Complex survey samples
  complex survey samples, 242, 243–244
  multilevel data, 222–223
  propensity score adjustment, 123
  propensity score matching, 78–79, 78*t*

DEFF adjustment, 245–246, 249, 250, 252–253, 254–258, 255*t*–256*t*, 257*f*, 259–260
Defining variables, 246–247
Definition, 142
Descriptive statistics
  matching weights, 160, 163
  multilevel data, 224*t*, 225*t*
  prognostic scores, 360, 360*t*
Design effect, 240
Design matrix, 181–182
Design-based approach, 239–241
Difference-in-differences matching, 8. *See also* Propensity score matching
Differences in means, 103. *See also* Mean differences (B); Standardized mean difference (SMD)
Disaggregated approach. *See* Model-based approach
Distributions, 175–176
Double robust matching weight estimator, 152–153, 165*f*
Doubly robust estimation, 170
Dual-matching method
  examples of, 227*t*, 229–230
  multilevel data, 217, 218–222, 231
Dual-model strategies, 120

# E

Educational Longitudinal Survey of 2002, 78–79
Effect estimation, 75–76
Effect size. *See also* Standardized bias (SB)
  balance diagnostics, 39*f*, 40*f*
  propensity score adjustment, 130*t*
Effects, 34, 35–36
E-M algorithm, 271
Error distributions, 175–176
Error variance, 372–373
Error-prone propensity score, 300–302
Estimands, 170–171
Estimation, 151–152

Estimation bias
  multilevel data, 230
  propensity score matching, 76
Estimation selection bias, 123–124, 125t.
  See also Selection bias
Exact matching criteria, 99–100
Expected mean difference, 163

## F

Feasible region-based sensitivity analysis approach, 326–335, 329f, 332t, 334f. See also Sensitivity analysis
Fixed-effect approach, 356–359
Full matching, 8, 37, 121. See also Propensity score matching; Subclassification

## G

GBM fitting process, 52–54, 53f. See also Generalized boosted modeling (GBM)
GBM statistical software package, 33–34. See also Generalized boosted modeling (GBM)
Generalizability, 108–109
Generalized boosted modeling (GBM). See also Boosted regression
  examples of, 62–69, 64f, 65f, 66f, 68f
  multiple treatments, 60–62
  overview, 49–54, 51f, 53f, 69, 70n–71n
  propensity score adjustment, 121
  propensity score estimation, 55–60
  treatment effects estimands, 54–55
Generalized estimating equation (GEE), 116, 119
Generalized propensity score, 270
Genetic matching, 7. See also Propensity score matching
Gibbs sampler, 276–277

%GMATCH macro
  matching methods, 22
  nearest neighbor matching, 23–25
Goodness-of-fit test
  matching weights, 154–155
  unobserved confounding, 307–310, 309f
Greedy matching algorithm, 7–8. See also Propensity score matching

## H

Hot deck procedure, 272
Hypotheses
  matching weights, 154–155
  propensity score adjustment, 122

## I

Ignorability assumption, 164
Imputation approaches, 272–277, 285–288, 285f, 287f, 289f
Indirect adjustment, 314–315
Indirect control, 305
Inferences, 232
Interactions, 97
Inverse probability weight (IPW), 149–150
Inverse-probability-of-treatment-weighted (IPTW) estimator
  complex survey samples, 239
  estimands, 170
  generalized boosted modeling, 69
  missing data, 268–269
  outcome analysis, 11–12
  propensity score adjustment, 117, 121, 126
  sensitivity analysis, 322, 325–326, 337, 341–342
Iterations, number of, 57–58

## J

Jackknife (JK) procedure, 240–241

## K

*k*:1 nearest neighbor matching, 22–27
Kernel matching, 8, 30. *See also*
    Matching methods; Propensity
    score matching; Subclassification
Kolmogorov–Smirnov test, 126–127, 127*f*
KS statistic, 57–58

## L

*l* method. *See* Least-squares estimates
Latent class indicators, 277
Latent class mixture model, 285–286
Latent class model, 288, 289*f*
Latent factor, 194–196
Latent growth model with a dummy
    treatment indicator (LGM-DTI)
    examples of, 202–213, 204*t*, 205*f*, 207*f*
    overview, 197–198
Latent growth modeling
    examples of, 198–213, 204*t*, 205*f*,
        206*f*, 207*f*
    latent growth model with a dummy
        treatment indicator (LGM-DTI),
        197–198
    longitudinal studies, 192–194
    multiple-group latent growth
        model with a treatment factor
        (MG-LGM-TF), 194–196
    overview, 191–192
    parallel-process latent growth
        model with a treatment factor
        (PP-LGM-TF), 196–197
Least-squares estimates
    examples of, 183–184, 183*f*
    RW method, 178–179
Level-1 matching
    examples of, 227–228, 227*t*
    multilevel data, 221–222
Level-2 matching
    examples of, 227*t*, 228–229
    multilevel data, 221–222
Linear model, 300–301
Linear programming methods, 321–322

Linear response surfaces, 180*t*
Linear sensitivity function, 340–342,
    341*t*, 342*t*
Linearization adjustment, 245, 252–253,
    256*t*
Local linear matching. *See* Kernel
    matching
Logistic regression
    complex survey samples, 247, 249
    generalized boosted modeling, 59–60
    imputation approaches, 272
    matching weights, 154–155, 157
    nearest neighbor matching, 22–23
    overview, 20–21
    pair matching, 146
    propensity score adjustment, 121, 122
    propensity score weighting, 32–33
    sensitivity analysis, 338
    unobserved confounding, 315*n*, 316*n*
Longitudinal data, 191–194
Longitudinal studies
    complex survey samples, 243–258,
        248*t*, 249*f*, 251*t*, 255*t*–256*t*, 257*f*
    examples of, 198–213, 204*t*, 205*f*,
        206*f*, 207*f*
    missing data, 289–292, 291*f*
    multilevel data, 231
    propensity score matching, 192–194
Love Plot, 93*f*, 102, 103

## M

M imputed covariate datasets, 107–108
Mahalanobis caliper matching, 7. *See
    also* Propensity score matching
Mahalanobis metric matching. *See also*
    Propensity score matching
    nearest neighbor matching, 23, 27
    outcome analysis after, 10
    overview, 7
    prognostic scores, 353–354, 364
Mantel–Haenszel approach, 36
Matched data, 10–12. *See also* Propensity
    score matching
Matched design, 98

Matched-pairs observational study.
  *See also* Matching methods;
  Observational study design
  estimands, 170–171
  outcome analysis alternatives,
    173–178, 174*t*
  overview, 168, 171–173, 184–185
  role of propensity score in, 168–169
  RW method, 177–184, 180*t*, 183*t*, 184*t*
Matching, caliper. *See also* Matching
    methods; Propensity score
    matching
  latent growth modeling, 201–202
  longitudinal studies, 193
  multilevel data, 230
  nearest neighbor matching, 24–25, 25
  outcome analysis after, 10
  overview, 7
  pair matching, 148
  propensity score adjustment, 124
  propensity score matching, 81–85, 83*t*
Matching methods. *See also* Matched-
    pairs observational study; Matching
    weights (MWs); Propensity score
    matching
  advanced matching methods, 28–31
  multilevel data, 227–230, 227*t*, 231
  nearest neighbor matching, 22–27
  observational study design, 169
  overview, 21–31
  prognostic scores, 353–354, 355–356,
    372–373
  propensity score adjustment, 115–116,
    118, 122, 124, 132–133
  propensity score matching, 81–85,
    83*t*, 84*t*
Matching weight estimator, 151–153,
    165*f*
Matching weights (MWs). *See also*
    Matching methods; Propensity
    score matching
  examples of, 155–164, 159*f*, 161*f*, 162*f*,
    164*f*
  overview, 141–142, 148–155, 165–166,
    165*f*
  pair matching, 142–148, 144*f*, 147*t*

*MatchIt* program
  balance diagnostics, 37–38, 39*f*
  coarsened exact matching (CEM), 28
  covariate balance, 103
  full matching, 37
  nearest neighbor matching, 22–24
  optimal matching, 30–31
  outcome analysis, 10
  overview, 21–22, 43, 44*n*
  subclassification, 34–35
Maximum likelihood (MLR) estimation,
    202
Mean differences after matching, 82
Mean differences (B). *See also*
    Differences in means; Standardized
    mean difference (SMD)
  propensity score adjustment, 129*t*,
    130*t*
  propensity score matching, 82
Medical research, 297–299
Methods in propensity score analysis,
    6–12
MICE package in R, 275
Mirror histograms
  matching weights, 158, 159*f*, 161*f*,
    162*f*
  pair matching, 143–145, 144*f*
Missing at random (MAR) data. *See also*
    Missing data
  misspecified imputation models, 285
  overview, 270
  simulation study, 278–279
Missing completely at random (MCAR)
    data, 279. *See also* Missing data
Missing data
  complex survey samples, 244
  covariate balance, 107–108
  examples of, 289–292, 291*f*
  imputation approaches, 272–277
  latent growth modeling, 200
  nonimputation approaches, 270–271
  overview, 267–269, 292
  with propensity scores, 269–270
  simulation study, 277–288, 280*t*, 281*t*,
    282*t*, 285*f*, 287*f*, 289*f*
Misspecification, 352–353

Misspecified imputation models, 285–288, 285f, 287f, 289f. *See also* Imputation approaches; Model misspecification
Mixed-effects logistic regression, 124
Model adequacy, 249–252, 251t
Model misspecification, 285–288, 285f, 287f, 289f
Model-based approach
  complex survey samples, 239–241
  missing data, 275–277
Model-based imputation methods, 275–277
Mplus codes
  latent growth modeling, 210–213
  multilevel data, 225–226
Multilevel analysis, 239. *See also* Model-based approach
Multilevel data
  bias, 220–221
  dual matching, 218–222
  examples of, 222–232, 224t, 225t, 226f, 227t
  overview, 217, 230–232
  prognostic scores, 356, 361–362
Multilevel random intercept model, 361–362, 373
Multiple imputation, 273–275
Multiple imputation combining rules, 107–108
Multiple regression, 117–118
Multiple samples, 77–86, 78t, 83t, 84t
Multiple treatments. *See also* Treatment conditions
  generalized boosted modeling, 66–69, 68f
  overview, 60–62
Multiple-group latent growth model with a treatment factor (MG-LGM-TF)
  examples of, 202–213, 204t, 205f
  overview, 194–196
Multiplicative adjustment, 245–246, 256t
Multistage sampling method, 237–238, 239
Multiway frequency analysis, 116

# N

Nearest neighbor matching. *See also* Propensity score matching
  matching methods, 22–27
  outcome analysis after, 10
  overview, 6–7
  propensity score matching, 81–85, 83t
Nonimputation approaches, 270–271
Nonoverlapping confidence intervals, 259
Nonresponse weight, 239–240
Not missing at random (NMAR) data, 269–270. *See also* Missing data
Notation, 142
Null hypothesis significance tests, 249

# O

Observational study design. *See also* Matched-pairs observational study
  covariate balance, 90–98, 93f, 94f, 95f, 96t, 99
  role of propensity score in, 168–169
  using propensity scores, 96–98
One-to-one matching. *See also* Matching methods
  longitudinal studies, 193
  propensity score adjustment, 121
Optimal matching. *See also* Matching methods
  full matching, 37
  overview, 30–31
  propensity score matching, 81–85, 84t
Optimal matching algorithm, 7–8. *See also* Propensity score matching
Outcome analysis. *See also* Outcomes
  alternatives to, 173–178, 174t
  issues in, 14–15
  latent growth modeling, 199–200
  on matched data after propensity score matching, 10–11
  matched-pairs observational study, 172
  after matching, 10–12, 14–15

## Subject Index

matching weights, 163, 164f, 165f, 166
observational study design, 169
Outcome effects, 131–132
Outcomes. *See also* Outcome analysis
covariate balance, 91–92
propensity score adjustment, 130–131, 130t
Overfitting, 352, 373

## P

Pair matching
matching weights, 142–148, 144f, 147t, 149, 158, 159f, 165
methodological issues with, 146–148, 147t
Pairwise effects, 60–62
Parallel-process latent growth model with a treatment factor (PP-LGM-TF), 196–197, 202–213, 204t, 205f, 206f
Parameter estimation
missing data, 271
RW method, 181
Parametric modeling, 20–21, 331–333, 332t
Percent bias reduction (PBR)
balance, 80
overview, 8–9
propensity score matching, 82, 84–85
Picked-points analysis (PPA), 170, 171
Point estimates, 279–284, 280t, 281t, 282t
Population average treatment effect for the treated (PATT). *See also* Average treatment effect for the treated (ATT)
matching weights, 142, 150
pair matching, 143–146, 144f
Population average treatment effect (PATE). *See also* Average treatment effect (ATE)
matching weights, 142, 150
pair matching, 143–146, 144f
Population-level propensity score model, 241

Post-hoc adjustments, 245
Predicted probability of treatment, 307
Predictors of outcome, 93–96, 93f, 94f, 95f, 96t
Primary sampling unites (PSUs), 240–241
Prioritized covariates, 97
Prognostic balance, 351–352
Prognostic scores
in clustered settings, 354–359
examples of, 359–371, 360t, 366t, 367f, 368t, 369t, 371t
overview, 348–354, 371–374
Propensity score adjustment
continuous and categorical outcomes, 121–135, 125t, 127f, 128t, 129t, 130t
outcome analysis, 12
overview, 115–118, 135–137
studies comparing methods of, 118–121
Propensity score analysis in general
assumptions of, 5–6
causal inference, 3–5
issues in, 13–15
latent growth modeling, 201–202
missing data, 269–270
overview, 3, 15, 49–50, 237
steps in, 6–12
Propensity score balance, 132–133. *See also* Balance
Propensity score calibration, 299–302
Propensity score estimation
complex survey samples, 247–249, 248t, 249f
covariate balance, 99
generalized boosted modeling, 55–60, 62–69, 64f, 65f, 66f, 68f
issues in, 13–14
matched-pairs observational study, 172–173
missing data, 269
overview, 6, 20–21
propensity score weighting, 31–32
subclassification, 35–36
Propensity score histogram, 39f
Propensity score jitter plot, 39f

Propensity score matching. *See also*
Matched data; Matching methods;
Matching weights (MWs)
  application of with 60 experimental
    trials, 77–86, 78t, 83t, 84t
  evaluation of the quality of, 8–9
  issues in, 14
  latent growth modeling, 200–201
  longitudinal studies, 192–194
  matching methods, 21–31
  outcome analysis after, 10–12
  overview, 6–8, 74–75, 85–86
  pair matching, 142–148, 144f, 147t
  propensity score adjustment, 122, 124
  research and issues relating to, 75–77
  resources for, 43–44
Propensity score model
  matching weights, 149, 157–160, 159f
  propensity score calibration, 300
  unobserved confounding, 310–311
Propensity score overlap, 41–42
Propensity score weighting. *See also*
Weighting techniques
  covariate balance, 98
  generalized boosted modeling, 59–60, 67
  multiple treatments, 60–62
  outcome analysis, 11–12
  overview, 31–34
  propensity score adjustment, 117, 118–119, 122, 126, 131, 135–136
  propensity score matching, 15
Propensity scores, 96–98
Pseudo-propensity score, 326–327, 332
*psmatch2* package
  balance diagnostics, 42, 42f
  kernel matching, 30
  nearest neighbor matching, 26–27
%PSMatching macro
  matching methods, 22
  nearest neighbor matching, 25–27
  radius matching, 29
*p*-values
  covariate balance, 103–104
  matching weights, 163
  sensitivity analysis, 321

## Q

Quadratic sensitivity function, 340–342, 341t, 342t

## R

R statistical software package
  balance diagnostics, 37–38, 39f
  covariate balance, 103
  full matching, 37
  latent growth modeling, 201–202
  matched-pairs observational study, 185–187
  matching methods, 21–22
  matching weights, 166
  missing data, 275, 291
  overview, 20
  propensity score estimation, 21
  propensity score weighting, 32
  resources for, 43–44
  sensitivity analysis, 323
  subclassification, 34–35
Radius matching, 7, 29–30. *See also*
Matching methods; Propensity
score matching
Random intercept multilevel model, 361
Random sampling, 78–79, 78t
Randomized controlled trials (RCTs), 4
Randomized experiments, 109
Randomized treatment, 98–99
Rank transformation, 179–181, 180t
Reduction, bias. *See also* Bias
  multilevel data, 217, 227, 227t, 231
  prognostic scores, 350, 353–354, 364–365, 373–374
  propensity score adjustment, 117, 118, 119–121
  propensity score matching, 77–86, 78t, 83t, 84t
Regression coefficients, 220
Regression estimates
  matching weights, 153
  propensity score adjustment, 129t, 130t

## Subject Index

Regression model. *See also* Boosted regression
  matching weights, 152
  outcome analysis, 10
Regression tree models, 51–52, 51*f*
Regression with propensity score adjustment, 15
Replacement
  longitudinal studies, 193
  propensity score matching, 75–76, 82
Replication methods, 241
Resampling procedures, 272
Robust Wilcoxon method. *See* RW method
Rubin Causal Framework, 91
RW method
  examples of, 182–184, 183*t*, 184*t*
  matched-pairs observational study, 177–184, 180*t*, 183*t*, 184*t*, 185–187
  software, 185–187

## S

Sample conditions, 74–75, 78–79, 78*t*
Sample size
  KS statistic, 58
  matching weights, 149
  propensity score matching, 85
Sample size ratio, 77
Sampling distribution, 146
Sampling errors
  dual matching, 218–219
  pair matching, 146
Sandwich error, 163
SAS statistical software package
  balance diagnostics, 41–42
  matching methods, 22
  nearest neighbor matching, 23–26
  optimal matching, 31
  overview, 20, 43
  propensity score adjustment, 124
  propensity score estimation, 21
  propensity score weighting, 32
  radius matching, 29
  resources for, 43–44
  subclassification, 35–36

Scatter plot, 285*f*
Selection bias. *See also* Estimation selection bias
  dual matching, 218–219, 220, 220–221
  multilevel data, 217, 220–221
  overview, 74
  propensity score adjustment, 122, 123–124, 125*t*, 131–132
Selection bias (B)
  overview, 4, 8–9
  subclassification, 8
Selection bias reduction, 15. *See also* Bias reduction; Selection bias
Sensitivity analysis
  examples of, 322–325, 324*f*, 333–335, 334*f*, 338
  feasible region-based approach to, 326–335, 329*f*, 332*t*, 334*f*
  methods and applications, 325–342, 329*f*, 332*t*, 334*f*, 339*f*, 341*t*, 342*t*
  overview, 320–322, 342–345
  propensity score estimation, 14
  sensitivity function-based approach to, 335–342, 339*f*, 341*t*, 342*t*
  unobserved confounding, 311–314
Sensitivity function-based sensitivity analysis approach, 335–342, 339*f*, 341*t*, 342*t*. *See also* Sensitivity analysis
Simulation design
  matched-pairs observational study, 174–178
  missing data, 277–288, 280*t*, 281*t*, 282*t*, 285*f*, 287*f*, 289*f*
Single imputation for covariates, 107–108
Software. *See individual software packages*
  latent growth modeling, 209–213
  matched-pairs observational study, 185–187
Specific outcomes, 12
SPSS statistical software package, 43–44
Stable unit treatment value assumption (SUTVA), 5–6

Standard bias reduction, 80
Standard deviations, 136
Standard errors, 129t, 130t, 136
Standardized bias (SB). *See also* Absolute standardized mean difference (ASMD)
　generalized boosted modeling, 64–65, 67, 68f
　overview, 8–9
　propensity score adjustment, 127, 128t, 132
　propensity score estimation, 56–57
　propensity score matching, 84–85, 86
Standardized difference (SDF)
　complex survey samples, 249–250
　matching weights, 154–155, 157–158, 159f, 160, 161f, 162f, 165f
Standardized effect size (ES). *See* Standardized bias (SB)
Standardized mean difference (SMD). *See also* Differences in means; Mean differences (B)
　balance diagnostics, 38, 39f, 41
　complex survey samples, 247, 249–250
　covariate balance, 95f, 103
　propensity score adjustment, 131
　propensity score matching, 82
Standardized regression coefficients, 367–368, 368t
STATA statistical software package
　balance diagnostics, 42
　coarsened exact matching (CEM), 29
　kernel matching, 30
　matching methods, 22
　nearest neighbor matching, 26–28
　overview, 20, 43
　propensity score estimation, 21
　propensity score weighting, 33
　radius matching, 29–30
　resources for, 43–44
　subclassification, 36–37
Statistical adjustments, 124, 126, 130t
Statistical inference, 151–152
Statistical significance testing, 80
Steps in propensity score analysis, 6–12

"Stopping rules," 58
Stratification. *See also* Subclassification
　complex survey samples, 252–258, 255t–256t, 257f
　prognostic scores, 352, 368
Structural equation modeling (SEM) framework
　latent growth modeling, 191–192
　multilevel data, 223–226, 224t, 225t, 226f
　multiple-group latent growth model with a treatment factor (MG-LGM-TF), 194
Subclassification. *See also* Stratification
　complex survey samples, 251t, 252–253, 253–258, 255t–256t, 257f
　covariate balance, 98, 99
　observational study design, 169
　outcome analysis, 11–12
　overview, 34–37
　propensity score adjustment, 116, 118, 120–121, 122, 126, 127, 134–135, 136
　propensity score matching, 8, 15
Subclassified design, 98
Substance Intensity Index (SII), 52–54, 53f
Surrogacy, 301–302
Survival outcomes, 12
Synthetic cohort design, 230–231

# T

Taylor-series linearization, 240–241
*teffects*, 27
Toolkit for Weighting and Analysis of Nonequivalent Groups (*twang*) package. *See twang* package
Transformations
　covariate balance, 97
　sensitivity analysis, 333
Treatment conditions
　covariate balance, 104–107, 105f, 106f
　generalized boosted modeling, 62–69, 64f, 65f, 66f, 68f
　more than two, 60–62

Treatment effect after matching, 23–24
Treatment effects. *See also* Average treatment effect (ATE); Average treatment effect for the treated (ATT)
  complex survey samples, 253–258, 255t–256t, 257f
  dual matching, 218, 220
  missing data, 268–269, 279–284, 280t, 281t, 282t
  multiple-group latent growth model with a treatment factor (MG-LGM-TF), 194–196
  prognostic scores, 365–366, 370–371, 371t, 372
  propensity score adjustment, 118, 130t, 133–134
  unobserved confounding, 307–310, 309f
Treatment effects estimands, 54–55
Treatment-by-strata factorial analysis of variance (ANOVA), 116
*t*-tests
  complex survey samples, 254
  covariate balance, 103–104
  propensity score adjustment, 116
*twang* package
  balance diagnostics, 38, 40f, 41
  generalized boosted modeling, 63–64, 64f, 65f, 66f, 67–69, 68f, 69
  overview, 43, 44n
  sensitivity analysis, 323
  treatment effects estimands, 54–55

## U

Unequal selection probabilities, 237–238
Unmeasured confounders, 322

Unobserved confounding. *See also* Confounding
  indirect control for, 302–305, 303f
  in medical research, 297–299
  overview, 296–297, 314–315
  propensity score as a diagnostic for, 306–311, 309f
  propensity score calibration, 299–302
  sensitivity analysis of, 311–314
Unweighted propensity score, 246, 248t, 251t

## V

Van Elteren approach, 36
Variance estimation, 146
Variance of a covariate, 153–154
%VMATCH macro
  matching methods, 22
  optimal matching, 31
*VWrfit* function, 185–187

## W

Weight as a covariate adjustment, 245
Weighted propensity score, 248t, 251t, 256t
Weighted regression model, 10
Weighting techniques
  covariate balance, 98
  outcome analysis, 11–12
  propensity score adjustment, 117, 118–119, 122, 126, 131, 132–133, 135–136
Within methods. *See* Across and Within methods

# About the Editors

**Wei Pan, PhD**, is Associate Professor and Biostatistician in the School of Nursing at Duke University. His research interests include causal inference (confounding, propensity score analysis, and resampling), advanced modeling (multilevel, structural, and mediation and moderation), and meta-analysis, and their applications in the social, behavioral, and health sciences. Dr. Pan has published over 50 articles in refereed journals as well as other publications. He also has served as an associate editor, guest associate editor, or editorial board member for professional journals including the *Journal of the American Statistical Association, Frontiers in Quantitative Psychology and Measurement, The Journal of Experimental Education,* and *Counseling Outcome Research and Evaluation,* and is the recipient of several awards for excellence in research, teaching, and service.

**Haiyan Bai, PhD**, is Associate Professor of Quantitative Research Methodology at the University of Central Florida. Her research interests include resampling methods, propensity score analysis, research design, measurement and evaluation, and the applications of statistical methods in the educational and behavioral sciences. Dr. Bai has published a book on resampling methods as well as numerous articles in refereed journals, and has served on the editorial boards of journals including *The Journal of Experimental Education, Frontiers in Quantitative Psychology and Measurement,* and the *Journal of Data Analysis and Information Processing*. Dr. Bai is a Fellow of the Academy for Teaching, Learning, and Leadership and a Faculty Fellow at the University of Central Florida, where she has been the recipient of several awards for excellence in research and teaching.

# Contributors

**Haiyan Bai, PhD,** Department of Educational and Human Sciences, University of Central Florida, Orlando, Florida

**Lane F. Burgette, PhD,** RAND Corporation, Arlington, Virginia

**M. H. Clark, PhD,** Department of Educational and Human Sciences, University of Central Florida, Orlando, Florida

**Tom H. Greene, PhD,** Division of Epidemiology, University of Utah, Salt Lake City, Utah

**Beth Ann Griffin, PhD,** RAND Corporation, Arlington, Virginia

**Rolf H. H. Groenwold, MD, PhD,** Julius Center for Health Sciences and Primary Care, University Medical Center Utrecht, Utrecht, The Netherlands

**Debbie L. Hahs-Vaughn, PhD,** Department of Educational and Human Sciences, University of Central Florida, Orlando, Florida

**Bradley E. Huitema, PhD,** Department of Psychology, Western Michigan University, Kalamazoo, Michigan

**Ben Kelcey, PhD,** School of Education, University of Cincinnati, Cincinnati, Ohio

**Olaf H. Klungel, PharmD, PhD,** Division of Pharmacoepidemiology and Clinical Pharmacology, Utrecht University, Utrecht, The Netherlands

**Scott F. Kosten, PhD,** inVentiv Health Clinical, Coopersville, Michigan

**Walter L. Leite, PhD,** Research and Evaluation Methodology Program, University of Florida, Gainesville, Florida

**Liang Li, PhD,** Department of Biostatistics, The University of Texas MD Anderson Cancer Center, Houston, Texas

**Lingling Li, PhD,** Department of Population Medicine, Harvard Medical School, and Harvard Pilgrim Health Care Institute, Boston, Massachusetts

**Xiaochun Li, PhD,** Department of Biostatistics, Indiana University School of Medicine, Indianapolis, Indiana

**Daniel F. McCaffrey, PhD,** Educational Testing Service, Princeton, New Jersey

**Joseph W. McKean, PhD,** Department of Statistics, Western Michigan University, Kalamazoo, Michigan

**Robin Mitra, PhD,** Mathematical Sciences, University of Southampton, Southampton, United Kingdom

**Wei Pan, PhD,** School of Nursing, Duke University, Durham, North Carolina

**Cassandra W. Pattanayak, PhD,** Quantitative Analysis Institute, Wellesley College, Wellesley, Massachusetts

**Brian C. Sauer, PhD,** Division of Epidemiology, University of Utah, Salt Lake City, Utah

**Megan Schuler, PhD,** The Methodology Center, The Pennsylvania State University, State College, Pennsylvania

**Changyu Shen, PhD,** Department of Biostatistics, Indiana University School of Medicine, Indianapolis, Indiana

**Christopher M. Swoboda, PhD,** School of Education, University of Cincinnati, Cincinnati, Ohio

**Qiu Wang, PhD,** Department of Higher Education, Syracuse University, Syracuse, New York